Dynamic Embodiment℠ of the Sun Salutation

A rare gem, this book demystifies our bodies' inner world and provides clear pathways to explore the wisdom of many generations of visionaries and seekers. A great resource for all. *Mariko Tanabe, Program Director and Certified Teacher of Body-Mind Centering®*

In reading **Dynamic Embodiment**[SM] **of the Sun Salutation** by Shakti Smith and Martha Eddy, I am struck by their clear and comprehensive presentation of the material. They interweave Yoga, Body-Mind Centering®, Laban/Bartenieff, and Dynamic Embodiment … It is thorough and profound. *Genny Kapuler, Certified Teacher of Iyengar Yoga, Alexander Technique, and Body Mind Centering®, NYC*

It's astounding how many healing portals into the body there are! This book is guaranteed to open you to new possibilities and potential in healing, growth, and self-awareness. Eddy and Smith offer a masterful and comprehensive synthesis from the ancient chakra system to current research and the experiential connection of the chakras to the endocrine system, nervous system, and the mind-body. This book is a valuable resource for self-exploration, and for health care practitioners looking for innovative ways to work with their clients. *Ellen Krueger, LMHC, LMT, BCPP, Director of Soma-Psyche Institute, NYC; Faculty at the Swedish Institute College of Health Sciences, NYC*

Readers are guided to take inventory and cultivate a ritual of self-inquiry into their 3-D body for courageous self-care. *Vivian Chávez, Associate Professor, Doctor in Public Health, San Francisco State University, CA*

As conscious yoga practitioners and business owners examine their degree of cultural appropriation and attempt to rebalance more respectfully, **Dynamic Embodiment**[SM] **of the Sun Salutation** addresses that adjustment on a holistic level. It is timely and an essential read for anyone looking into their blindspots and hoping to awaken. *Scarlet S. Johnson, www.mvyogabarn.com, Chilmark, Martha's Vineyard, MA*

Eddy and Smith draw on their profound understanding of the interconnections between yoga and other movement modalities, healing arts, and wellness. Though nominally about the yoga sequence called surya namaskar, the book is in fact an in-depth resource on anatomy, philosophy, human movement, the endocrine system, and somatic awareness as they apply to yoga. *Peter Ferko, Peterferko.com, Teacher Trainer and Yogiraj of ISHTA Yoga, NYC; Author of* The Genius of Yoga *and* Yoga for Artists

This is a comprehensive and carefully laid out guide to expand and spark one's imagination, curiosity, explorations and understanding of "body-mind" in yoga practice … This book provides broad support for establishing an embodied asana practice and designing classes that are life-affirming and empowering. *Roxlyn Moret, CMA, ERYT-500, RSME, Licensed Teacher of BMC, Embodied Breath Yoga teacher, NYC*

What a resource! The wise, substantial, and deeply researched material will enhance the work of any movement teacher and practitioner. As a movement teacher, working with people of all body types, levels of trauma, and emotional expression for over 25 years, I'm thrilled to bring this knowledge to my students in training and to my own personal learning and continued study. Anyone in the Conscious Dance modalities has a new book on their reading list! *Toni Bergins, Creator of JourneyDance*[TM]*, The Remedy Expressive Arts Program, and the Embodied Transformations Coaching Method, MA*

When a lifetime of personal and professional experience, as well as research, inspiration, and intuition, culminates in a revolutionary approach to our bodies, hearts, and minds … we are truly given a gift to light our paths. *Dr Linda Burham, Naturopath and Author, Santa Fe, NM*

Do you know when you hear a word or a phrase, and your body reacts to it, like it's been called its real name? This book is like that: it gives us a new language, giving weight to the somatic, and helping us connect to it. This book is … a fresh approach to body-mind integration. *Michael Hayes, LMT, Founder of Buddha Body Yoga*[TM]*, NYC*

I've experienced and witnessed the impact of movement on human health, the human spirit, and the human community. After reading this book, I'll never be able to practice the "familiar" Sun Salutation again in a superficial or routinized way. *Ronald Lavine, DC, RSMT, AskDrLavine.com, Doctor of Chiropractic, Princeton, NJ, and NYC*

This book will make a valuable contribution to the field, and offer much to inspire practitioners and teachers of both yoga and somatics. *Linda Hartley, MA, BMCA, RSMT, CTP, DipPsych, www.lindahartley.co.uk/*

This innovative, pragmatic text integrates yoga principles with somatic research as a valuable contribution to literature on balancing the body, relating chakra energy vortexes with the functioning of the endocrine system. *Sondra Fraleigh, PhD, Professor Emeritus, State University of New York, Director, www.eastwestsomatics.com*

Dynamic Embodiment℠ of the Sun Salutation

Pathways to Balancing the Chakras and the Neuroendocrine System

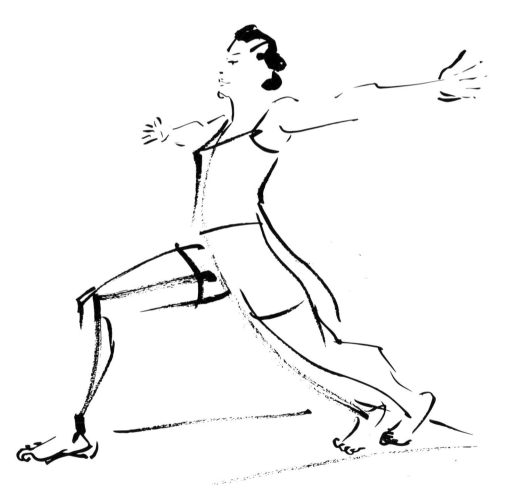

Martha Eddy ◆ Shakti Andrea Smith

HANDSPRING
PUBLISHING

Forewords Eleanor Criswell ◆ Per Erez

HANDSPRING PUBLISHING LIMITED
The Old Manse, Fountainhall,
Pencaitland, East Lothian
EH34 5EY, Scotland
Tel: +44 1875 341 859
Website: www.handspringpublishing.com

First published 2021 in the United Kingdom by Handspring Publishing Limited

ISBN 978-1-912085-99-6
ISBN (Kindle eBook) 978-1-913426-00-2

British Library Cataloguing in Publication Data
A catalogue record for this book is available from the British Library
Library of Congress Cataloging in Publication Data
A catalog record for this book is available from the Library of Congress

Body-Mind Centering® and BMC® are registered services marks of Bonnie Bainbridge Cohen. Dynamic Embodiment^{SM} and DE^{SM} are service marks of Martha Eddy.

Notice
Neither the Publisher nor the Authors assume any responsibility for any loss or injury and/or damage to persons or property arising out of or relating to any use of the material contained in this book. It is the responsibility of the treating practitioner, relying on independent expertise and knowledge of the patient, to determine the best treatment and method of application for the patient.
All reasonable efforts have been made to obtain copyright clearance for illustrations in the book for which the authors or publishers do not own the rights. If you believe that one of your illustrations has been used without such clearance please contact the publishers and we will ensure that appropriate credit is given in the next reprint.

This book is a guide for personal exploration and is in no way meant to substitute for any type of medical advice - allopathic, Western, Eastern, Indian. It can complement a healing protocol. Ultimately all movement ideas are to be visited with gentleness allowing your body responses and related sensations to guide you.

Commissioning Editor Sarena Wolfaard
Project Manager Morven Dean
Copy editor Glenys Norquay
Designer Kirsteen Wright
Indexer Aptara, India
Typesetter Amnet, India
Printer Bell and Bain, UK

Book printed in Minion pro 11.5/13pt

Contents

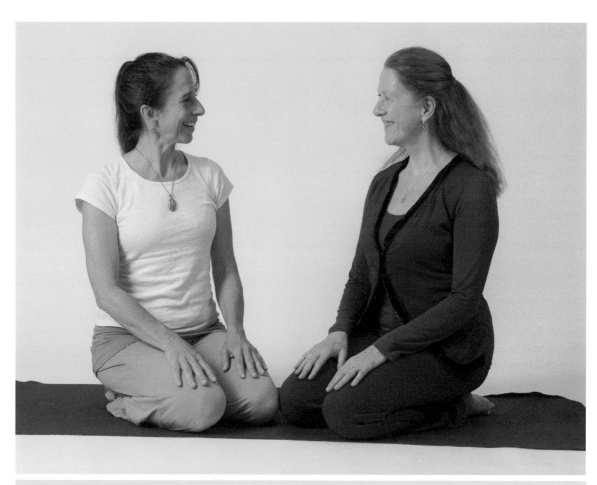

Shakti and Martha. Photo by Serge Cashman.

About the Authors

Dr Martha Eddy, CMA, DEP, CTBMD, MFLCI, RSMT, EdD, author of *Mindful Movement: The Evolution of the Somatic Arts and Conscious Action*, is the Founder and Director of Dynamic Embodiment^{SM} Somatic Movement Therapy and a co-founder of two non-profits, Moving For Life and Moving on Center, which bridge somatics with social change. She has served on the faculty of Columbia, Princeton, and New York Universities, and as President of ISMETA, the somatic field's professional association. Since 2019 she has worked as the Geraldine Ferraro Fellow of Social Justice through Movement for Marymount Manhattan College. She began practicing yoga and the Sun Salutation in 1977 with Bonnie Bainbridge Cohen during Hatha yoga classes taught by Jeannie Erlbaum. By 1984 she was the primary faculty member at the School for Body–Mind Centering® to teach the nervous system, the endocrine, and the motor development courses. She instantly applied this knowledge to her practice of Sun Salutations, establishing it as a central ritual within Dynamic Embodiment and her system of dance education – BodyMind Dancing. This 45-year practice of infusing Dynamic Embodiment principles into moving through the Sun Salutation has sustained her through injury and health challenges. She has further developed this knowledge with Shakti Smith and is thrilled to share it with you.

Shakti Andrea Smith, RSME, RYT, LMT, DEP is a Registered Somatic Movement Educator, Registered 500-Hour Yoga Teacher, Licensed Massage Therapist, Polarity Practitioner, Sound Healer, and Founder of Prema Soma Healing Arts in New York City. She served on the faculty at the Swedish Institute College of Health Sciences and at Movement Research, and developed the courses Integrating Chakras Into Your Bodywork Practice, Movement for Bodyworkers, Medicine Dance, and Nature Connection. A long-time member of ISMETA and Yoga Alliance, Shakti is an instructor of Contact Improvisation and Authentic Movement, and has been teaching and practicing the Sun Salutation for 35 years. She has developed a somatic approach to yoga that integrates shamanic earth-based practices, developmental movement, and awareness of the chakral/neuroendocrine bridge. She empowers others with this self-healing practice. As a social worker and psychotherapist in training, she looks forward to continuing to bring these healing modalities to populations on the frontiers of social change.

About the Artist

Stewart Hoyt is an interdisciplinary artist and an ecstatic presence practitioner who dances, designs, and builds art in Brooklyn, NYC. A Yale-trained artist and a pioneer in the second wave organic farming movement, he built two green homes and a gray water recycling system in the style of John Todd in the Northeast Kingdom of Vermont. *Stewarthoyt.com*

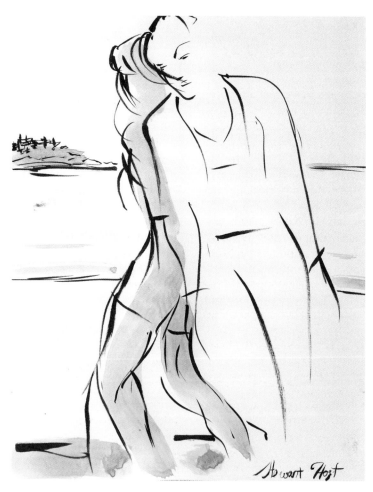

Shakti and Teresa at Popham Beach, by Stewart Hoyt.

Foreword by Eleanor Criswell

I have been teaching the Sun Salutation off and on for over 45 years: first, in the Psychology Department's Psychology of Yoga class at Sonoma State University and later during the Somatic Yoga training program of Novato Institute for Somatic Research and Training. Students regularly experienced this series of yoga postures, done as a posture flow, as enlivening and enhancing to their yoga practice. *Dynamic Embodiment*^{SM} *of the Sun Salutation: Pathways to Balancing the Chakras and the Neuroendocrine System* is a greatly expanded approach, a somatic approach, to the ritual of the Salutation to the Sun.

There is a somatic revolution occurring in the world, propelled by people of all ages who want to be in touch with their embodied selves. They are living in the world by way of mind/body integration, trying many approaches to embodiment. They want the health and holism that come from this integration. Martha Eddy and Shakti Andrea Smith, along with this book, are helping encourage this revolution.

Somatics is a term coined by Thomas Hanna to name the mind-body disciplines. I first met Eddy in the 1990s when she invited me to be on the Advisory Board for ISMETA – our somatic movement professional association. Smith, Eddy, and I are all connected through this field and organization. I teach Hanna Somatics and somatic approaches to yoga. Smith has been teaching somatic yoga for decades, specializing in integrating earth-based (Shamanic) practices and investigating their merging with embodiment of the chakras and neuroendocrine system; as a social worker she will be exploring how to bring this work to new populations. During much of Martha's life, she has been living with embodiment and somatics. She first trained in Body-Mind Centering® (BMC®) with Bonnie Bainbridge Cohen when she was 19 years old and has studied many somatic disciplines.

The book brings together science and metaphor. It is an embodied approach to understanding your body – specifically your neuroendocrine glandular system and nervous system – in the context of the Sun Salutation. The chakras can be stimulated deliberately with certain practices or they can be awakened naturally by yoga practice. The chakras have been associated with the nerve plexuses: locations in the body where the nerves come together and then branch out. The endocrine glands have also been linked with the chakras. In this book, the Sun Salutation is practiced with a focus on the chakras and the blending of these two systems.

Heavily inflected by BMC®, it is experiential learning at its best. It brings in BMC® knowledge as support for many of the concepts. Eddy and Smith help the reader see the Sun Salutation in some new ways. The ritual is done emphasizing the neuroendocrine glands, helping one to understand the neuroendocrine system more deeply. They also guide an enhanced understanding of the chakras – energy vortices located in the subtle body.

A unique characteristic of this book is how it is written from a holistic perspective rather than in a third-person, left-hemispheric way: it is written somatically. It also pays homage to the ritual aspect of the Sun Salutation, honoring a return to nature, and adopts a social justice perspective. Anecdotes by Eddy and Smith illuminate different concepts, and illustrations – both photos and drawings – are included throughout. The style is lively and inclusive, supporting the reader to teach these practices with their students or clients. It would be luxurious to work through it as a textbook in a class.

It is an honor and a pleasure to be able to contribute this Foreword. Enjoy!

Eleanor Criswell Hanna, Ed.D., C-IAYT
How Yoga Works: An Introduction
to Somatic Yoga
July 2021

Foreword by Per Erez

The practices described in this book by Dr Martha Eddy and Shakti Andrea Smith poignantly illustrate the ritualized movement practices of Surya Namaskar. The Salute to the Sun, as it is known, powerfully affects our functioning at the biological, psychological, and social levels. The yoga tradition has long understood human functioning and evolutionary development as a basis for working with the body–mind–spirit complex. They can help us determine which areas of our lives require our attention and intervention.

As one aspect of the tradition, Sun Salutes can foster somatic intelligence, social cohesion, and self-agency. When practiced with clarity and including our desires and needs, these practices can become a part of our personal journey of self-discovery. This work explores that process in a very down-to-earth way.

Written in part as trail guide for the beginner, the book shows how the postures of the Sun Salute series, the chakras, and the connections with the neuroendocrine system offer a complete toolkit for intentionally improving all aspects of your life. Adept yogins, somatic movement enthusiasts, and veteran teachers will also find intriguing personal inquiries into psychophysiology in the book. These readers will find much to consider about the way in which our human ability to move in space, hormonal balance, and ailments correlate with our mental outlook. The information offered has wide application, regardless of the reader's walk of life and previous background.

Dynamic Embodiment[SM] as an approach to the practice of yoga is the condensation of the writers' explorations of over 70 combined years of practical knowledge and deep immersion in integrative and complementary medicine and somatic education, as well as yogic history, anatomy, and

systems of thought. The work is a dance, weaving together thoughts from ancient Greek ideas of the Platonic solids and "spatial harmony," to specific considerations of how glandular processes, sound, colors, shapes, and psychological states of mind may all have connections worth investigating for our well-being.

These insights are anchored by mindful engagement and immersion in the essential practice found in the Sun Salute, familiar to most physical yoga traditions around the globe. The Dynamic Embodiment teaching principle of "observing, supporting, and providing options (OSO)" really helps to holistically ground the practice.

The authors articulate a first-person somatic process orientation where you decide to focus your attention based on your own unique needs, even if someone else facilitates the exploratory process. The result draws together both feminine and masculine elements, leading to a deeper understanding of our human nature without limiting the ways of knowing ourselves in any way.

I resonate strongly with this somatically grounded process orientation, which, like many professionals, I learned by trial and error. My personal practices with Surya Namaskar eventually led to my certification as a yoga teacher, professional yoga therapist, and Hanna Somatic Educator. When asked to write a Foreword for this book, I was delighted to find that my own teaching for the last 30 or so years echoes much of what I found to be so well articulated in these pages. I see that I have a lot in common with the views shared in this work – practically, experientially, and professionally.

Our physical, energetic, emotional, and mental states, as well as our openness to innate happiness (sometimes called spirit), are core expressions of what it means to be a whole human. As outlined in

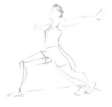

this manual, the practice of Sun Salutes can refine our understanding of our lived human experience. Thus, this book is in many ways a crucial bridge for this particular time in our history. As yoga and more modern concepts such as somatic education are combined and integrated, we may find answers that offer direly needed insight into our current issues. Of course, solving systemic problems that have festered for decades won't happen from doing Sun Salutes alone. Yet the authors envision an important subtle influence, where being dynamically embodied can have both individual and global ramifications and include interesting insights into how this might aid us in current times.

"We have 99 problems," as the saying goes, but being embodied is not one of them. In fact, the book suggests that it might very well help us address issues such as the erosion of modern healthcare systems' ability to manage ailments; the widespread political tensions and economic turmoil we see globally; and the pandemic recovery efforts still in the process of unfolding. Working with these issues in an embodied way is seen as a means to create resiliency for future decades. Furthermore, finding a deeper relational connection might curtail (what many see as the ever-widening) racial and gender divisiveness evident in the large-scale demonstrations of recent years; the "Me too" and "Black Lives Matter" protests are emblematic here. All of these suggest that fundamental change is required in human societies.

And of course, the precipice that serves as a backdrop to these human societal structures on the verge of breakdown is the ecological planetary collapse, pointedly awaiting whether we continue the compartmentalized thinking that prevails currently in the way we address our bodies and minds. The macrocosm is the microcosm, and vice versa.

In light of all this, a resounding return to rhythmic repetition, like that featured in the Sun Salute flow, might be what each of us individually needs to get "as big as we are" and grow, both inwardly and outwardly, towards a new homeostasis. Although simplistic, the Salute to the Sun as an ideal and practice might be a means to help create the critical change needed to generate new social and environmental rhythms, so desperately needed by our planet at this time. This process, honoring the circadian rhythms internally, could connect us to the planet's movement, our inner subtle energy, and the realms of deep individual psychological insights.

It is common in particular circumstances to craft ceremonies where Sun Salutes are repeated 108 times as a deep healing process for cleansing, for honoring the past, and as a reset for the future. I'm hopeful that practicing the holistic-minded approach here, as evidenced by the authors' wisdom within these pages, can help us build a somatic movement practice for ourselves as a worthy structure for making the kinds of changes humanity requires to thrive in the future.

So ma om,

Per Erez, C-IAYT, AHSE
Director of Somatic Interventions
Mind Body Co-op
Owner, First Person Healing Arts Studio
Chicago, IL, USA
July 2021

Preface

Martha's Story

The Sun Salutation has been a part of my life for over forty years. When I was in undergraduate school I went to my first yoga class with Bonnie Bainbridge Cohen in South Amherst, Massachusetts. It was taught by Jeannie Erlbaum, long-time teacher of Hatha yoga. My college dance professor introduced us to two forms of somatic movement education that became formative. One was Laban Movement Analysis (LMA) with Irmgard Bartenieff and the other Body-Mind Centering® (BMC), created by Bonnie Bainbridge Cohen. I also studied sciences, danced regularly, and was becoming a feminist. For recreation, I did organic farming and studied herbal medicine.

It felt good, and special, to debrief yoga classes with Bonnie, who helped us source resonant power in our bodies. My second BMC workshop was on working with the endocrine glands in an embodied way. With BMC we explored vitality and meaning, whether practicing yoga poses, dancing, flying on trapezes, or going about daily life. I joined a cadre of students who took part in the early explorations and development of BMC, which has become a philosophy and methodology of cellular consciousness and human evolution. Private sessions in BMC with Bonnie also helped me release the intensity of my inner-city upbringing and hyper-sexualized teen years. Movement as a healing force, together with strengthened identity as an independent woman, helped me develop "protective resiliency" – my ability to kick or to yield as needed.

I loved yoga – it was a calm, centering experience. The mood was straightforward, humor-filled, and deep all at the same time. We learned to meditate, chant, and follow Sanskrit incantations while we practiced asanas, yoga postures. Jeannie guided me to various yoga retreats to learn meditation practices.

In 1980, I was given Shaktipat and the name Daya-Devi (by Chidvilasananda).

While I had always been "sensitive" – declared "the psychic one" in my family by local Espiritistas – the Kundalini opening of Shaktipat was profound and set me on my path of daily meditation, reinforced by my family. My sister was a teacher of Transcendental Meditation and our parents were deeply spiritual, forward-thinking ministers and community activists in Spanish Harlem, where we were born and raised.

Movement was central. I found my personal way to Spirit through yoga, dance, and somatic movement. I also chose to do the Sun Salutation as a key movement prayer most days. Various friends were exploring higher consciousness. When I returned to New York City I delved into the art of Ki movement, now Shin Budo Kai, with Imaizumi Sensai, and also traveled to Japan to study Ki-Aikido with Tohei Sensai. These are all forms of moving energy.

The scientist in me wanted to further understand movement and energy. Graduate studies at Columbia University in Applied Physiology and doctoral research in Movement Science with the School of BioBehavioral Studies gave me another lexicon for bodily experience. Love of exploration and of scientific investigation informs this book.

A key concept that threads through these pages is one I developed while shaping the theories and practices of my system of Dynamic Embodiment Somatic Movement Therapy. I posit that engaging in dynamic spatial pulls through the specific areas of the body serves as a way to stimulate the glands. This concept brings together the influence of one principle from each of my two primary teachers' work: Bainbridge Cohen/BMC taught that "glands can be stimulated by movement and vocalization," and Bartenieff/LMA that "the body can be harmonized by exploring ways to balance spatial forces" and through clarifying "spatial intention."

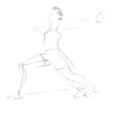

Serendipity also led me to "Tensegrity" amongst Rolfers in the 1970s and it stuck with me because my brother had built a Geodesic Dome in Vergennes, Vermont, in the late 1960s. As a high-school student, he used the Tensegrity model of dynamic forces from Buckminster Fuller. Then Virginia Reed, former President of the Laban/Bartenieff Institute, brought her plastic fluctuating Tensegrity model to a Laban Space Harmony class in 1980 and talked about how Bartenieff also loved the Tensegrity model of human movement. I have been using this concept ever since. Tensegrity underlies how fascia creates structural support for the body, posture, and human movement. Both (Ida) Rolf and Bartenieff focused on fascia and its health as critical to alignment and movement. It is thrilling to see the intersections of all of our movement approaches now. Over a decade ago I sponsored a workshop for Dr Stephen Levin, the person who coined the term Bio-Tensegrity, the application of Tensegrity concepts to biology. I recently spoke on this history and related concepts at a forum of Dr Levin's community – Bio-TensegriTEA (<https://www.youtube.com/watch?v=Dbpy3U2SHik>, August 14, 2020).

All of these threads weave together in the development of Dynamic Embodiment Somatic Movement Therapy and explain how I have remained motivated to practice the Sun Salutation, with new angles and experiences, daily for decades. When teaching Dynamic Embodiment Somatic Movement Therapy I met Shakti Smith, who matched my passion for yoga, BMC, DE, herbs, and mysticism, and brought her own expertise. We have woven much more through our explorations together. It is exciting to share this journey with you.

Martha Eddy, CMA, CTBMD,
DEP, EdD, MFLCI, RSMT
Founder and Director of
BodyMind Dancing &
Dynamic Embodiment SMT
Director of Programming and
Research www.MovingForLife.org
DrMarthaEddy.com
July 2021

Shakti's Story

I first did yoga as a child at an experimental school called the Bundy Art Gallery school in Warren, Vermont. I vividly remember doing tree pose in the high country meadow, as well as balancing in crow when I was four or five years old. From the beginning, my practice was intertwined with nature. As a teen I did some yoga with my father, who regularly went to Kripalu Center and learned from GuruDev. During my first year at the University of Vermont I studied yoga. I was pretty excited, as this was 1986 and yoga was not yet popular in the mainstream. In this class, along with my studies in Voice and Theatre, I began to understand the importance of breathing, following the teacher's instructions to use more of the torso in the breath, not just the belly or just the chest. Fueled by this experience I began doing Sun Salutations regularly. They were an important part of traveling with friends: starting the day with Surya Namaskar, the Salute to the Sun, was a necessary way of centering when on the road. These sacred moments in community cemented this practice as an intrinsic part of my life. I have been practicing and teaching Surya Namaskar now for 35 years.

In 1990 I was introduced to Contact Improvisation (CI) at a Jam on the island of Maui, in Hawaii, where I lived for a year to study meditation; soon after, I was introduced to Authentic Movement and Body-Mind Centering® (BMC®) at radical Burlington College in Vermont, from Luanne Sberna and Sara McMahon. These three forms (BMC, CI, and Authentic) went hand in hand and became central to my life and teaching. BMC was a part of most Contact Improvisation warm-ups, and when I began teaching intensively, in 1995, I drew heavily on BMC and its study of developmental movement to assist dancers and non-dancers alike, to learn the multifaceted form of Contact. I discovered that, if I made developmental movement part of the warm-up, all of the students became more coordinated and body-smart, leading to safe and sophisticated dancing. Even beginners were better able to grasp the complex workings of the form. People learned better, more quickly, and more easily. I saw the joy

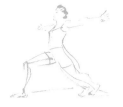

Preface

come into their faces as they became more coordinated and had fun engaging in the dance. For many, learning Contact Improvisation was learning how to play again.

When yoga became more of a focus in my life, somatic practices were a way to soften the smartly specific and strong Iyengar method that I was learning. I studied with Eileen Muir in western Massachusetts while I worked as Manager for two years at the Earthdance Living Project, famed in the movement world as a home for Contact Improvisation and other movement arts. This is also where I met Martha for the first time.

Since moving to New York City, I have had the great pleasure of studying anatomy, BMC®-style, with Genny Kapuler, BMC and Iyengar yoga teacher, and a special group of students in her home and studio. For thirty years I have studied anatomy – from college to massage school, multiple yoga trainings, and many years of Thai Bodywork Training with Kam Thye Chow in Montreal. I first experienced the chakras when I lived at the Findhorn Community in Scotland in 1989, and furthered my studies with Tim Yandow of the Barbara Brennan School of Energy Healing and with Yogiraj Peter Ferko and Yogi Master Alan Finger of Ishta yoga. With Ana Ameryich, student of Sarah Tomlinson (who learned with Harish Joshi), I studied yantras through ceremony, drawing, meditation, and chanting in New York City. With Suren Shrestha I learned Tibetan energy healing and bodywork with singing bowls. Ellen Krueger brought new subtlety and depth to my understanding of the chakras at the Soma-Psyche Institute; later I had the pleasure of teaching chakras with her at the Swedish Institute College of Health Sciences.

With Martha Eddy and Bonnie Bainbridge Cohen I began integrating glandular and developmental awareness more fully into yoga. In classes with Martha, I was able to deepen into my poses in striking ways. I have found that the gland and organ focus grounds the energetic practices of yoga for my students. It makes it more real. My yoga practice found new depth during my ten-day Vision Quest in the mountains of New Mexico with Sparrow Hart in 2017. During this time, spirit spontaneously moved through me while I was practicing Surya Namaskar outside in nature, showing me how to create space inside the body and heal in concert with the elements.

The Sun Salutation is the practice that I have found myself coming back to, again and again, for thirty-five years now. It is a ritual that lasts through time. I have found that when one has a spiritual practice, it can be the forum through which spiritual openings can happen; and when this practice is also a physical one, these openings are grounded in the present reality of our bodies and our lives.

Shakti Smith, RSME, RYT, LMT, DEP
Prema Soma Healing Arts
Somatic Movement Educator,
Yoga Teacher, Energy and
Bodyworker, Sound Healer
July 2021

Salute to our Teachers and Acknowledgments

Salute to our Teachers, our Elders

Shakti and Martha salute:

Irmgard Bartenieff
Bonnie Bainbridge Cohen
Jeannie Erlbaum
Genny Kapuler
Eileen Muir
Peter Ferko
Ellen Krueger
Tim Yandow

We dedicate this book to our elders.

We have come to love listening to our elders, appreciating their wisdom. Some of the women we respect most are leaders in the somatic movement world, like Irmgard Bartenieff and Bonnie Bainbridge Cohen, each of whom rejects the marginalization of the esoteric, of dance, and of women, and embraces all people as valuable on the earth. Writing invites the unknown. Embracing awareness of movement and posture, or any difficult change of habit, often takes place through integration and application of the combined knowledge that we inherited from our teachers – whether ancestors, family members, educators, therapists, or friends who touched our lives. As we worked together on this text, surges of liberty, activism, and dance each emerged. So here we are, 35 years later, happy to share what lived in our notebooks for years.

Acknowledgments

There are numerous people that Martha and Shakti would like to thank for helping bring this book into being:

Dana Davison, for her informed care and knowledge of the material, as she assisted both of us with her technical and style editing. Shakti gives heartfelt thanks for her steadfast belief in and support of this project from the beginning.

Sarena Wolfaard, for having faith in the vision and purpose of this book and bringing together a wonderful team at Handspring. Thank you, Morven, Glenys, Wendy, and Kirtsteen.

Stewart Hoyt, for his beautiful drawings done live, of Shakti and students in her yoga classes, that grace almost every page. Thank you to the yogis and yoginis that he drew at Wendy Newton and Peter Ferko's The Table yoga studio in Brooklyn, including Sarah, Martha, Phebe, Sally, and Peter Anthony.

Serge Cashman, for capturing the moments with his stellar photography, and for opening up Unit 108 Yoga studio in Brooklyn to us during the pandemic for a photo shoot. Thank you to Michelle and little Hunter for joining us there and working and playing to find the right developmental images.

The yoga teachers, from all over the world, who teach at Unit 108 and whose images are in these pages: Krista, Asher, Isabelle, Rinchen, Karen, Lupe, Serge, and Sara.

Thank you to Hrana Janto for her artwork, and to her and Dave Sheppard for permission to use

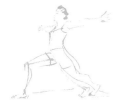

Salute to our Teachers and Acknowledgments

the full-color Shakti chakra drawing in Chapter 2. Thanks also to Marghe Mills-Thysen, Teacher of BMC® and Feldenkrais Practitioner, for her drawings of the arm bones to help depict the scapula–fingertip connections. Shakti is grateful to Jeff Volk for his assistance with the Cymatics section and giving us permission to use the fantastic images. She also thanks Kyle Buller for his generous contributions to and assistance in editing the section on entheogens. Shakti thanks Peter Ferko for making sure we correctly quoted Yogiraj Alan Finger, and gives deep thanks to him for the most powerful Chakra yoga teachings of her life.

Shakti also wants to thank her many anatomy teachers, including Genny Kapuler for her special and layered way of teaching that has impacted her own greatly. Shakti thanks from over the years the great teachers of yoga, herbalism, energy work, sound healing, and shamanism who influenced her life, teaching, and healing work – their wisdom has found its way onto these pages.

Thanks to Bonnie Bainbridge Cohen for her ongoing luster for discovery and decades of inspiration and love; and for spending hours on the phone with Martha to assist in presenting Body-Mind Centering® in its true light, and for sharing some nuggets that are being published here for the first time.

Martha and Shakti thank each other.

Shakti thanks her partner, Stewart, for his love, support, and cooking while she wrote and arranged for production of photos and images.

Martha thanks Blake and Kaya Middleton for their willingness to share Martha with her computer and their excitement about this book coming to fruition.

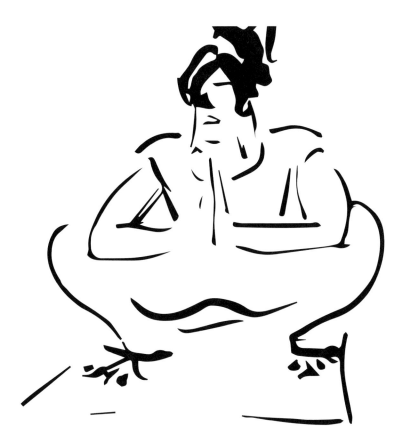

Introduction

Orientation

*Dynamic Embodiment**SM of the Sun Salutation* is a guidebook that walks you through practices of the Salute to the Sun, also known as the Sun Salutation. The traditions primarily influencing this guide are Iyengar, Ishta, and Hatha yoga.

This book focuses on engaging with yoga using a somatic approach, called Dynamic Embodiment^{SM} (DE^{SM}), developed in the 1990s by yoga practitioner Martha Eddy. It is co-authored by longtime Yoga and Somatics teacher Shakti Smith, who is also a Dynamic Embodiment Practitioner (DEP). Together the authors aim to share how some specific somatic approaches to practicing the Sun Salutation can result in more ease, no matter how you are feeling each day. For those who teach, the aim is to support you in conveying this easeful and dynamic approach to others.

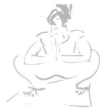

Introduction

A major goal of this book is to assist you in meeting your body and mind health goals and those of your clients and students. The DE Somatic Movement approach (DE) brings physiological and spatial perspectives to working with the chakras and our glandular energies. Both authors have personally been using these as the center point of teaching yoga to movement therapists, dance educators, cancer patients, and women of all ages working through health and hormonal issues, as well as older adults and people with injuries. It provides inroads for making yoga positions more comfortable and sustainable.

This book shares how the Sun Salutation serves as a container for glandular balancing. By learning "different angles or lenses" for your practice, you can discover how DE supports musculo-skeletal alignment, organ health, and optimal endocrine functioning. This approach is embedded in how the human body organizes itself to learn early foundational movement (prenatal through to toddlerhood) and how these movements impact on the "neuroendocrine" system. This neuro-developmental glandular approach to the Sun Salutation is important for physical, emotional, and spiritual impact. It is an "even more" embodied approach to practicing the Sun Salutation.

A major thrust is to describe health imbalances impacted by glands and chakral issues and to work with recuperative yoga in new ways, adding more subtlety to how to support comfort and ease. You can gain more perspective on what to do when yogic or endocrine work brings on intense feelings – from trauma triggers, Kundalini overwhelm, and hormonal flooding to basic life confusion. While the main focus of the book is on personal glandular experience, it also takes into account cultural contexts and the upheaval and challenges that arise from societal forces, acknowledging that different bodies have different experiences and therefore varied responses to yoga and to movement in general. Intermittent references to the oppressive forces in many societies lead to a need for resources in social somatics, such as *Cultural Somatics* (Menakem 2017) and *Generative Somatics* (Haines 2019), and work with the "Socially Conscious Body," a construct of Carol Swann's. These assist in the healing of personal wounds or those emergent from intergenerational trauma. A new concept being presented in the DE approach to the Sun Salutation is that adults can be supported by recalling, relearning, and reliving the developmental movement of early childhood movements.

As background to this fresh approach to yoga, a history of the purpose and evolution of the Sun Salutation is shared, followed by multi-layered guidance for using this ritual in personally tailored ways. The focus is on the embodiment experience, taking time to feel the body, whether in stillness or movement, and to gain access to physical resources within the body that come from your glands – your endocrine system – as well as from your brain – your neural system. This combination of neural and endocrine activation relates, in DE, to the time-honored experience of the chakras.

A predominance of the perspectives and knowledge in this book is drawn from the "new" wisdom of somatic education as it relates to ancient yoga and one hundred years of the Sun Salutation practice. Somatic education is often sourced from Asian, African, and Indigenous movement practices (Eddy 2002, 2016), and merged with western science to awaken neuroplasticity and activate psychoneuroimmunology – how the mind and stress affect immunological functioning (Pert 1997, 2007). In DE this interactive health includes the impact of neuroendocrine control. A major focus is to explain how the brain and entire nervous system, as well as hormones (the chemicals secreted into your bloodstream by the endocrine glands), can be gently stimulated or calmed, and thereby regulated.

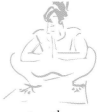

DE principles teach how to carefully engage in embodiment of different bodily tissues, using movement, sound, sensation, and spatial awareness. Used within the poses (asanas), this can be an effective inroad for stimulating and balancing glands (Bainbridge-Cohen & Mills 1980, Hartley 1995, Eddy 2020). These DE perspectives on holistic movement guide you as reader/mover/teacher/therapist to better understand the experience of moving through the Sun Salutation with bodily consciousness. Throughout these chapters, the aim is to clarify the postural alignment of the skeletal system, activate support from "the inner body," and integrate the imprint of our early childhood movement experiences (developmental movement), especially as taught in Body-Mind Centering® (or BMC®), the work of Bonnie Bainbridge Cohen. If someone has a bodily challenge, muscular, skeletal, organ, and endocrine attention can help to find safer ways to move like babies and children often can – arching backwards, folding over, resting into small shapes, stretching into big steps, moving into resting positions, bowing, and stretching. Each vital action of the Sun Salutation can become more easeful with neurodevelopmental endocrine support.

In DE the movement transitions between the asanas are taught from both a neuroendocrine and a developmental perspective. Skeletal alignment is one way to reduce joint stress, discomfort, and pain. Additionally, accessing "inner body focus" by contacting the endocrine glands, with some reference to the organs, supports lightness and fullness. How each of these "layers" can be used when practicing the Sun Salutation emerges in a progression. However, you can return to any specific part of the book whenever needed. The knowledge and modifications shared are to help you to experience new ways of moving, which in turn you can use to guide people. You can learn and teach how, through practicing neurodevelopmental

movements, almost anyone can re-enter the comfort and purity of the Sun Salutation actions, as if children. Over the course of this book, these choices become more familiar and easier.

Throughout this book, the desire is that each person who wants to continue to practice the Sun Salutation through the hills and valleys of life – injuries, illness, or stress – can do so. When dealing with pre-existing pain, a new injury, exhaustion, or stress, it is important to rest and go easy. Indeed, a central premise of the DE approach is to rest often, especially when tired. Focusing on the glands also supports asanas and posture, which is enhanced by integrating with neurodevelopmental movement. By practicing from these points of view, you and your clients will (1) access issues that underlie the causes of pain, (2) have guideposts for experimenting with adaptive positions, and (3) learn techniques for balancing the hormonal systems. The following explains how this is done.

How the Layers of Learning Unfold

Chapter 1 explains the overall approach and underlying theories of DE and somatic education.

Chapter 2 provides a history of yoga and Sun Salutation, as well as the history of the chakra system. You are introduced to the relationship of the chakras to the nervous system and glands, to "Working in Threes," a safe way of working, and also to Kundalini connections.

Chapter 3 describes each of the 14 glands as taught in BMC, discussing the physiology and the hormone secreted, and offering meditations, movements, types of touch, and vibration as used by DEPs to bring balance. You receive "calls to action." With each gland, you are invited to: Locate, Sound (Vibrate), Energize (Touch or Movement).

Chapter 4 is dedicated to an overview of the chakras, describing how chakral energies can be contacted by themselves or by moving through the related glands. This journey through the chakras is supported by sound, moving from the root to crown chakra, approached with glandular and/or chakral attention.

In Chapter 5, the practice of the Sun Salutation is outlined and guided. Charts depict how the Sun Salutation can be approached with glandular and/or chakral attention. Additional tips are added from another somatic system – Bartenieff Fundamentals (BF), the work of dancer and physical therapist Irmgard Bartenieff, also a student of Qigong.

Chapter 6 is dedicated to understanding that each person's movement at any age in life is based on what was learned and practiced *in utero* and during the first years of life. In Body-Mind Centering®-influenced somatic movement approaches, each of these patterns is considered to be further influenced by, and to act as an influence on, hormonal development. A third set of Sun Salutation tips/guidance is added here, bringing in the lens of developmental movement, how our early childhood and animal-like experience influences movement.

In Chapter 7 the focus is on alignment and how each joint in the body bears weight, impacted by gravity, posture, and our habits of use. These asanas, movements, and meditations in many cases are similar to recuperative yoga. The DE approach provides further adaptations of the Sun Salutation. Caring for each joint is supported by focusing on the glands/chakras or developmental movement. Specifically, tips are given for how to continue your practice even if you have an injury or limitation in your range of motion.

Chapter 8 discusses how the glands play a part in health challenges. Four common syndromes that are signals of imbalance within westernized cultures have been selected: (1) dealing with the pressures of work stress and related exhaustion, (2) sleep disorders and related syndromes – menstrual, mental unrest, health issues, (3) weakened immune systems and toxicity in the environment, and (4) managing energy. The goal is to learn to locate, breathe, vibrate, and energize the pineal, adrenal, thymus, and thyroid glands safely, with the goal of supporting the successful management of these issues.

Chapter 9 addresses how you can teach yoga focusing on the anatomy and movement of the glands or chakras as a key curricular focus. You learn more about how to explain the Sun Salutation practice and why working from a DE perspective is useful. Lessons are shared to inspire and ignite. The goal is that everyone will keep moving with ease and joy for years to come.

The final chapter, Chapter 10, moves beyond movement interventions for glandular imbalances with brief stories about and knowledge of the power of supportive herbs and healthy lifestyle – the needs to eat, rest, meditate, and think consciously. Also included is a small section on entheogens.

Introducing Broader Perspectives and Purposes

A value that is underlying the entire book is the importance of working toward a healthier society, undoing policies that create inequalities, and striving for more intimate and caring connections within and with others. Individual health can be related to a concern for health equity worldwide. This construct also assumes that desire for community health helps each individual. A second construct is that by attuning with your own body as you gain embodiment skills you are supporting your self-care through bodily relationships and healthy behaviors. In many cases this vulnerability and development of strength can be a model for social and environmental justice – cultivating a positive relationship with self, with

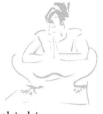

other people, and with the earth. To honor these values, *Dynamic Embodiment*^{SM} *of the Sun Salutation* ends with the continued goal to work toward overcoming inequities. The importance of nature is celebrated with a four-day unit on *outdoor yoga* – connecting with the originating resource of yoga and the Sun Salutation – moving with awareness of the earth and the sun!

Encapsulation

DE is a three-decade-old somatic movement system that brings together the theories, practices, and philosophies of Body-Mind Centering® with the Laban/Bartenieff work, along with two other foci – movement science and social justice. When invested with the somatic awareness of DE, each of the reasons for the practice of the Sun Salutation takes on more layers of meaning. As you expand your somatic sensitivity you too are able to:

1. Enjoy the experience of nuanced sensations that allow you to adjust your movement in order to know yourself better and to protect your body from injury.

2. Discover the glands and chakras by choosing how to move your body in or through space, and how this can support your movement efficiency.

3. Learn about early childhood movement and how the Sun Salutation is so much like the movement of children and animals – as in mimicking "cobras" and "dogs." These movements reactivate the learning processes of early development to refresh the nervous systems. Practicing any movement with neurodevelopmental guidance can also stimulate the underlying connections to the brain and glands (Bainbridge Cohen 1993, Hartley 1995).

4. Find the connections between thinking, feeling and the hormonal system.

5. Expand your mental picture of where you source your movement and moods from – specifically, which gland supports meditation, sleep, silence, expression, inner strength, breath rhythm, emergencies, anger, saying yes and no, feeling sexual, and experiencing centeredness on the planet (to name some).

6. Relate these movements and sensations to what is meaningful in your life – experiencing relief from stress and pain, finding joy and pleasure, and having fun.

How Dynamic Embodiment^{SM} and This Book Work – Separately and Together

In *Dynamic Embodiment*^{SM} *of the Sun Salutation*, principles of somatic movement are aligned with specific activities that can be tailored to you or your family, your friends, or your students and clients. Throughout the book, it is suggested that you witness how your Sun Salutation practice impacts you from a perspective of current cultural and psychophysical occurrences as well as from a more traditional focus on self and on bonds with nature. Your health and attitudes transmit to the people around you, including your students. Finding your own vitality, feeling how it is impacted by social forces, and knowing how to strive for world health while rejuvenating yourself are critical for you and for your students/clients/patients. Taking time with nature is a powerful resource and moving the Sun Salutation with somatic awareness, "natural intelligence" (Aposhyan 2007), can foster these

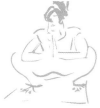

deep connections between body, mind, and place, being on and of the earth (Olsen 2002).

You are encouraged to revisit chapters when you want to better understand how to:

- Reactivate the glands and hormones and chakras (Chapters 3 and 4)

- Reinvigorate your posture and moving alignment using precise musculo-skeletal terms and activities (Chapters 5 and 7)

- Re-experience the purity of early childhood, and revisit or activate conscious sensation of the nervous and endocrine systems to help you perform each pose with more ease (Chapters 6 and 8)

- Refresh your practice for teaching or deepen your holistic lifestyle by discovering lesson plans or lifestyle tips (Chapters 9 and 10).

You, as the reader, can focus on integrating the tools from this book either for personal practice, when attending classes, or in teaching all or parts of the Sun Salutation to individuals or groups.

Setting Goals for Your Sun Salutation

Once you have decided to explore the Sun Salutation as a ritual, there are choices to make about which focus to bring to it, and why. To deepen your practice, it is helpful to ask yourself: What are your goals in doing the Sun Salutation? You can even ask: What do you expect to learn from a book, and specifically this book? You might just be curious – that is great. Or you might have specific physical, mental, or spiritual goals. This book is meant to engage with your own desires and pathways for meeting your goals.

To determine an answer to the question "What are your goals?", take a moment and do some "free-flow" writing about practicing the Sun Salutation. You can start by completing one or all of these sentences:

- I am intrigued by the Sun Salutation because….

- I practice it because….

- I choose to see what emerges. This is what I imagine…. (add in images that work for you – being in water, supported by spaciousness or breath etc.)

Stop reading here and write or audio-record yourself using the prompts above.

- Continue reading once you have written, read, and reflected on your sentences.

You may have already answered the following questions. If not, feel free to answer them now:

- What do you know about the Sun Salutation (nothing, a lot, or a little)?

- Do you already practice it? If so, in what contexts (how often, where, with what thoughts going through your mind)?

- What goals do you have, if any, in setting out to practice the Sun Salutation?

- What intimidates you about it? What resistances do you have?

- What do you love and want to preserve about your movement and/or yoga practice?

Honor what emerges and find someone to talk about it with if you want to hash anything out.

Taking Care: Being Careful But Not Too Cautious

Throughout this book there are specific cues for moving through the asanas within the Sun Salutation. You learn to adapt it for different

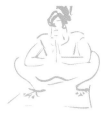

goals and for different conditions. It is important to be careful, but being overly cautious can curtail your exploratory spirit. It is ideal to learn how to experiment with movement within a "safe-for-you range."

Perhaps you have an orthopedic pain – joint discomfort or a recent injury. You will read how to adjust many of the movements for different joint-related issues. Or you may have a hormonal issue. While this knowledge does not substitute for medical advice, our goal is to share the power of the Sun Salutation in stimulating the glandular system and the power of bringing awareness to the glands and their related hormones in performing the Sun Salutation, plus potential impacts on specific health challenges.

Movement coordination is important, and this is addressed through the "developmental approach." These concepts are reflected in charts of the Sun Salutation, which often follow this pattern – starting out simple and whole and then becoming more layered. These provide quick visual reminders of the different lenses for experiencing the Sun Salutation, whether looking at early childhood movement development, including prebirth and infant experiences, or the related connections of joints and glands that impact postural habits that began in youth and may still be operative today. In the teaching section you receive guidance about when to use which resources: asana, glands, chakras, or developmental movement, depending on what your goals are.

Embodied Reading

By moving through and with the chapters of this book, the Sun Salutation can be a journey into multiple lands – the domains of bodily alignment, of balancing the synergy of muscles to feel expansive in space, of finding hormones as resources, of embodying the volume of organs inclusive of emotions, and by remembering early childhood movement. These domains work together to stimulate or calm glandular energy. They can be ramped up or dampened down as needed to avoid injury, preserve energy, or awaken to different feeling-states.

Learning becomes strongest when practicing the activities in this book by applying the concepts in daily life. In Chapter 7 tips are provided to experiment with the Sun Salutation in a manner that is gentle for the specific joints: for instance, protecting the knees, supported by spaciousness in the kidneys and adrenals, and helping the upper body, with more awareness of the posture and "breath of the heart" and lungs and the power of the thymus and thyroid. You may want to use this as a workbook to study with a partner or group.

Again, everything in this book can be learned for your own health and exploration or for teaching others. It makes somatic sense to start with yourself. And, if you like specificity, it can be helpful for you to know what your own personal health, educational, and professional goals are and to approach the learning with focus.

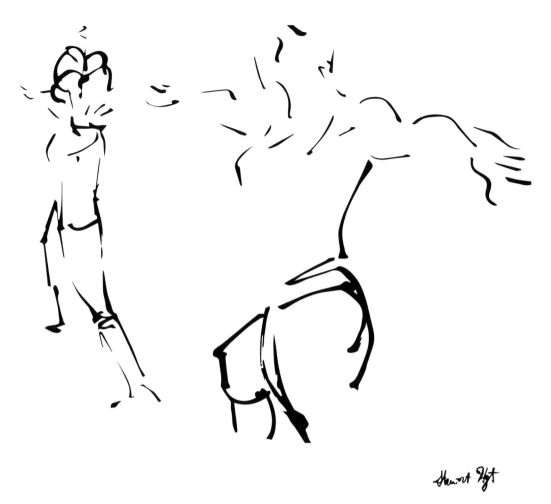

1 Somatic Awareness and Dynamic EmbodimentSM – Components that Support the Sun Salutation

Somatic Awareness

Somatic awareness aims to awaken bodily choices, change deleterious habits, and improve coordination, comfort, and ease through growing skills in listening to body cues. A next step is to apply this awareness to your movement. Many people need support to exercise without discomfort and/or meet their individual health goals. Forming new positive habits takes practice and new perspectives. Somatic awareness provides fresh perspectives by paying keen attention to bodily sensations, whether in stillness or while moving. To notice new sensations, it is often best to "take a bodily inventory" while standing or sitting in a position or doing a movement that is familiar. Dynamic EmbodimentSM (DESM) celebrates the importance of rituals, like the Sun Salutation. A movement ritual sets a base for becoming more conscious

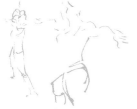

of movement and of changes. Somatic awareness intensifies what you become conscious of within the body-mind.

In order to become somatically aware there are two main methods – self-study (exploring sensations alone) or learning with a guide (in a group or one to one). Both methods require the use of our "hidden senses," two senses that you may never have learned about in school. The primary senses for somatic awareness are those that direct your focus inward in order to feel your body. These are called proprioception and kinesthesia. Proprioception is being able to know your own body shape (what joints are bent or extended and to what degree) and your level of muscular tension. Proprioception also underlies kinesthesia – the ability to sense the body while moving. The kinesthetic sense includes being able to know body shapes and tensions (proprioception) while also including perceptions of movement that come from the

vestibular organs of equilibrium (also known as the semicircular canals/labyrinths) found inside the inner ear.

Interoception is a newer term, which relates to internal perception, originally referring to sensing the autonomic nervous system impacting organs, fluids, and glands. It is now also being used to include self-awareness of musculo-skeletal posture and movement. Its opposite is exteroception, which refers to the five senses that many learned as schoolchildren – tasting, touching, smelling, hearing, and seeing. In teaching children, DE educators identify five internal senses as well, now totalling ten senses (see Fig. 1.1). They include the abilities to feel one's shape, level of tension, posture, being off-vertical in falling or tilting, and at what pace a movement is happening – starting and accelerating on the way to stopping by slowing down. The first two, perceiving one's own body tension and form, are proprioceptive. The last two, awareness of falling

Sensing the World – Exteroception

Sight

Taste

Hearing

Smell

Touch

Sensing Yourself – Interoception

Stand Tall

Body Shape

Stop/Start

Tilt/Fall

Tension

Figure 1.1
The ten senses as taught at the Center for Kinesthetic Education, NYC. Copyright ©Martha Eddy
www.wellnessCKT.net

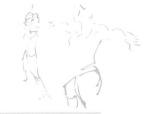

off vertical or accelerating and decelerating, are kinesthetic. Standing tall is a combination of all of these four sensory elements.

Another aspect of somatic awareness is how outer sensory information and inner sensory information can support one another. Working with a somatic expert, or with the experiences and ideas in this book, will bring awareness not only to the sensations of the musculo-skeletal system but also to the autonomic nervous system as well as surroundings.

The autonomic nervous system is the part of the nervous system which governs the behavior of the parts of our bodies that you don't have to feel or think about in order to function – they are automatic and therefore involuntary and "subconscious." It includes the low brain – the brainstem and cerebellum that have everything to do with heart rate, breath, balance, and primal emotions (especially in relationship to the vagus nerve) – as well as the limbic system, where our emotions and pain are regulated. The vagus nerve is an important regulator of the breath, heart, guts (microbiome), and other autonomic functioning. Polyvagal theory includes additional pathways to the eyes, mouth, and face as well. Positive, compassionate interaction with others can help modulate "vagal tone." This helps to balance moods and emotional state through co-regulation (Porges 2011).

> **Common Features of Somatic Movement Training**
>
> Through a lifetime of embodied study and ten years of cross-case anthropological research, Eddy (2009, 2016) located these features as common in all somatic training:
>
> - Slowing down in order to feel the inner body
>
> - Breathing deeply
>
> - Releasing tension, often lying down, moving in as easy-going a way as possible
>
> - Sensing the body's three-dimensionality
>
> - Practicing new movements to change habits, sometimes referred to as "novel coordination" (Batson & Wilson 2014, Eddy 2016).

Novel Coordination and Repetition

Engaging with novel coordination means doing something new with your body. When someone guides you with words, visual teaching (demonstrating a movement, whether online or in person), or touch, this can be referred to as Movement Re-patterning or Movement Re-education. "Re" is used because most people learn these movements as babies and children, and yet with life's challenges and sedentary ways many cultures have lost the naturalness of these movements. Almost everyone needs to reproduce these building blocks of movement. Somatic movement practitioners (educators and therapists) can help with this process.

No matter what the goal, almost every human can benefit from tapping into the self-awareness that somatic education cultivates. The main tool for that embodied self-awareness is proprioception. The proprioceptive sense is a deeply embedded tool of the soma – the living body. It is the ability to feel sensation and take care of oneself, whether consciously or through unconscious self-regulatory responses.

Somatic knowledge always exists but people are often not aware of this resource. By paying attention to the soma, the living body, awareness of the body increases, and insights gleaned from the body can be a link to diverse mental

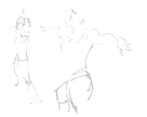

states and emotions. You can gain somatic awareness on your own, but an outside view can help. Whether enlisting a mirror or a person (who ideally compassionately mirrors), you are provided with new insights. When doing this type of consciousness-raising with a skilled practitioner or a friend you can also discuss questions like: What did you perceive differently? What changed in your body, if anything? What allowed for the change of perception or sensation? A skilled somatic movement practitioner is trained to guide you into deeper realms (of body, mind, or emotions) safely. Gleaning information from our bodies is done best when practicing everyday movements or routines that are familiar. The Sun Salutation is a great ritual for practicing somatic awareness.

Dynamic Embodiment^{SM} as a Somatic System

To engage with the Sun Salutation using DE is to engage in somatic movement. Somatic movement refers to moving with body-mind awareness. The DE approach expands multi-dimensions of consciousness by deepening self-awareness and cultivating meaning and purpose from awakening the body-mind connection within cultural frameworks.

DE is relational. It acknowledges that personal awareness occurs in the context of interacting with nature and with other beings. DE's primary entry point of conscious awareness involves witnessing movement preferences or habits and recognizing them as part of functional or expressive behavior. Embedded in this acknowledgment is a recognition that both personal and cultural influences are important. There is also an understanding that life could be more joyful if societal pressures (or oppression) and/or personal attitudes or behavior can change.

Movement preferences are known to have roots in our early childhood development, which are influenced by experiences such as parenting, family dynamics, the setting of one's home, and related cultural values and societal conditions. One's personal movement style reveals one's personality and traits, including habits that may or may not be serving.

Inner physiological systems and states of being affect how one sits, stands, or moves. These physical interactions relate to moods and emotions. Posture, movement, habits, and moods can be addressed powerfully through the DE approach. This is done through your own self-exploration, and being guided by neuromotor and anatomical knowledge, along with imagery from nature and the cosmos, all within a current moment context.

Description, History, and Purpose

DE is a form of somatic education and movement therapy developed by Eddy, who educates Dynamic Embodiment Practitioners (DEPs) to be eligible for registration as Registered Somatic Movement Educators and Therapists. DE lessons use somatic movement, skilled touch, and conscious dialogue to bring health, vitality, consciousness, clarity, and creativity into people's lives, whether learning as individuals or in groups. Using various philosophical foundations, knowledge bases, developed skills, and approaches of DE, one goes deeply into the body and uses spatial awareness and movement observation to find a multiplicity of lenses (inside and outside, upside down and right-side up) for attuning with self, others, and the planet. It also includes powerful investigation into one's quality of movement (e.g. strong, light, free, or tense) and where in the body those motivations come from. DE uses both novel coordination and repetition, often

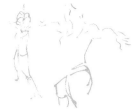

in the form of movement rituals, for learning and for meeting goals.

The process of engaging in conscious dialogue about what is often unconscious is a key feature of DE. Asking what bodily sensations "are saying" or mean can be helpful on one's life path. In DE, one also asks "Somatics for What?" Ultimately, DEPs seek to move beyond gaining awareness for oneself into taking awareness into ACTION. This can include standing up for one's gut feelings or lying down for a deep rest in order to be ready for the next wave of stimulus that life brings.

Begun in 1990, and originally named the Somatic Movement Therapy Training (SMTT), this program was the first training to use the term *somatic movement* in its title. It is also the first to merge the two potent somatic lineages of Irmgard Bartenieff, who created the Laban/Bartenieff Movement Studies curriculum after her studies with Rudolf Laban, and Bonnie Bainbridge Cohen, the founder of Body-Mind Centering® (BMC®). DE applies the work of these three unique mover–thinkers, Bainbridge Cohen, Bartenieff, and Laban, to everyday life and movement through an emergent lens – the lemniscate of highly contemplative inner focus with the outward focus of moving through space to build relationships and engage across people, groups, cultures, and environments.

When the term *somatic movement* started to be used in the titles of more programs, Eddy renamed it Dynamic Embodiment Somatic Movement Therapy Training (DE-SMTT) to differentiate from the others. DE reflects the integration of its major influences. The biology of all tissues of the body is taught experientially to enhance **embodiment** using BMC's keys to consciousness. This embodied learning is contextualized within the Laban/Bartenieff paradigm that says all of life and body use is **dynamic**. This is seen in the powerful variability of human behavior as expressed by diverse movement styles, which can be observed by noting how the body moves in space with unique qualities and shaping. Laban/Bartenieff recognizes that there are always a multitude of behavioral choices existing along diverse continua (e.g. being quick or slow, moving up to down, small to large, narrow to wide, with arms or legs). DE is now a 30-year-old somatic movement system with practitioners around the world, each of whom works in unique ways with this DE-merger of the theories, practices, and philosophies of BMC, BF, and Laban Movement Analysis (LMA).

Teaching Methods: The Use of Ritual and Repetition in Learning

It is often the unity of being involved with a holistic psychophysical process that is healing in and of itself. When one is first learning a new movement coordination it is difficult to also pay attention to oneself. DE values finding a movement sequence that is simple enough to remember and become centering but stimulating enough to expand neural pathways by activating new sensations and spotlighting them in one's awareness. Movement with awareness can be a lead-in to asking questions of the body that, in turn, provide support for "internal self-regulation" – giving the body time and space to engage in the healing it wants to do. Often it is important to get out of the body's way; engaging in familiar and pleasurable movement provides that framework. It gives enough mental space to also notice bad habits so that you can inhibit them. With the reflection process you can also identify new positive goals. Some variability within the ritual is great for pleasure and keeping one's focus.

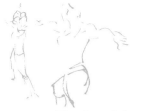

Chapter 1

The Sun Salutation is a powerful yet simple series of movements that many people choose to practice often. This repetition is a perfect vehicle for deepening one's somatic awareness. DE recognizes that the basic postures are reminiscent of infant and early childhood movement, the very movement that originally opened up neural pathways. Revisiting them keeps these pathways active. Revisiting the movements within the Sun Salutation with new information and awareness opens up new levels of consciousness.

> **Why Dynamic Embodiment^SM and the Sun Salutation? A RITUAL Allowing for Embodied Neuroplasticity**
>
> In DE the Sun Salutation has been taught as a ritual for integration of new somatic knowledge and a place to come home to, to check in with oneself. Why else use the Sun Salutation? There are many reasons.
>
> - This ritual from the yogic tradition has been an important part of the authors' lives even before DE existed.
>
> - Over the decades it has served as a ceremony of "awakening to the day," an archetypal prostration prayer, and/or a daily ritual of returning to self, attuning with "where the/my body is at."
>
> - Within the context of DE the daily practice becomes a type of lifelong somatic journey. It serves as an opportunity to link body and mind, and to self-regulate or recharge through movement awareness. It provides both centering and new information.
>
> - It can serve as a template within which to compare somatic sensations as they change from day to day, week to week.
>
> - Through the practice of these particular movements there is opportunity to rehearse and thereby deepen one's neural connections.
>
> - One can do this exploration while maintaining a universal appreciation of the grandness and mystery of life.

Honoring the Lineage

As yoga has much respect for lineage, DE also recognizes Body-Mind Centering® (BMC®), Bartenieff Fundamentals of Movement (BF, a neurodevelopmental approach to human movement awareness, efficiency, and expression), and Laban Movement Analysis (LM) as a large part of its history. DE is an amalgam of these three systems. BF is rooted in LMA, which is a comprehensive framework for understanding and talking about human movement in great detail. Each of these different somatic systems emphasizes different aspects of movement behavior.

Body-Mind Centering®

BMC® is a somatic movement system developed in the early 1970s by Bonnie Bainbridge Cohen. In her recent book (Bainbridge Cohen 2018) BMC is described as having three pathways – Embodied Developmental Movement, Embodied Anatomy, and Embodied Embryology. Not many somatic systems address or have a language for the awareness of the inner body, such as the consciousness and movement of each organ and each endocrine gland. BMC does. It even teaches how to move from the fluid rhythms of the body and how attuning with the rhythm opens you to what aspect of consciousness it represents. Time is spent moving with a specific body system (e.g. organ, gland, fluid, skin, ligaments, soft tissues) and then discussing the personal and collective experience of moving with awareness of each of these distinct body parts. What part of consciousness

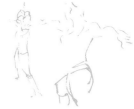

does this body region elicit? BMC also uses awareness of neurocellular development and neuroendocrine awareness as important facets of the embodiment process.

A Taste of Bainbridge Cohen's Story

Bonnie Bainbridge Cohen, a dancer, occupational therapist, and student of more than a dozen somatic systems, was also influenced by the art of Katsugen-undo as developed by Noguchi Sensei and the study of yoga with Yogi Ramaiah. She practiced Katsugen-undo while living in Japan in the late 1960s/early 1970s (Eddy 2002). Katsugen-undo teaches how to access the autonomic nervous system through movement. This discipline, together with her long yoga practice begun with Yogi Ramaiah, opened her experience to the potential movement initiations from organs and the autonomic nervous system, referred to as "organ support" (as in postural support) or "organ movement." Organ support impacts posture by establishing internal volume through somatic awareness. Organ movement is when movement is initiated from deep within the body, accessing the smaller deeper muscles and the quality of internal yet voluminous activity. This can be seen in belly dancing, which sources movement from deep within the body. Different organs elicit different degrees of depth and volume, as well as qualities of movement.

Neurocellular Perspectives and Neuroendocrine Awareness

The developmental process is that of growing bodily and in consciousness throughout the lifespan. BMC has the most in-depth set of theories, amongst the somatic systems, about neuromotor development or neurodevelopmental movement. Through exercises, somatization, and discussions of consciousness as a felt experience anyone can engage with movement memories from infancy, childhood, or adult life.

From the BMC perspective developmental movements are neurocellular – meaning that they are based on a foundation of awareness that predates the development of the nervous system through embryological movements. Development and anatomy meet in BMC when exploring neuroendocrine processes. In studying BMC one also learns a theory of how the different parts of the brain are stimulated by different baby movements (from *in-utero* through to cross lateral movement) as well as Bainbridge Cohen's theory of Equal and Opposite Reflexes (Bainbridge Cohen 1993, Eddy 2016). While learning how primitive reflexes become integrated in our volitional movement one learns there is also simultaneous activation of the glands and hormones.

BMC's neuroendocrine awareness has long recognized the potential for nerves or glands to initiate or support movement and their power in dictating behavior (Bainbridge Cohen 1993).

Other Neurological Influences

The concept of amygdala hijacking (Goleman 1995) and the connection with adrenaline and cortisol coursing through the body during a trauma experience is one example. Another is the ability to calm oneself down using deep brain resources like finding physical or emotional balance by moving from the cerebellum or high-level brain activity as in the frontal lobe. This example is just one of many embodied resources of BMC. Other resources used in BMC since the 1970s include moving in the rhythm of the cerebro-spinal fluid to calm the brain, breathing into specific parts of the body that are holding traumatic memories, and understanding how to feel into and move from

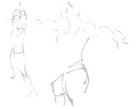

other parts of the body. This is supported by the work done with revisiting embryological and specific infant movements as a stimulus for different regions of the low, mid and high brain, and their relationship to the endocrine system.

The above examples imply that the nervous system is not the only system that impacts behavior and behavioral choices – the hormonal system (the endocrine gland system) does as well. Indeed, both the nervous and endocrine glandular systems are thought to govern feeling and responses – behavior. BMC has taken into account the unconscious, autonomic functioning of the body for almost six decades borrowing the term neuroendocrine from Dr Temple Fay long before it became popularized. Bainbridge Cohen also believes in cellular consciousness, with an awareness that the embryo is a living being, making choices even before having a nervous system. Philosopher Maxine Sheet-Johnstone espouses a similar idea, that a cell moving away or toward another volume demonstrates consciousness.

Activating the Glands Requires Spatial Awareness

When meditating, one is often guided to 'sit tall'. This is of course good for posture. It is relevant in this book as well because good posture aligns the glands. In BMC one way to activate the glands is to experience each one by locating it, breathing into it, feeling its substance or three-dimensionality, and either vibrating it or vocalizing from it. In DE suggestions are to locate, breathe, volumize, and energize. As one feels the expansiveness of each gland, the possibilities for occupying more space and moving through space become easier.

Understanding that awareness of the space around the body supports the body also can be used to awaken glandular energies. Much of

Bainbridge Cohen's current work (Bainbridge Cohen 2020) invites resting into space as well as "allowing space to move the body." This can start as an image: imagine the space under your leg can be engaged to pick up your leg. With enough practice the ease of movement that comes from using this image becomes a reality. One example of activating the endocrine system is to feel each gland in relationship to the space around it, by "taking out the slack" and literally feeling "support from space."

Bartenieff Fundamentals and the Complexity of Space

Bartenieff Fundamentals® of Body Movement emerged from the work of Irmgard Bartenieff (1900–1981), a woman who studied and then worked with the movement scholar also known as the father of German Dance Expressionism, Rudolf Laban, in Berlin, Germany, in the early part of the 20th century.

A Taste of Bartenieff's Story

Bartenieff escaped Germany during the rise of Hitler and the Nazis and came to New York City in 1936. Unable to find work as professional dance performers, she and her husband, Igor Bartenieff, went back to school in their mid-thirties and became physical therapists. While working as a physical therapist treating polio patients at Albert Einstein Hospital, she was invited to use her skills and methods, which integrated with her Laban knowledge, with psychiatric patients as well. Her successes helped to launch the somatic (mind-body integrated) field of Dance Therapy. As one result of this multidisciplinary expertise, Bartenieff developed a series of principles, concepts, and movement activities throughout the 1930s–1970s to teach movement efficiency and enhance

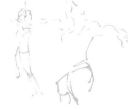

movement expression. Her system, Bartenieff Fundamentals, is considered one of the first systems of somatic education. During this time she also developed the world-renowned curriculum for observing human movement (Laban 1948) called Laban Movement Analysis, now often referred to as Laban/Bartenieff Movement Studies (Bartenieff 1980, Fernandes 2015, Bradley 2008, Studd & Cox 2019).

Fundamentals for Movement Efficiency

Bartenieff's somatic system includes exploring and learning to identify in others the embodiment of the following concepts: Spatial Intent, Breath Support, Core Support, Effort Life (dynamic changes in movement), Shape Support (postural changes), the importance of accessing efficient Weight Shifts, and using the Rotary Factor in human kinesiology, as well as paying attention to the Organization of Movement and its developmental constructs. This involves noticing what early childhood patterns of movement occur in any movement, no matter what one's age. Bartenieff's choice to observe the developmental organization of movement in adults was a break-through in understanding how important developmental movement is throughout the lifespan. The language that Bartenieff and her team established to discuss the developmental progression of body organization includes the following six patterns: Breath, Core–Distal, Head–Tail, Upper–Lower, Body Halves, and Diagonal. These organizational patterns reflect the neurodevelopmental framework of her training as a physical therapist, and her choice to have her adult patients move these patterns was a natural evolution of her training as a dancer. Movement must be practiced.

Bartenieff went on to identify over a dozen exercises that were critical to learn to walk again, which helped her polio patients succeed. Six of them are referred to as "the Basic 6 exercises." Another critical concept that she drew on from her own teacher, Rudolf Laban, is that of "spatial intent." Spatial intent is basically knowing where you want to go. Having a road map for where the body can go helps. Laban developed that map.

Laban Movement Analysis and Space Harmony

Rudolf Laban is considered the father of German Expressive Dance, and was the creator of a written notation and related language for describing human movement. As developed by Irmgard Bartenieff, Laban Movement Analysis (LMA) teaches how to observe unique body part use, movement dynamics and relationships, with awareness and respect for how the mover negotiates environmental influences. It is an experiential learning process that also leads to being aware of one's movement qualities as well as one's presence in space. This dynamic framework describes what is unique about each individual – the special ways a person performs a task or expresses an emotion. Laban also developed movement scales that are part of a larger system named Space Harmony and were taught in his schools throughout northern Europe.

A Taste of Laban's Story

Laban lived through the turn of the 20th century and was considered a Renaissance man. He was part of the "free love movement," was involved with vegetarianism, studied as an architect, and became a crystallographer, dancer, and human movement expert who devised a comprehensive system for describing human movement. As Laban came to identify descriptors for many

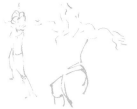

components of movement, he created his notation system, which is analogous to a musical score. It is often called Labanotation. In analyzing movement, he taught hundreds of people to describe what they saw using these parameters: what body parts are moving through space and with what qualities of movement? He took time to develop principles of movement and an entire language for movement description. Four primary Laban principles state that there are constant interactions in any movement between a) mobilizing and stabilizing forces, b) exertion and recuperation, and c) internal and external experience, and d) also state that the functional and expressive aspects of any movement are interrelated. He also got thousands of people dancing together for a common purpose, including union member workers for Labor Day events. The large events were called "Movement Choirs."

Mobility and Stability in Space

When studying mobilizing and stabilizing forces within movement, Laban developed a body of scholarship called Space Harmony. He found that the harmony of moving in space comes from systematically moving through balanced pathways. He developed movement scales, which can be thought of as rituals much like the Sun Salutation, to be practiced both for invigoration and celebration of life, and to check in somatically. Also like the Sun Salutation, practicing movement scales balances the muscles of the body. What fully distinguishes them is the need to maintain a cognitive awareness of where you are moving in space. This practice awakens sensitivity to the space you occupy and how your body feels while moving there and once you arrive. In that way you become more aware of how you stand in space and how you move from place to place. Practicing the Space Harmony scales

or exploring your own movement within these sacred forms enlivens your "spatial awareness," whether standing still or moving.

Space Harmony

In studying LMA, one learns to move through space using spatial scales in much the same way that musicians practice musical scales (Dell & Crow 1977). Moving in harmonic sequences through space, one can become aware of exactly where the pathways of movement are in space, as well as the shape of the crystal that the movement is tracing. This can be visualized when you think of a mime depicting a wall in front or to the side of a space, using the movement of his or her hands. When speaking, there is a constant painting of pictures with the hands whenever gesticulating. A Laban Certified Movement Analyst (CMA) has insight into what type of world you are painting with your movement and enough links into the possible psychophysical meaning of the gestures in order to start a good conversation.

Space Harmony includes many concepts – pathways that body parts travel along, "traceforms" as the pathways that gestures leave in imaginary space, cardinal directions that make up your kinesphere: up–down, right–left, forward–back plus levels, planes, diagonals, and zones: front and back areas, side to side. The kinesphere is the space you can extend out to without taking a step.

Movement Scales

Laban created sequences of movement inside each of the different crystalline forms (Dell & Crow 1977). They are practiced with the whole body to understand how to maximize the harmony of the body by moving through space in a logical progression. Laban situated these scales inside the sacred polyhedron so they provide a symmetry supporting the logic of

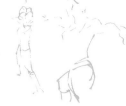

the body. For every crystalline form there is an inner scaffolding and an outer shell. The scales constantly move out on the periphery, or also move through the center of the form, or move between forms.

The interconnectivity of human movement and place is palpable when the mover chooses to pay attention to the fact that movement happens in space. The sensory intensity of "knowing where you are in space" increases when experiencing how one's bodily movement has a cause and effect, by perceiving the pressure changes in space. This awareness is amplified when invoking the sacred forms: tetrahedron, octahedron, cube, icosahedron, and dodecahedron. These are the symmetrical polyhedra known as Platonic solids, which can be found in nature, geometry, and movement. They can serve as organizers of movement if one practices seeing them as existing inside and outside of the body. This practice, of Space Harmony and its related scales, involves using these imaginary maps for physical movement in the space around the body (without taking a step) and moving from point to point, from one spot to another. When moving in the scales one is moving through the shapes of these sacred crystals, creating a crystalline form around one's own body.

Harmonizing with Space – Tensegrity

At the Laban/Bartenieff Institute in the late 1970s, faculty member and former President Virginia Reed taught about "tensegrity." The word was developed by architect Buckminster Fuller, based on concepts he used to create the geodesic dome. The basic premise is that balanced spatial pulls can create support for structure. These are *tensile* forces establishing *integrity* of structure: hence tensegrity. This concept has also been applied to the body and further developed by Dr Stephen Levin, who coined the term "biotensegrity" (Scarr 2014, Eddy 2020). In biotensegrity models, it

is believed that a healthy structure improves biological functioning. This is the premise in applying spatial awareness to working with the glands, while moving.

Reed also shared the work of author Lawrence Blair (1976), whose book *Rhythms of Vision* conveyed how colorful crystalline shapes lent their specific energies to different chakral regions. She had us explore the combinations of Laban's scales being performed inside imaginary sacred crystals (the five Platonic equal-sided polyhedra; see Fig. 1.2) using the concept of tensegrity together with invoking the colors and energy described by Blair (Eddy 2020). Laban did drawings and wrote poetry that was published in a book called *A Vision of Dynamic Space* (Laban with Ullman 1984) which harkens to this integration.

Laban's dimensional scale lives inside the octahedron. Internally, one can breathe along each of the cardinal dimensions – vertically, horizontally, or sagittally – of the octahedron. You can also move outwardly through space along these axes imagining you are inside the "crystal house of the octahedron." The Sun

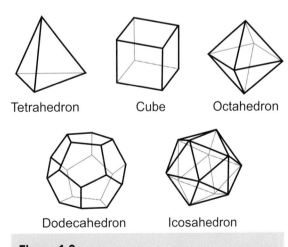

Tetrahedron   Cube   Octahedron

Dodecahedron   Icosahedron

Figure 1.2
The five Platonic solids, sacred forms/crystals/polyhedra.

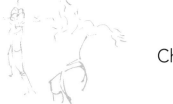

Salutation is most often aligned with the cardinal directions, living inside the octahedron and icosahedron. When you start to tilt, fall, or become off-vertical, this movement shifts to only occupying the icosahedron, a more multifaceted and dynamic form.

The sacred forms are also referred to as the Platonic solids, since Plato developed a philosophy based on them. These polyhedra have been recognized as special from antiquity. They are correlated by Plato with the four elements (earth, air, fire, water) and also are a part of the field of geometry. Their names, from simple to complex, are: tetrahedron, octahedron, cube, icosahedron, and dodecahedron. In Figure 1.2 you can see the five sacred forms, symmetrical and polyhedral.

Blending the Influences and Adding Distinctive Features

These three influences – LMA from the early 1900s, BF from the 1950s–1970s, and BMC from 1960s until today – have shaped a core part of DE. In addition, Eddy brings her background as a scientist, a dance artist, and an advocate for social justice to DE and the DE Approach to the Sun Salutation. Like BMC, DE maintains two main strands of study – that of embodiment through awareness of each and every part of the body and attuning with our bodily roots, our early developmental history. DE also adds scholarly research and social somatics components. A primary goal of the work is to make it as accessible as possible to all people – through working with children, parents, classroom teachers, and visual and performing artists as well as other scientists and medical professionals. Her additional systems, Moving For Life Dance Exercise for Cancer Recovery and BodyMind Dancing, are examples of expansive outreach and applications of the DE work.

Embodied Physiology

Embodiment is supported through two different inroads – by exploring anatomy and physiology experientially, and by exploring the dynamic qualities to express different emotions and to accomplish varying tasks. These dynamics of the effort that goes into moving (minimal or intense) have to be resourced from somewhere! DE looks to the different tissues of the body to find the sources of those varying qualities of movement. This is our access route to the chakras, through understanding our strong glandular activity and how it moves us. Explore how to use the Sun Salutation to regulate our vital energy forces by learning about the multifaceted nature of spacious movement.

The Neurodevelopmental Approach

The second strand is about exploring early experiences – embryonic, birth, and learning to coordinate the body during the first 12–24 months after birth. Each person came into the world through a different journey – that of the biological family and related genetics, that of the people who raised you including their current culture choices, and that of the larger cultural/societal context including experiences of advantage and disadvantage.

The throughline of the BMC work parallels concepts from BF, both involving an understanding of how movement is organized into patterns based on which body areas are moving and which are stable. BMC goes deeply into embryological development and encourages the practice of infant to toddler movement that is common amongst most people. Eddy saw correlations in the embodiment of the "organizational movement patterns"

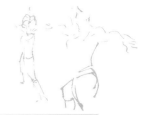

Chart 1.1		
Dynamic Embodiment^{SM} Developmental Stages Comparison Chart		
Developmental organization of body part relationships: Bartenieff's Body Organization, Bainbridge Cohen's Basic Neurocellular Patterns, Eddy's NeuroDevelopmental Organization. These are all stages of perceptual-motor development.		
	Bartenieff Fundamentals	**Body-Mind Centering**	**Dynamic Embodiment**

	Bartenieff Fundamentals	Body-Mind Centering	Dynamic Embodiment
	Body Organization (Bartenieff) Or one can refer to "Patterns of Total Body Connectivity" (Hackney 1998), which echoes the DE improvization of eliciting the connectivity and resulting state of mind particular to each stage. These six stages are not to be confused with Bartenieff's Basic 6 exercises.	Basic Neurocellular Patterns (BNP) Formerly referred to as Basic Neurological patterns; cellular reflects newer embryological study (Bainbridge Cohen 2011)	NeuroDevelopmental Organization (NDO) of perceptual-motor coordination and expression
1	Breath	Breath (cellular and lung)	Three-dimensional Breathing (begins with conception)
2	Core–Distal Connection (condensing and expanding from feet, hands, head, and tail)	Navel Radiation (radial navigation initiated by umbilicus)	Whole Body (torso and limbs) Coordination (going towards and away; begins *in utero*)
3	Head–Tail Connection	Spinal Patterns	Head–Spine Coordination (practiced *in* and *ex utero*)
4	Upper–Lower Connection	Homologous Patterns	Symmetrical Upper–Lower Coordination
5	Body Half Connection	Homolateral Patterns	Right–Left Body Half Coordination
6	Diagonal Connection	Contralateral Patterns	Contralateral Quadrant Coordination

Dynamic Embodiment uses the following language when working with children and educators to teach more about space and geometry as well: three-dimensional breath, whole-body coordination, head to tip of the spine coordination, upper–lower symmetrical body half coordination, right–left body half coordination and cross-lateral quadrant coordination.
Other taxonomies include the following words, listed in developmental order by stage number:
1. respiration
2. contraction–release, or grow–shrink
3. caudal–cephalic
4. bilateral symmetry
5. unilateral or lateral symmetry or ipsilateral, sidedness
6. opposition, cross-lateral, asymmetrical

From Eddy, M. (2015). The ongoing development of "Past Beginnings": neuro-motor development somatic links with Bartenieff Fundamentals, Body-Mind Centering® and Dynamic Embodiment^{SM}. Updated from 2012: Somatics Journal

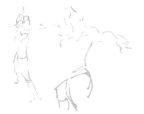
identified by Bartenieff and the BMC physical exploration of the early movements of infants. Eddy brought to light how BMC and BF need to be understood separately to recognize the nuances of infant and adult idiosyncratic personal movements, along with their strengths and need for support.

The neurodevelopmental component shared by both BF and BMC and taught in DE brings all people onto an equal footing. In DE one is taught to also view early childhood development with consideration of the imbalances of societal forces – how conditions of class, race, and ethnicity impact resources available to a family or neighborhood. DE brings awareness of how people with disabilities have contributed to the creative problem-solving of how to most comfortably negotiate space in the activities of daily living and in the arts, no matter what "patterns of coordination" are available.

Research, Bio-Medical Science and Holistic Health

DE adds a research perspective to all units of study. The types of research link to Eddy's expertise in applied physiology, motor learning, curriculum development, violence prevention, exercise science, dance science, and somatic movement. Together they result in a strong focus on injury reduction – including injury to the body or the mind. Other unique features of DE come from Eddy's own life-long training, including elements of Upledger and Biodynamic Cranio-Sacral Therapy and Vodder Lymphatic Drainage. Aspects of these systems are integrated with DE methods as appropriate for enhancing conscious movement. DE also draws from her work as a founding member of the International Dance Science and Medicine Association and as an award-winning dance educator. Holistic

health and wellness concepts are further supported by Eddy's study in holistic healing from 1980 to 1990 with leaders in the fields of herbal medicine, naturopathy, consciousness studies, and energy medicine.

Including Social Somatics

Social Somatics is the examination of self that shapes "a socially informed body," understanding its relationship to culture, class, gender identity, sexual orientation, race, and physical ability, as well as personal history. "Social Somatics understands that the individual *soma* is not separate from its experience in the social context that shapes it. The exploration of Social Somatics is the relationship between our inner embodied experiences and the social systems that shape our lives… Unlike conventional Somatics, Social Somatics consciously activates awareness of our social bodies to transform internalized, relational, structural and cultural conditions that impede wellness for everyone" (from Zea Leguizaman and Sam Grant being quoted by Carol Swann in Eddy 2016).

DE applies all of its principles within a "social somatics" context. This means it seeks to align with environmental and social justice, bringing a somatic perspective to these movements. DE aims to work toward equality of access to holistic health information and practices for all. Moving For Life, free somatic fitness classes for elders and people with cancer, is one example of community outreach based in DE principles. Each DE student is encouraged to tune into and align with personal aesthetics, value their own physical aesthetic, and cultivate unique approaches to the work. Another value is to strive to reverse socially oppressive policies, while taking somatic consciousness into everyday life including interactions and organizations.

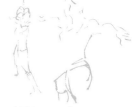

Layers of Who We Are: Culture and Somatics

The DE concept of "Being as Big as We Are" is about claiming space. It is both a bodily and, potentially, a cultural concept. DE teaches the BMC concept that how muscles perform is hugely impacted by the inner body. The inner body includes the positioning and tonus of the organs, glands, and circulating fluids (controlled by the autonomic nervous system). A goal is to learn how to shift the awareness of its function and expression from being unconscious to becoming conscious. DE espouses the belief that there is more musculo-skeletal efficiency when being supported by the healthy working of the nearby organs and glands, and much of that is predicated on having basic needs met, and having access to emotional, physical, and spiritual support.

A cultural and global concept is that all people have varying degrees of these supports. People in the Global Majority (Indigenous peoples and those with Black and Brown bodies, often living or having their heritage in the Global South – south of the equator) have often been greatly disadvantaged regarding economic support due to white European colonization. On the other hand, western cultures of the "Global North" have often turned to the music, dance, and movement life of cultures in the Global South for health and to find harmony and resilience. This irony is evidenced in looking at the roots of most American music and in seeing how many northerners are benefitting from yoga. Another example is the search for holism that is still alive in Indigenous cultures and importing it and sometimes appropriating it. Many white-bodied groups stole land, ideas, and even people from other cultures and then further diminished their worth by maintaining oppressive systems that also include not

teaching accurate history, or uplifting values and ownership from these cultures.

Resmaa Menakem (2017) makes a case for Black people having developed cultures of resilience through strong emotional, physical, and spiritual practices. White people are often attracted to these cultural attributes but have historically sought to control them. His work in Cultural Somatics asks each person – whether a white, or Black, Indigenous, Person of Color (BIPOC), or even "blue-bodied" individual (in uniform for policing, military, and other "security systems") to become conscious of harms done/received, trauma experienced, or chronic oppressive forces of this lifetime or inherited through generations. Next the mandate is to transform behavior that either ignores these harms and preserves the status quo, or is so reactive it simply retriggers the harm. Without this change we are all exacting a toll on each human being. None of us is free until all of us is free. One way to acquire the resiliency for building equitable societies is to recognize injustice and trauma, to learn self-care, and to do so within cultures of respect. As a predominantly white-bodied community, DE participants are encouraged to build these cultures, which also appreciate the historical roots of yoga and the global roots of somatic work, reaching across racial lines to learn from people who are too often referred to as "others."

The Dynamic Embodiment^{SM} (DE^{SM}) OSO Model

DE uses the ritualized practice of sequences that relates to early infant movement such as exist in BMC (Series 1 and 2), neurodevelopmentally based movements from BF (the Basic 6 exercises), and the seated and standing versions of developmental sequences from DE (Relax to Focus©), as well as the Sun Salutation.

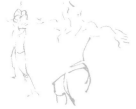

Chapter 1

Each of these is simple enough to learn, varied enough to be stimulating or even challenging if desired, and quiet enough to allow for varying one's attention with each round of it. The Sun Salutation is a quintessential blend of all of these – involving both child-like and animal-like movements that are simple yet stimulating and can be done at whatever pace suits the goal. It has a long history of being meaningful for many people.

These experiences can be explored within the central framework of DE, a model for working with clients, groups, and organizations developed by Martha Eddy, called the OSO model (Observe, Support, Optimize Options). OSO aims to empower people to practice keen awareness skills, and to apply the insights gained to move with a sense of connection, belonging, or support in order to behave with conscious choice of options. Underlying these steps is a philosophy to interact compassionately with others and that choice helps liberate from oppressive forces. DE supports individuals and groups to somatically focus on "self-observation" and to use this awareness for personal growth, interpersonal interaction, and social good.

DE practitioners are trained to be keen observers of their clients and students using the lenses provided by both LMA and BMC. An important DE goal is to cultivate an "internal non-judgmental witness" and to engage this witness, whether moving, thinking, or acting. Discoveries in self-awareness can be mysterious, murky, confusing, difficult, or even painful, as sensations or emotions. This is where the need for support comes in. People need to feel a sense of belonging. Support can be emotional or physical and both are ways to experience connection. Once one feels "connected" internally – within the body – and externally – with others and the environment, then one can also feel the choice to be creative,

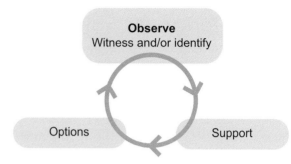

For self-care ⟶ & others
Observe:
What do I/you do?
Tactile
Proprioception
Visual
Auditory
Gustatory

Support:
What works now?
What feels good?
What is supportive?

Options ⟶ Change
Options: Play, creativity & what choices?

Figure 1.3
Dynamic Embodiment^SM OSO cycle of personal and social care.

playful, and engaged in the world, to find what is motivating. Experiencing that one has options provides freedom of mind. Practice of these options encourages neural pathways and cellular consciousness, critical to being able to readily adjust when interacting with others or within any aspect of life's pursuits. Part of the practice is to make meaning from what is discovered from the body sensation and emotions and relate them to everyday experience. All inner awareness, whether experienced as positive or negative, needs to be balanced with outer awareness.

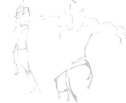

The Dynamic Embodiment^{SM} OSO Model: Observe=> Support=> Optimize Options

- Keenly OBSERVE using all senses in order to acknowledge and accept another's behavior (remaining non-judgmental).

- Sensitively provide mind-body-spirit SUPPORT – identifying and appreciating strengths and providing care for under-resourced parts or aspects of the self.

- Explore diverse OPTIONS in behavior. OPTIMIZING options involves exploration, variation, a child-like attitude of a beginner's mind. This creativity leads to us feeling free to make choices. Employing different strategies provides opportunities for new sensory experience to integrate and new movement–behavioral choices to emerge. This model works for movement of the body and expansion of the mind. It also is a metaphor for opening to a wide range of emotional expression.

Dynamic Embodiment^{SM} in a Nutshell

DE is a somatic movement system that builds a deep understanding of how to access body sensation and ground within the process of experiencing the body, a sentient process often referred to as embodiment. DE includes how to become aware of social influences on individuals and groups (a social somatic perspective that considers the impact of oppressive forces), and how to broaden behavioral choices to enhance communication and appreciation for others. When societal forces allow one to access numerous possibilities for movement expression/non-verbal communication one can both (1) come to appreciate oneself and most others, or at least be conscious of what is different

from one's own experience enough to interact with it boldly, and (2) have more choices – new ways to respond. The OSO model is all about self-discovery, connection, and accessing choices. DE involves recognizing patterns of behavior, supporting what is working well, providing compassion for what is challenging, and experiencing that there are resources for making it safe to be caring and "in connection." Once one is feeling strong enough, the next goal is to challenge one's habits of self, of culture, of society, or of nation that represent a monolithic point of view and to shift toward knowing there are a set of choices. This final step involves practicing novel coordination – new patterns – by engaging with various movement/behavioral possibilities in one's life.

Components that Support the Sun Salutation

The Sun Salutation provides a powerful structure for improving movement efficiency, health, and vitality. Practice of the Sun Salutation in the spirit of DE invites you to tap into the body wisdom of each of the different physiological systems, to observe or "get a daily read on" one's current state, and to make personalized movement choices that optimize balanced energy and health. When practicing the Sun Salutation regularly using DE as a somatic ritual, one can compare sensations in each layer of one's being – in the nervous system, muscles, bones, organs, fluids, and endocrine glands. Each elicits a different energy, or movement quality. By noticing the change in the quality of movement you become more conscious of yourself and of your behavioral choices. DE also encourages engagement in this practice with awareness of any other emotional or social factors that are present.

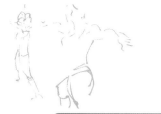

Chapter 1

Bringing It All Together – Dynamic Embodiment[SM] and the Sun Salutation

DE recognizes the power of ritualized movement sequences as a framework for deepening self-awareness through comparing and contrasting day-to-day experience. DE uses the observation of movement *dynamics* to inform *embodiment* – for instance, in how to work with the glands, neurodevelopmental movement, and chakral energy during movement – and finds it is easiest to be aware during movement rituals. The Sun Salutation is a great practice for developing more consciousness, somatic awareness, while moving.

The Sun Salutation is a great choice since almost everyone who has taken a yoga class has learned at least one version of it, as it has been taught within yoga asana classes for decades. Yoga derives from the Global South (cultures south of the equator where the Global Majority live) and has spread throughout the world with a huge impact on the Global North (cultures north of the equator where the Global Minority live). It encapsulates actions that are classic movements within daily life (many from early childhood): standing, reaching upwards, balancing while arching the spine, bowing, lunging as in taking a large step, taking weight in the arms and feet, whether bent or straight-legged,

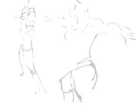

folding into the body center, and gesturing around the heart. Each of these can also be seen as a prayer or prostration that distinctly connects with caring. In aligning with the sun and placing hands on the heart, one can invoke reverence for that which is greater than the single human person. In bending down or folding into the earth there is an element of prostrating to it, which can be another type of reverence. It is interesting to think of taking a step backward or forward as a respect for our ability to move in relationship to the planet. The sequence involves doing actions and reversing them, which allows for a balancing of muscles, in and of itself a type of movement repatterning. It is also a way to practice movement choice. These movements can involve whatever level of attention is desired. There can be a focus on health, on physicality, on energy flow, or on gratitude, to name a few. As a ritual, the Sun Salutation can be a fitness routine or a sacred practice. Even these approaches can be practiced in a variety of ways, from a specific tradition or several traditions, alone or amongst others. Many people maintain a movement practice with a teacher or guide, someone with expertise who can support them. Others instinctively are able to journey solo. They are most likely already kinesthetic learners or not focused on new approaches. With the DE approach to practice the Sun Salutation you learn to pay attention to a myriad of bodily resources, honoring your sensations, and determining what shifts and nuances might help in meeting your life or health goals.

In a time when people are searching for the 10-minute, then the 7-minute, and even the 5-minute workout, the Sun Salutation provides a "workout" that has been circulating globally for years, AND that, if desired, can also serve as a prayer or meditation. With the DE approach, the practice can release stress and

bring not only musculo-skeletal vitality, but also glandular/hormonal balance and energy.

Embodying the glands through BMC's developmental approach includes locating body parts plus an understanding of careful skeletal positioning, brain-activating developmental movement, and related hormonal balancing. DE then adds in the spatial and dynamic investigation that comes from LMA, as well as integrating broader social somatic contexts such as the impact of lifestyle, cultural, and intergenerational influences.

Each of these systems in DE interacts for movement and efficiency and expression. This is another key tenet of DE – which stems from LMA and BF – that enhancing our movement function enhances our movement expression (and vice versa). In DE one goal is on "being as big as you are" relative to the Sun Salutation, which involves claiming full body space as a method of glandular balancing. One can enrich the performance of the Sun Salutation through being aware of how bodies occupy three-dimensional space. Laban/Bartenieff studies go even further, echoing the energy work of Lawrence Blair (one of the earliest writers about the chakras from a western perspective) by seeing our movement inside of crystalline forms. This energy may be culled from the choice to harmonize with being alive on earth and awareness that our planet is also part of a greater whole, the solar system.

Relating Body-Mind Centering® to the Sun Salutation

One premise from BMC in the DE approach to practicing the Sun Salutation is that the locations in the body where the nervous and endocrine systems meet, the neuroendocrine centers, are the nexus that can also be experienced as the chakras. Hence, chakral energy can be felt through experiential learning of anatomy and physiology.

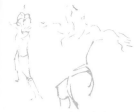

Glandular energy can be strong since it impacts the entire body. Another BMC premise is that hormonal intensity/chakral energy can be grounded through moving with initiation from the skeleton, which provides containment and grounding through the bones. One example is by learning the glandular qualities while practicing the building blocks of early infant movement. Another BMC idea is to bring attention to the glands to discover ease and lightness in your movement. The Sun Salutation has been selected by DE as an elegant movement ritual that works well to balance glandular intensity and support more efficient movement.

The form of the movement helps to contain and balance the volatility of the hormone-releasing glands. Adding knowledge of neuro-developmental movement leaves the cortex freer to calm down impulses from hormonally flooded blood flow. Learning to somatically sense and interact with the nervous system awakens subtle cues before stress or illness is rampant. This is somatic neuroendocrine balancing. The Sun Salutation, done with a neuroendocrine lens, can serve as a "safe container" for practicing glandular balancing and chakral flow.

Bartenieff Fundamentals and the Sun Salutation

Bartenieff concepts and principles that are most helpful in a DE approach to the Sun Salutation include establishing spatial intention and becoming aware of bodily interconnectivity. Taking time to establish spatial intent means determining where you want to go. In a static pose this means knowing how different body parts best relate to one another. Another way to say this is to know where each body part needs to be positioned in space, in relationship to one another. There are several body connections that are especially important to learn to engage:

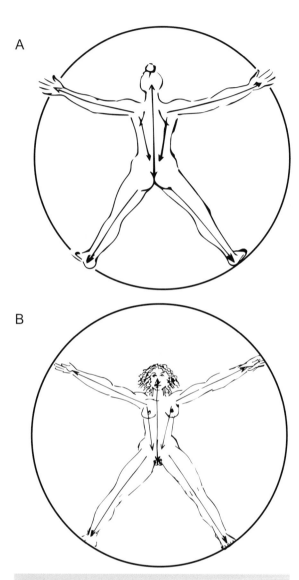

Figure 1.4
Bartenieff body connections, by Stewart Hoyt.

- The head to the tail

- The two shoulder blades (scapulae) to the sacrum

- The wing of the scapula to the fingertips

- The heels to the sit bones.

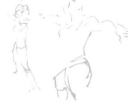

In addition, the trochanter (outer bony knob of the thigh bone) connects through the pelvic floor to the opposite trochanter.

With the enhanced sensory awareness of these connections the practice of any movement becomes clearer and more efficient.

Laban's Space Harmony and the Sun Salutation: Tensegrity Awakens Chakras and Glands

The Sun Salutation can be practiced as a type of Space Harmony. This is done by feeling the spatial tensions – the polarities from one end of the body through the body center to another (e.g. hand through torso to the opposite leg and foot). There are different spatial tensions or pulls. Some are mobilizing – when a pull overcomes your stability and causes you to move or even fall. Others are called counter-tensions or counter-pulls and are stabilizing. When you have equal counter-pulls in the body you can stay in a pose for a long time and minimize the muscular effort in doing so.

An additional benefit is that the glands are activated by this expansiveness and then bring additional energy to the movement. During the Sun Salutation being aware of the spatial intention and activation of spatial pulls or counter-pulls supports both the moments of stillness and the transitional movements.

The Sun Salutation specifically moves along the edges of the sagittal plane (sometimes referred to as the plane of the wheel). It includes movements that stretch out to the edges of personal space. The wheel can move from front low, front high, back high, and back low points in space, or vice versa. It is a narrow space, looking into the future and the past and also connecting with the heavens and the earth – up and down, as well as forward and back. There are definitely opportunities

both to highlight their tensile components and to deviate from it. Sometimes the deviation is simply a recuperation – widening out, taking in the horizon, twisting. Engaging "spatial pulls" provides space in the joints, enlivens movement by awakening choices within the sacred forms, and is experienced by many people to stimulate glands. Using spatial pulls is coached throughout this book, to guide you to activate the glands, especially during the Sun Salutation.

The places in space that are important to the Sun Salutation are place middle, back high, forward middle to place low, back low, back low to middle and forward low, low, back low toward forward middle, back low to middle and forward low, place low to place middle, high or back high, place middle. As you explore the sagittal plane – the plane of the wheel – you can discover what directions feel easiest or most challenging to you and whether keeping a tether line to its opposite is helpful in any way. It often brings lightness to have balanced counter-pulls. These pulls stabilize and so in order to move, allow one direction to take over and follow the spatial intention to keep moving. As you are moving forward or back with some up and down you may need to work to reduce side-to-side movement unless you choose to be in a wide sagittal plane.

The Sun Salutation as a Social Somatic Practice

The Sun Salutation is important as a physical practice, a ritual in which to feel glandular balancing, and can be used as a somatic assessment. Moving through the Sun Salutation invigorates. With the addition of neuroendocrine and neurodevelopmental perspectives it is possible to activate the body with new resources – paying attention to how the body is

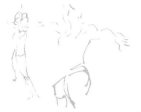

structured and being extremely specific about the sources of energy that run through it. These impact physical and mental well-being. Regular practice allows you to note "where you are at" on any particular day. It is also useful to put the practice into a social context.

The Sun Salutation is a resource that almost everyone can have, once learned, for free.

Having gratitude for the yogis of India who developed the practice, based on strong body wisdom, is one form of honoring. Checking in with the societal forces that impact each day also awakens awareness of different experiences based on power and privilege.

For instance, it is a privilege to be able to have access to space (especially clean open space), time (ideally when solitude is available for at least 3–5 minutes), and knowledge of the form that makes it safe to do, no matter what the specific constraints of your body. Each body has its challenges (Eddy 2016, 2017). For some bodies, more adaptations from the classic Sun Salutation are needed. This is an exciting prospect – it reflects human creativity and adaptability. Humans often learn the most from people who need to change or create something to make an aspect of life viable. When this creativity is shared, without over-pricing it, everyone can benefit.

Practice Examples

Observation, Support, and Optimizing Options with the Sun Salutation

Structured movement performed as rituals is both a place of learning (opening up neural pathways) and a place of reflection (including noticing new somatic awareness). The Sun Salutation is taught as part of DE as a ritual that is a place to return to, gain comfort from, and "check in" about one's bodily status. The specific movements in the Sun Salutation are simple enough to give a wide berth for exploration so that any person can feel successful. It provides an elegant clarity, a chance to move in easy everyday-like movements – stepping, bending, reaching while also being challenging.

As part of the DE approach to practicing the Sun Salutation, the invitation is to recognize how the Sun Salutation can be an opportunity for each part of the OSO cycle. You can discover how to be observant for self-awareness, experience support, and explore new options while engaged in the Salute to the Sun practice.

Observing: Perceiving Body Signals Is Easier Within a Centering Ritual

In order to observe one's own behavior with a somatic lens it is important to slow down and feel centered. In DE exploring familiar movement in a repetitive or ritualized way becomes a form of both centering and grounding that allows for self-observation. The Sun Salutation can be deeply centering because if one takes time to learn the ritual, then the movement control becomes subcortical. When you know a simple movement pattern well, you spend less energy thinking about planning and executing the movement. This gives the brain the capacity to be self-monitoring. And if the activity is calming, the chances are you can be more self-loving as well. If one chooses to infuse the practice with meaning and awareness, it shifts from being a purely physical practice to becoming a psycho-physical experience. For some people this process also opens up or deepens a spiritual path.

Observing the Emotional Brain: What Are You Thinking and Feeling as You Move?

Whether one comes into the day with anxiety or "off-rhythm" due to cramps, or exhaustion, or

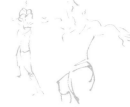

with readiness and excitement, or "relaxed alertness," life is being governed by the action of the glands – the endocrine system. The Sun Salutation as a ritual can be a check-in about overall well-being including mental and emotional states. When first learning the Sun Salutation it might be a cause of some anxiety if it is either a physical or a mental movement challenge. Once it is learned, and hopefully with satisfactory support (see next section) that makes it comfortable to do, it can serve as an emotional barometer.

For instance, when one discovers a reduction in ability to perform any part of the sequence, an inner judge may take over and be self-critical. It is important to counteract that. Having new ways to do the same movement is one solution. In the case of the Sun Salutation, the focus is on finding more space in the body and relating to the environment through feeling gravity (yielding), pushing, and also reaching and pulling. Feeling inner and outer spatial support is a resource to discover and embrace new postural habits and spatial pathways. DE recognizes that either moving or imaging tensile structures within the body enhances posture and movement. Different spatial frameworks allow for a flow of life energy through the glands, fostering ease of movement. This work is enhanced by practicing the Laban harmonic scales through space. From this perspective, the Sun Salutation can be perceived as a Harmonic Spatial Sequence that emphasizes spinal flexion and extension in the sagittal plane (indicated by these points: forward and up, forward and down, back and down, and back and up).

Another, equally important, observation is about mental attitudes. Recognizing that one is being hard on oneself is an inroad to learning to be gentle with oneself regarding expectations. In the DE Sun Salutation practice, no matter what you have brought to consciousness

about your life story, guidance is suggested to remain open to the range of shifts of mind and/or changes of body that you might experience when moving or maintaining a posture with profound embodiment. For example, when you experience energy moving in your body, you might feel the bones shift in your spine and hear them making sounds. What do you feel about this? What do you want to hold onto or let go of from this experience? What are you noticing about attributes of your life that may be repeatedly causing compression in your joints or in your muscles? These recognitions serve as a pathway to finding new resources, support.

Support: Learning, Adjusting, Embracing

DE espouses a belief that one of the best ways to change patterns, reduce pain, and act with consciousness is to locate and name what is working well in life, and in one's movement. After "taking inventory" with a "somatic check-in" during the Sun Salutation, you have more information about what is going well in your body, mind, and emotions, and where you might be calling for support. In DE support is given to both (1) what is working well by acknowledging and appreciating anything and everything you are comfortable with and (2) once this positive and nurturing rapport is established with yourself or your student, you can move on to finding support for what feels unclear or uncomfortable.

Exploring Movement, Free Dance, Movement Rituals, and the Sun Salutation

The principles of DE are conveyed through guided movement, movement exploration, and dance explorations. This is a time to learn new information about the body, and the body-mind connection, as well as to discover

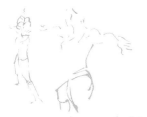

one's own habits. Everyone who studies DE engages in movement and dance, no matter their skill level, their inhibitions, bodily challenges, or conditions, doing so with respect for cultural beliefs. Indeed, everyone is invited to bring their cultural traditions into classes or sessions.

DE suggests engaging in rituals like the Sun Salutation in order to learn what needs to be adjusted in one's bodily alignment and effort, and mental or emotional focus. With that information one can find support for any area using tools such as breath, contact with the ground, chair or wall, gentle adjusting movements, and toning. In the DE approach to practicing the Sun Salutation, time is also spent on debriefing the experience. Discussions ask: What was challenging? What was surprising? What was comforting? What did you do to adjust it? What felt new? What is something that would help you remember what worked for you?

Gaining Support for Challenges

Within the Sun Salutation it is easy enough to have a day when one is stiff or not able to move fluidly. If one has had an illness, surgery, or another sort of stress, specific parts of the body become rigid, stuck, or inhibited. Support for these areas is critical. Both BMC and DE have been using props such as small or large pillows, balls, and towels to provide comfort to body areas within asanas for decades. There are now many products that are available to help provide support. They include toe separators, special socks, bolsters, egg-shaped balls, and yoga blocks of different sizes and textures, among many others. The key idea from DE is to truly embrace the support by feeling the contact with one's body and allowing one's weight to give in to the support, enlisting the force of gravity as a type of massage. With support one can find new movements, which further relieve tension and can also be fun due

to the physical novelty, new pleasurable sensations, or resulting joy or lightness. Restorative yoga is a great resource for dealing with bodily challenges. DE brings in resources from within the body – more support for musculo-skeletal alignment as well as from the inner body – the organs, fluids, and glands.

Options: The Sun Salutation as Ritual Allows Movement Repatterning, Awakening the Brain

Bringing the subtle shifts of attention to different lenses within DE provides a variability that is important for pleasure, focus, strengthening, and (re)awakening brain pathways. In order to expand brain pathways – whether through the growth of nerve pathways in the peripheral nervous system or with the interneurons of the brain – action MUST repeat. There is research that states that the action can be explored with mental rehearsal only; however, the physical body doesn't derive as strong a physiological benefit from visualization alone. The repetition of physical movements both carves out the new pathway and sets down the myelin sheath, the fatty protection which serves the body like the rubber around an electrical wire. This creation of new neural pathways is known as neuroplasticity. Movement is an extraordinarily important stimulus for neural development.

If you are in a rut or feeling sluggish or as if you are aging too rapidly, it is important to learn something new. This is important for keeping the brain fresh. Movement with thinking is a powerful combination (McCracken 2020). For adults, going back to moving with baby movement can be one of the most effective new (or remembered) experiences for stimulating the brain (Bainbridge Cohen 1993, 2018; Bartenieff 1980; Eddy 2016; Feldenkrais 1989). Babies gain perspectives on

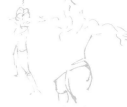

the world by exploring environments physically, practicing a new behavior until it becomes automatic.

These early childhood developmental movements can provide support for your practice of the Sun Salutation. During infancy and into adolescence the glandular and related hormones are set into gear by neurodevelopmental movements. Diet, movement, and attitude all affect hormonal balancing. Having insight into what the glands do for our bodies and how to use proprioceptive awareness of the glands can support glandular balancing for health, joy, and pleasure. Knowing what types of movements activate or relax each specific gland is what can be practiced within the Sun Salutation. This information can also be extended to modifications or other asanas.

There can be a problematic side to repetition, however. Unconscious repetition of bad habits just thickens a pathway. If you are engaging in repeating an action with poor joint alignment or challenged spinal posture you may be deepening a negative habit, one that could be deleterious for your health (or that of your students). A new stimulus is needed to break it up. DE's somatic verbal or tactile cueing helps students to avoid alignment misuse and other challenges by sharing new anatomically based information and reminding them to somatically "check in." Having a movement ritual frees the brain for being able to coordinate checking in at the same time as moving.

While neuroplasticity explains a lot and offers great potential for growth, there will most likely always be aspects of our lived experience that remain mysterious. This is particularly true of human emotions and relations. For instance, rituals can be thought of or experienced as scary by some people. It may even be that the constancy of action feels boring or cultish. In DE you are reminded to get more information when you feel stuck, and

knowing the origins of yoga and the multiple pathways that yoga has taken gives one choices about if and how to engage with the Sun Salutation. You know that the Sun Salutation can be practiced as part of spiritual expression or as a health-supporting mind-body activity. The primary sacred aspect of the movement sequence is to revere the sun, greet the day, and re-arrive from sleep with awareness of being on the planet. The need to connect with nature for basic health reasons is well founded in science (Ducharme 2019).

Conclusion

The Sun Salutation is sacred and yet it can be treated as if mundane. Yoga is what one makes of it – what is taken in and what is left out define your experience of it. Using tools from DE offers you different ways to focus your practice and helps you to let go, breathe, sound, rock, and move more consciously through the Sun Salutation and related poses.

To transmit an understanding of the complex interplay of bones, joints, organs, and muscles, it is best to fully occupy space. DE teaches this through "being as big as you are." Engaging in somatic movement means taking time and using awareness to maintain positive postural positioning. It means finding the confidence and resources to embrace living fully in one's body on this planet. The influences of Space Harmony, Bartenieff's spatial intent and Bainbridge Cohen's spatial consciousness invite actively moving, thinking, and interacting with spaciousness. This requires awareness while moving. This can reduce joint injury when specifically adjusted for long- or short-term pain or disability, by finding both spaciousness in the body and support for the surrounding space. Engaging to find space by activating bodily spatial pulls, in posture or when moving, also activates the glands and, in turn, the chakras.

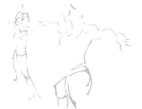

Chapter 1

These are glandular responses to movement that may also address various types of psychophysical imbalances. While spaciousness often begins in the core, the torso, with breath, it also extends out through the limbs. If you become conscious of your ongoing development as a human, you will revisit this core support and its connections to your limbs as well as to your adult movement. By becoming aware of your neurological patterning and its shifts and changes throughout life, you can find how reflection back to *in utero* and the neonatal and infant/toddler experience of coming to standing (if able to) through the first years of life supports current experience. A wide variety of psychophysical gems can be discovered in this exploration that allows for revisiting how to get down on and up off the floor during the Sun Salutation.

What makes this work unique is that as you bring more awareness to the sensations of your body, you are "unveiling consciousness," to quote Arthur Avalon (1974). If you consciously identify what is already powerfully embedded in your body while doing the Sun Salutation, you may experience the existential sensation of living in space. Another benefit of the DE approach to saluting the sun is finding pleasurable lightness and grounded strength. A predominance of somatic systems – from the Alexander Technique to Embodied Yoga – has found that when embodying space, especially symmetrically by widening, lengthening, and deepening, many people also awaken to powerful feelings of openness and lightness, as well as centeredness. These feelings are generally enjoyable and freeing, mood lifters.

Learning new coordination can sometimes be stressful and yet that stress is what helps us grow. Doing something familiar allows that stress to drop away. Rituals are familiar and provide a container for familiarity. The DE perspective also asks each of us to create a positive learning climate – to be non-judgmental, to simply observe our experiences and cultivate curiosity instead of judgment. This is an approach that asks the mover to learn compassion toward himself, herself, or themselves and not to get too comfortable or complacent. There is much about oneself to "mine" within a ritual. This book points to different ways of digging into bodily, mindful, emotional, and social issues as you practice the Sun Salutation. The Sun Salutation can also be a potential inroad to feeling connected to all beings, a transformational state.

What are the next steps for you? Join in exploring more about the Sun Salutation itself as well as about the glands, the chakras, and early childhood movement, and see what emerges. Learn how the glands support movement in the first years of life and how they relate to each of the postures. Re-experiencing the neurodevelopmental aspects of the Sun Salutation interwoven with glandular support helps you find ease, experience greater balance, and embrace the DE principle of "being as big as you are." When you expand in space, you experience more of your power. Each person is unique and will have a different experience! Let's continue by learning more about the Sun Salutation. Its history gives us more context for embodied engagement.

To the Reader

What are your goals?

- Strength?
- Avoiding injury?
- Growing awareness of self/inner focus/ somatic awareness?
- Doing so through "organ support"?

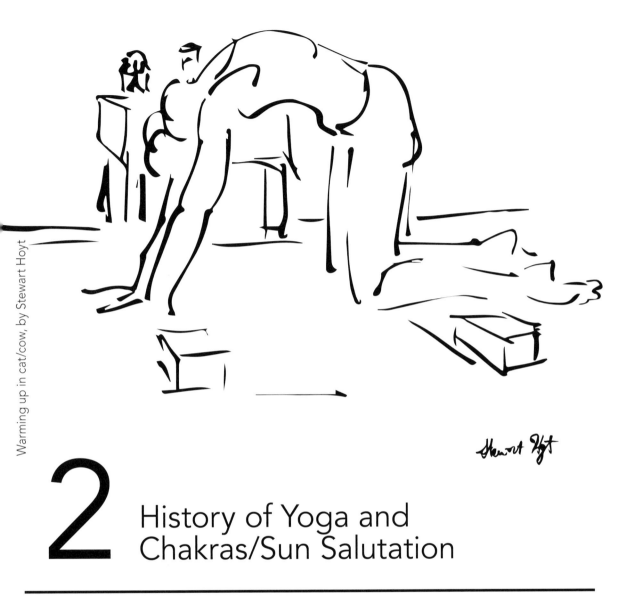

2 History of Yoga and Chakras/Sun Salutation

What is Yoga?

Yoga is an ancient practice, born in India, that is followed all over the world today. It is thought of as a physical practice in the west, but the asanas, or postures, are just one-eighth of the complex teachings for wellness and evolution of the whole being – body, mind, and spirit. Donna Farhi calls yoga "a technology for arriving in this present moment"; it is

the handbook for cultivating awareness. And the scholar George Feuerstein summed it up beautifully with "Yoga is the most sophisticated spiritual tradition in the world. It is also the oldest continuous endeavor to map the path from the valley of spiritual ignorance to the peak of enlightenment, and it offers the largest assemblage of practical tools for self-transformation and self-transcendence" (Feuerstein 2003). In this book that "one-eighth of

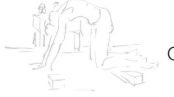

the practice," the asanas of the Sun Salutation, is central. However, the full yogic traditions encompass much more. Please know that "how you are with this practice" – how you interact with and embody the postures – can help heal and grow your thinking, your psychology, and your emotions. The postures are "centering practices" that bring us into deeper states of insight, reflection, and meditation.

Ashtanga is the Sanskrit term for the eight limbs of yoga as outlined in Patanjali's Yoga Sutras, written around 200 BCE. We have already visited the first branch, Asana. The other seven limbs are:

2. *Pranayama*, breathing practices.

3. and 4. The *Yamas* and *Niyamas*, "Ten ethical precepts that allow us to be at peace with ourselves, our family, and our community" (Farhi 2000). The Yamas are towards the outer, or our environment, including *ahimsa*: non-violence; *satya*: truthfulness; *asetya*: non-stealing; *bramacharya*: restraint or moderation; and *aparigraha*: non-greed or freedom from attachment. And the Niyamas are towards the self: *saucha*: purity; *santosa*: contentment; *tapas*: self-discipline; *svadhyaya*: self-study; and *isvara pranidhana*: surrender or dedication to God/dess.

5. *Prayahara*, withdrawal of the senses from the outside world.

6. *Dharana*, concentration.

7. *Dhyana*, meditation, awareness.

8. *Samadhi*, "a state of super-consciousness brought about by profound meditation, in which the individual aspirant becomes one with … the Universal Spirit"

(Iyengar 1979) or "the return of the mind into original silence" (Farhi 2000).

The Sun Salutation

In the United States and in dozens of nations around the world, one may be referred by a friend, a colleague, or even a doctor, to go to a yoga class to help improve conditions like poor posture, a bad back, hurt neck, or overall stiffness. In India, it is just as likely for someone to be referred for a glandular issue such as a problem with the thyroid. In India there is an understanding that yoga affects the unseen, or more subtle, physical glandular system, as well as the organs, glands, and nerves, not just the muscles and bones as in the west (Anand 2013).

Whereas yoga dates back at least 5000 years, the Sun Salutation, Surya Namaskar, is a modern invention. This is surprising for many yoga practitioners, for in this short time, this ritual, this linking of poses, has taken on ancient and archetypal significance for many. It is meaningful to face the sun in doing it, just as the door to the Native American sweat lodge faces east (where the sun rises), and if you choose to engage with it in a sacred manner. It has a sagittal orientation – it is geared toward one singular focal point, the sun, which is in front – and this movement represents greeting the dawn or disappearance of the new day. There is also a lunar version, Chandra Namaskar. The Moon Salutation is a more "inward-drawing" set of poses, quieting and restorative, created in the 1960s in the United States.

Yoga's longevity is well documented in writing via Pantanjali's Yoga Sutras, dating back 4000 years, and from 5000 years ago in the Rig Veda, "the oldest literary collection in the world" (Feuerstein 2003). Many of the poses that are classic to modern practice,

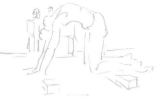

like headstands and virasana, a seated yoga pose, are documented in paintings from the 1600s. There is also a set of yogic drawings from 1600–1604 that depict virasana and garbhasana (physical poses or asana), sitali breath (a moon or cooling breath), headstand, khumbhaka (breath practice), and nauli kriya (a purification practice, rolling of the stomach) (Diamond 2013).

Now, fast forward to when the Sun Salutation was born – in 1929! This birth was fully documented in Washington DC in 2013 at the Smithsonian Museum's Arthur M. Sackler Gallery multimedia presentation of "Yoga, The Art of Transformation – the world's first exhibition of yogic art." Its invention is attributed to Pratinidhi Pant, a raja (energy/fire) and bodybuilder, as part of a health reform project. This was during a time when Indian doctors and bodybuilders were publishing, in a nationalistic context, about yoga, bodybuilding, health, and happiness. Before that there was a revival of Indigenous medicine in the late 1800s and early 1900s that merged modern medicine with yogic drawings of the chakras and subtle bodies (Diamond 2013, p. 277). During this continuing rise of nationalistic pride, the Surya Namaskar (translation: Salute to the Sun) was published in 1929 in a magazine as an indigenous bodybuilding practice. It was billed as "10 Steps to Health" (Diamond 2013). When it was originally introduced, it was shown as ten poses, done consecutively. The "flow" of Surya Namaskar happened later, as it was not until 1938 that Krishnamacharya and Iyengar made a film of one pose flowing into the next. This is perhaps the first linking of postures, the first yoga flow practice.

The history described so far has been about yoga in its Hindu context, but yoga also developed over the centuries within the traditions of Buddhism and Jainism. (See original films from Krishnamacharya at https://www.youtube.com/watch?v=8XF4sCV6aUY; and Iyengar at https://www.youtube.com/watch?v=LUvOuik-g4c.)

Yoga in Hinduism, Buddhism, and Jainism

The Sun Salutation was born out of the Hindu branch of yoga. But to understand yoga more holistically, let's explore its development a bit more. The Buddha was a Yogi, and he was, by the time he sat under the Bodhi tree, a Yoga Master. Vardhamana Mahavira, the founder of Jainism, was also a Yoga Master (Feuerstein 2003). All three traditions offer a way to "withdraw the senses" and realize one's essential self. Over the millennia many traditions have affected and helped to develop yoga. In Mark Singleton's book *The Roots of Yoga*, he cites 100 texts in its development including ones in Pali (Thai), Tibetan, and Persian; he also claims that yoga has Sufi (Muslim) roots (Singleton 2017).

The Chakras and the Glands and Nervous System

With the yogic practice the focus is on the seven major chakras. These chakras are energy bodies or vortices that stem from the energetic spine, or *sushumna* in Sanskrit. Together, they act like an electrical transforming station, taking energy in at the top crown chakra, from the cosmos, and transforming it down in vibration with each chakra, making it available for that area of the body. The chakras are within the body, and they move outward from the spine to the skin, and into the field of energy around the human body (see Fig. 2.1).

In books and art, the chakras are represented by lotus flowers with many symbols within them. Enter into this symbology and look at

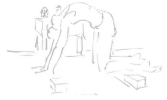

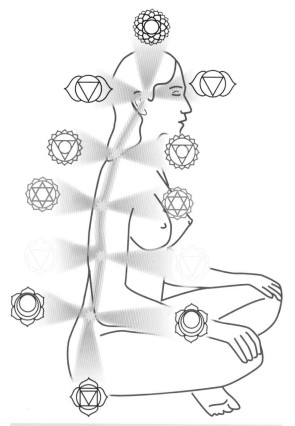

Figure 2.1
The chakras, moving from inside to outside the body.

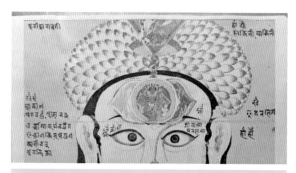

Figure 2.2
Brow chakras, Rajasthan, 18th century (author unknown).

some of the pieces. Understanding these symbols will help you navigate the literature as well as your inner map of the chakras in your own body.

In a diagram of the chakras, each of the seven major chakras is represented by a lotus flower. This can be seen as a flower, or as simply a circle with petals around it. The section of a centuries-old painting in Figure 2.2 shows two petals at the third eye chakra.

Interestingly, the number of petals tells us the number of nerve pairs. This informs us that Yogis have been aware of the nervous

system connection for hundreds to thousands of years, without the development of modern medicine. Each petal represents a nerve pair, and a nerve pair is also a bundle of 48 nerve branches. So at the third eye, we have two bundles, or nerve pairs. Each of the major chakras is at the location in the physical body of a larger number of nerve pairs. The drawing in Figure 2.3, from 1899, shows a similar location for the chakras and nerve bundles. There are paintings dating back 500 years showing these chakra petal diagrams, and writings going back 4000–5000 years.

From the Body-Mind Centering® (BMC®) perspective, the chakras are where strong glandular energy and nerve plexus meet. The glands transport information electronically via neurotransmitters, which excite or inhibit neuronal firing at the target cell of muscles, glands, or other nerves, thereby impacting almost every cell in the body. The glands can be seen as the physical bridge to the chakras – the connector between the physical and energetic bodies. With the electric nature of the brain, spinal cord, and nerves and the physical placement of the glands along the spine and nearby powerful nerve plexus, the glands are the natural bridge between body and energy.

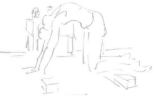

The glands aid you in having a physical experience of the energetic chakral field. By working with the endocrine system and the chakras, Dynamic Embodiment^{SM} (DE^{SM}) guides a grounding of "the subtle" in the body. The work brings the physical and energetic bodies together.

In the earliest Yogic texts like the Upanishads only four or five major chakras are listed. Arthur Avalon, also known as Sir John Woodroffe, in his 1919 book *The Serpent Power: The Secrets of Tantric and Shaktic Yoga*, speaks of five major chakras, with the upper two, Ajna and Sahasrara, seen as minor chakras. It is really only in the past 50 years that seven major chakras are cited within the human body. Less ancient sources added two or three, and by the New Age in the 1970s seven major

chakras had arrived, with hundreds of smaller chakras being known to exist throughout the body (see Fig. 2.4).

By the late 1800s, as part of a revival of Indigenous medicine in India, the chakras and subtle bodies were depicted in medical drawings showing their relationship to the physical anatomy. In 1929 Dr Vasant Rele published *The Mysterious Kundalini*, the first book connecting the chakras to the nervous system instead of the endocrine system. In DE these two systems are intertwined.

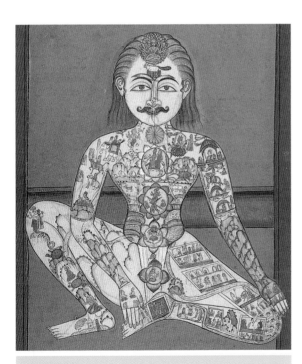

Figure 2.3
Sapta Chakra, 1899.

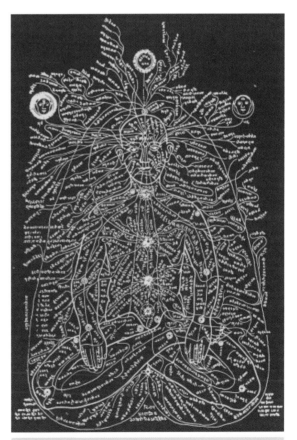

Figure 2.4
Hundreds of chakras, old Hindu drawing of nadis (energy lines) and chakras.

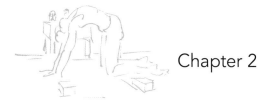

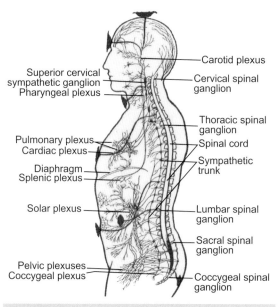

Superior cervical
sympathetic ganglion
Pharyngeal plexus

Carotid plexus

Cervical spinal
ganglion

Thoracic spinal
ganglion

Spinal cord

Pulmonary plexus
Cardiac plexus

Sympathetic
trunk

Diaphragm
Splenic plexus

Solar plexus

Lumbar spinal
ganglion

Sacral spinal
ganglion

Pelvic plexuses
Coccygeal plexus

Coccygeal spinal
ganglion

Figure 2.5
Chakra positions in supposed relation to nervous plexuses, from Charles W. Leadbeater's 1927 book *The Chakras*.

In the late 1800s and early 1900s Indian doctors began to take a renewed interest in publishing on the chakra/nerve/gland connection. This was embedded in the Indian empowerment movement, part of India re-establishing its own identity apart from the British, by showcasing its own unique heritage.

In the 1920s Indian studies were done showing the medical benefits of yoga, including measuring the effects on blood pressure from the headstand, and the benefit of fish pose on the thyroid (Diamond 2013, p. 279).

Alan Finger, creator of Ishta yoga, tells the story of the Rishis, many thousands of years ago, going into deep states of meditation. It was in these states that they saw, felt, sensed the chakras and their qualities. These qualities were translated into the colors and symbology

that are still used today: Yantra with color, shape (square, oval, star), animals, and number of petals. The symbols, placed at the center of each lotus, are called yantras, visual geometric images used to aid in meditation in Tantric yoga. The petals indicate the number of nadis in that area of the body, and Finger also explains that the petals each represent a different sound, of which there are 52. In yoga, this age of the rishis was a different Yuga, or time. In this yuga it was easier for everyone on the planet to sense things like these chakral essences (Finger 2005).

Today those petals can be thought of as indicating the number of nerve pairs at each chakra and recalling the links to color, shape, and animals as well.

Yoga and the Glands and Nerves

India's yoga benefits both the nervous system and endocrine glands. The understanding is that with these both healthy, the body is able to respond to the demands of life, and continue to function normally. If these systems (nervous or hormonal levels) are not balanced then many disorders result, ranging from fatigue to depression to obesity. "The different asanas systematically stretch and tone all the peripheral nerves, helping to strengthen them and stabilize neurochemical transmission ... tone the sympathetic and parasympathetic nervous systems, which ... regulate our voluntary and involuntary functions (response to stress to flow of gastric juices) ... the asanas also massage and stimulate all the endocrine glands" (Lidell 1983, p. 185). DE's approach to the Sun Salutation parallels this information, giving us a map for embodiment to bring the glands and nervous system into our western practice of yoga.

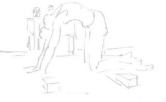

Somatic Movement and Yoga and the Glands

The perspective of Somatic Movement Therapists and Educators includes inhabiting the glands with awareness. This experience affects the mind and emotions, enhancing presence. Each has a particular energy or expression that can be felt. For example, connecting with the adrenals (yours or someone else's) somatically (with awareness and/or physical/energetic touch) can calm and lessen anxiety and give a sense of spaciousness.

The Power of Embodying the Kidneys and Adrenal Glands

I (Shakti) was in an improvisational dance class in 1995 or so, at Earthdance, where the class of 30–40 was almost literally bouncing off the walls. The energy was exciting, even frenetic. I think it was spring, and the first day of classes in a five-day event, a Contact Improvisation jam. Twenty minutes or so into the morning class, the teacher, long-time Body-Mind Centering® practitioner Ione Beauchamp, stopped the dance class. She guided us into pairs, and had us place our hands over our partner's kidneys and adrenal glands while seated or in child's pose, for 3–5 minutes each. After switching roles we then continued with the dance class. I remember experiencing the energy of the room as completely changed. There was still a lot of it, but there was now a spaciousness and calm holding or rather permeating the room as we continued with our group and partner dance explorations. This has always stayed with me, and inspired me to guide many private clients and yoga students into similar hands-on adrenal gland experiences.

A keystone to embodiment is discovering where in the body different types of consciousness live. BMC works with physically sensing or at first imagining the quality of a tissue, whether it be muscular, skeletal, fascial, fluid, organ, fat, or nerve. BMC also invites the mover to discover how all cells have access to glandular consciousness. As mentioned earlier, the neuroendocrine system is known to touch almost all cells in the body and may indeed touch every cell directly. Once an embryo becomes a fetus every human cell has the potential for a neuroendocrine relationship. Furthermore, there is a crystalline nature to the neuroendocrine system that will be discussed in detail in future chapters. This tensile force expands in multiple directions with an impact that is yet unknown. What is known is that attuning with our hormonal waves, as well as all parts of our nervous system – whether reflexive or highly analytic, makes the extremely pervasive neuroendocrine system critical to decision making, including self-regulation, mood shifts, and actions. Often enough, decisions may be made without a conscious alignment between one's body, the goal, and the environment, which can lead to poor choices. Learning to align these forces is an important aspect of an embodied approach to yoga.

Working in Threes

In DE one can explore glands in this way, within the context of dance/movement classes, experiential anatomy classes and sessions, self-care, and client treatments. DE has long embraced the BMC glandular practice of regularly working with glands above and below to ensure energy flow and balancing. The concept evolved over time, through the teaching of DEPs Shakti Smith and Dana Davison, to more specifically call the practice of working with a minimum of three

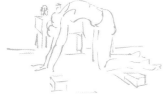

Chapter 2

glands and/or chakras at a time "Working in Threes." This triadic flow aids in integrating the work into the entire chakra and glandular systems by generating flow through different areas of the body. It is always good to generate support from below, in the lower body, before working with a particular gland or chakra. Why? This work can release or generate a lot of energy. Connecting with the energy is supported by also feeling the physical anatomy above and below, creating a channel that allows any energy generated to flow into the rest of the system. Grounding techniques, such as feeling our feet, breathing deeply, or putting one's head on the floor in a forward bend, aid us in holding this increase in energy, and can lessen the spacey-ness that can happen physically and in the brain from such expansion. This energy balancing also prevents exaggerations or distortions of energy that could happen when working with just one chakra or gland.

Experiencing the glands and chakras in this somatic way deepens the practice of the Sun Salutation. Practicing awareness of these systems brings your mind's focus into your own body. This is a powerful way to embody your practice. You are harnessing the power of your mind to focus, and dropping into your body. The complexity of the material demands your presence. This helps you shake off decades of being in just your head. It is anti-anxiety training. The rewards are numerous. Being in your own body. Feeling your power. The movement practice lessens the collective fear that sometimes drives many westerners "out of the body" and "into the head."

There is more detail on the chakras in Chapter 4. Whether practicing traditional or somatic yoga you may learn that each chakra has a sound – a bija (or beej, seed) mantra, as well as a yantra (an image), and a color that you can work with to balance it. Each chakra

Chart 2.1		
The Seven Chakras Presented in this Book		
Chakra	**Sanskrit Name**	**Anatomical Location**
1st	Muladhara	Pelvic floor
2nd	Svadhisthana	Below navel
3rd	Manipura	Solar plexus
4th	Anahata	Heart
5th	Visudha	Throat
6th	Ajna	Forehead
7th	Sahasrara	Crown

is connected with one or more glands. The glands can also be stimulated by "sounding" (there will be more on sounding in Chapter 3) and "felt into" energetically. Working with these areas helps you to balance, especially if you choose to get to know your body, to become embodied. This state of embodiment is a form of grounding. As you ground you may find that your thinking clears – you get less spacey, and brain fog can dissipate. As you embody, you become more present, which lessens anxiety, and enables you to more fully live your life.

Kundalini Energy/Energy Rising within the Body/Energy Release

Energy naturally moves from one chakra to another, up and down the length of the spine. As we have seen, this energy spine is called the *sushumna* in Sanskrit, and the two spiraling strands of it that move in a way similar to DNA are called Ida and Pingala. There is a ball of energy coiled at the base of the spine, called

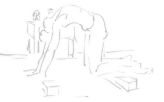

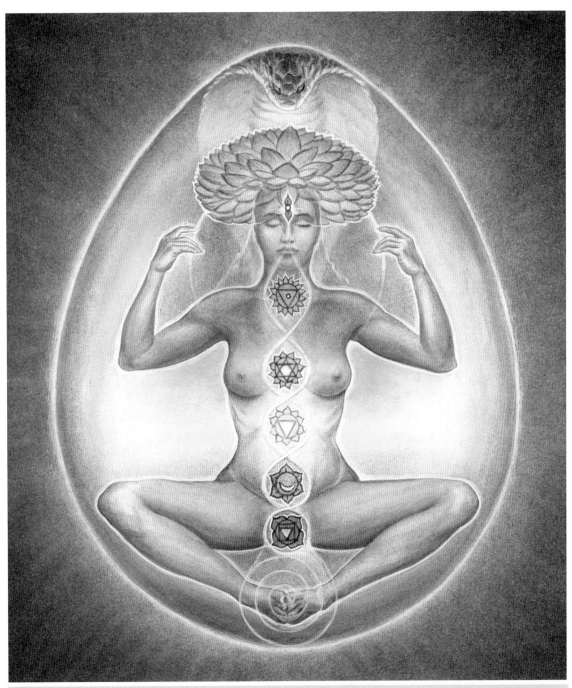

Figure 2.6
Shakti, by Hrana Janto. Permission generously given to us by the artist. Shared by courtesy of Dave Sheppard and Hrana Janto, *www.hranajanto.com*

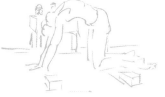

Kundalini energy. Often this energy is symbolized as a snake (see Fig. 2.6). It can release in small and big ways, especially during practices of meditation and yoga, spiritual dance like sufi whirling, and sometimes in women from the intense experience of giving birth. Its movement can be triggered by the presence or touch of someone already with awakened Kundalini energy – a spiritual teacher or guru.

This movement of Kundalini energy is from the base of the spine up. Humanity can also receive energy from the world and the universe, via the crown of our heads. This energy moves down through the body. The body has a North and South Pole, like the earth, and receives energy from both directions. This energy moves through all bodies naturally, and can also be directed intentionally through practices like Qigong and Tai Chi.

Many healing practitioners will be familiar with the phenomenon of their body beginning to rock in small circles as they do energy work with clients. This also is energy moving. A Reiki healer's initiation can start a wave or current of energy moving through the body from above through the crown, as can sitting in a meditation hall with a high-vibration teacher.

Energetic releases often happen in bodywork. The practitioner's hands and intention facilitate the movement of energy through the client's body. When stuck or stagnant places are found, the body releases energy in the form of heat or unconscious movement (the flickering of a finger, shaking of a leg); these can be light releases, clearing of energy from the life lived in a day. They can also be stronger ones which can be accompanied by an unconscious urge to move, shake, or tremor. There are specific practices like Tremoring and Reichian bodywork, as well as the Trauma Recovery strategies in Somatic Experiencing that work with this type of release to help unwind trauma stored in the body. Jim Gordon, the first Director of the United States Commission on Complementary and Alternative Medicine (CAM), has been teaching that method for decades, including with refugees of war (Gordon 2019).

Energy moving through the body can also be experienced in yoga practice, during meditation, or when near crystals or in other high-vibration environments like temples or churches. A Kundalini opening can be a subtle experience like the above, or it can shake through the body like tremoring, with stops and starts as the energy comes upon blocks it can hiccup. And in the case of Shaktipat with a Guru or a Kundalini opening that happens in meditation, the opening is often more rapid and intense. The experience can be even more dramatic.

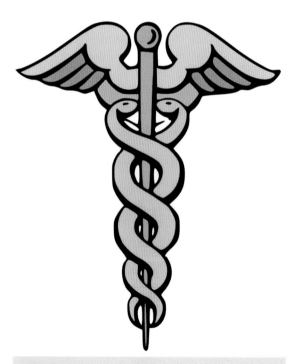

Figure 2.7
Caduceus, by Rama, 2004.

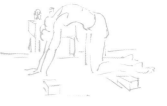

Shakti's and Martha's Personal Stories: Kundlalini Stories

When I (Shakti) was 25 I experienced a Kundalini opening during a ten-day silent Buddhist vipassana retreat. Fifteen years later I had an equally powerful Kundalini opening while sitting at the feet of a spiritual teacher. I've been investigating how to be with, and ground, this energy ever since. Menopause has made me even more fine-tuned to energy, while also exacerbating the uncomfortable aspects of Kundalini rising (heat rising to the brain during meditation practice, which leads to irritability and circular thinking).

Martha experienced a Kundalini opening during a Shaktipat initiation with a Hindu Guru during a meditation retreat in 1981. It was a physical dropping into a place of peace. It was so timely and profound that she was inspired to meditate from that moment on, to visit this place again and again. The experience has grown to becoming a blue light meditation as well.

People who experience energy moving through their bodies often experience increased sensitivity to sound, light, and smells. There can be more pleasure experienced with these senses, or also increased discomfort. Grounding really helps balance these shifts and changes.

If you are experiencing an increase in energy circulating through your system, try walks in nature to ground, eating fewer stimulants and more grounding foods. Quiet time alone may help, along with anything that helps you feel your legs and feet. You may also want to learn clearing practices and develop cleaner living. These dietary shifts can be supported by enhancing your "nature connection." Learn more in Chapter 10.

Also helpful will be practicing the Sun Salutation in this DE style – of bringing the mind into the body. This is called "conscious movement." Its physical benefits include grounding and stretching of the body and the energetic meridians held within. Feeling and reflecting during this ritual movement of the Sun Salutation sequence will help you find your center – physically and spiritually. DE values that, during or after any major stimulus, there is also time given to resting. This quiet somatic state gives your body and being a chance to digest experiences, to integrate and settle.

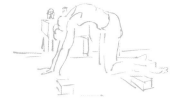

Chapter 2

Seated Chakra Bubble Meditation

 Sit in "easy pose" (sukhasana), lotus (padmasana), or half-lotus (ardha padmasana). Take a few moments to feel your connection to the earth, sensing the bones and muscles of your legs that are rooting your 1st chakra and your whole chakral system to the earth.

 Breathe in red light at your pelvic floor. Inhale; see a bubble of red light in between your pubic bone and tailbone. Exhale; see that light moving up your spine and sushumna into your 2nd chakra below your belly button, the color shifting to orange. Breathe into the orange light, seeing it fill your reproductive system.

 Now see it becoming a bubble of light as you inhale, and as you exhale, breathe that bubble up into your solar plexus, seeing it become yellow. Breathe in, seeing this yellow light fill your diaphragm, pancreas, kidneys, and adrenals.

 Breathe in, seeing a yellow bubble of light form; exhale it up into your heart, seeing it turn green. Visualize this light filling your heart space, emerald green light saturating the area from your sternum to your back body.

 Inhale and see a green bubble forming; exhale it up into your throat, and visualize it turning blue: a nice cooling blue light filling your throat, the back of your neck, your thyroid.

 Inhale, seeing the blue bubble form again; exhale this bubble up into your third eye. See it turning an indigo blue or violet color, and spreading out to fill your pituitary, the bottom of your brain to your occiput in the back.

 Inhale, seeing the bubble again rising up to the top of your head, blossoming into a flower with petals in every color of the rainbow unfolding over your shining skull, their tips caressing your heart and your upper back. Breathe in and out three more times as you sit with this image in your mind's eye. Now gently caress with your fingers down your face and head, and sweep your hands down your torso to your legs to ground this energy. Use soft fists to tap your legs all the way down to your feet. Enjoy the clarity and balance you may be feeling.

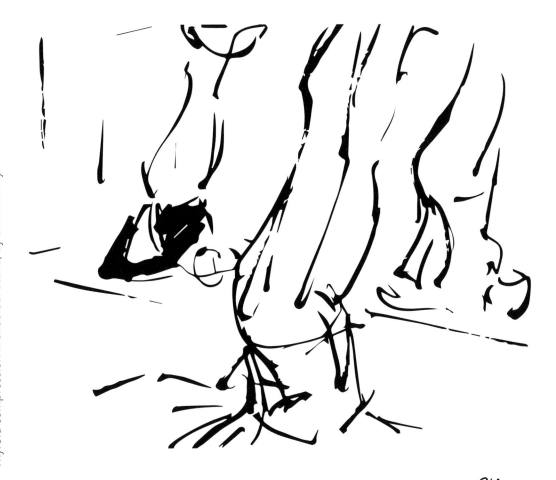

Thyroid compression in shoulder stand, by Stewart Hoyt

3A The Nervous System, Glands, and Neuroendocrine System

Introduction: The Neuroendocrine System

Understanding the anatomy and physiology is an important inroad to this embodiment.

Embodying the chakras involves blended energies of the nervous system and the endocrine glands, which is referred to as the neuroendocrine system. These two systems bring together a wide range of life activity, integrating subcortical and cortical brain responses with the emotional and spiritual life of the glands. This joined system can have intense impact and allow for a variety of behavioral choices.

The nervous system is a decision-making or control center for our life experience and our bodies, and also provides awareness of the "body-mind." It is an information center that is electrical, and known for its capacity for discrete informational exchange. For instance, one

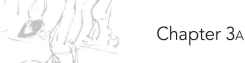

nerve – from neuron to axon and dendrite – can exchange information in a specific area of one finger, one organ, or one cell. What makes the nervous system distinct from the glandular system is that electrical signals traveling through the nerves go to a specific part of the body – to specific muscles, bones, or organs, or from those sites through the nerves sending messages back to the brain. This is different from the hormonal action of the glands. When a gland releases a hormone the person's entire mood, rhythm or behavior is impacted. These represent two different types of decision-making processes.

In high contrast, the endocrine hormonal responses are generalized throughout the entire body. The glandular system is "systemic" because the glands release hormones into the bloodstream through ductless glands that act through the entire body. By virtue of being carried in the blood, hormones impact diverse areas of the body while in transit, as well as their destination – the target cells. When hormones are "coursing through the blood" everywhere in the body they can, sometimes instantly, change one's entire mood or emotions. Glandular rhythms also vary. This is because the hormone release often acts in cycles, each gland having a unique rhythm – night and day (pineal), energy level (thyroid), monthly menses (ovaries), quick response to feeling or being attacked (adrenals) are examples.

Neuroendocrinology is the study of interactions between the nervous and endocrine systems (Martin 2001). The nervous system operates through electrical impulses and neurotransmitters (which excite or inhibit neuronal firing); the endocrine system acts in response to hormones, which are chemical messengers. In general, hormones act fast because they spread out through the entire body quickly through the bloodstream. Their impact also lingers for longer than nerve stimuli, because it has circulated so fully and then it takes a while for the blood to cleanse itself

of the hormones. And as one experiences the unified interactivity of the glands, a relationship to earth, emotions, spirit, and cosmos may emerge. From a Dynamic Embodiment[SM] (DE[SM]) perspective, the combined energetic force of the neuroendocrine system opens pathways through the body that are quite powerful – they create chakral energy.

The History of Neuroendocrine Awareness

According to *Merriam-Webster's Dictionary* the term neuroendocrine is defined as "of, relating to, or being a hormonal substance that influences the activity of nerves" and was first used in 1922. However, neuroendocrine tumors were identified in cancer research in 1870. For years the scientific community kept the study and even medical professions of endocrinology and neurology separate. The neurologist Temple Fay popularized the term in the 1930s. Bainbridge Cohen discovered his writings and shared it with BMC students in the 1980s.

Dr Fay was a huge proponent of the neuroendocrine experience. Fay lived from 1895 to 1963 and is considered one of the most skilled neurosurgeons of his day. He founded the Neurosurgical Service at Temple University Hospital in Philadelphia in 1930. Fay was a Cofounder and former President of the Harvey Cushing Society, which is now the American Association of Neurological Surgeons. He is also known for being a pioneer in the field of therapeutic hypothermia. Much of Fay's research focused on helping cancer patients relieve pain using extremely cold environments. His work also underlies much of the protocol development of the Doman–Delacotto method, the system that began the first synchronistic "movement repatterning" of teams of therapists to help people with motor coordination and spasticity problems.

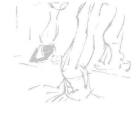

Defining and Locating the Neuroendocrine Cells

The neuroendocrine system is where the nervous system and endocrine system meet. The nervous system is composed of the brain, spinal cord, ganglia, and nerves. Neural cells communicate directly with one another (and with cells of sensory and effector tissues) by means of electrical impulses traveling along nerves and supported by neurotransmitters.

Oxford Dictionary (2020) refers to neuroendocrine simply as being "both neural and endocrine in structure or function." However, in the medical community there are definitions such as this one: the neuroendocrine system is made up of special cells called neuroendocrine cells, which are like nerve cells (neurons) receiving messages from the nervous system but they respond hormonally. Neuroendocrine cells are found in almost every organ of the body. The neuroendocrine cells scattered throughout these organs are often referred to as the diffuse neuroendocrine system. They are mainly found scattered in the gastrointestinal (GI) tract (including the small intestine, rectum, stomach, colon, esophagus, and appendix), the gallbladder, the pancreas (islet cells), and the thyroid (C cells). Neuroendocrine cells are also commonly found in the lungs or airways into the lungs (bronchi), as well as the respiratory tract of the head and neck. There are neuroepithelial bodies in the bronchopulmonary tracks. The pituitary gland, the parathyroid glands, and the inner layer of the adrenal gland (adrenal medulla) are made of mostly neuroendocrine cells. Other sites of neuroendocrine cells include the thymus, kidneys, liver, prostate, cervix, ovaries, and testicles – some are deep to the body's interior and others are more superficial. Even the skin has glandular components and of course has a huge neural network.

Integrating Somatic Influences

DE merges movement strategies and principles from the work of Laban, Bartenieff, and Bainbridge Cohen, using LMA, BF, and Body-Mind Centering® (BMC®). Neuroendocrine embodiment explorations include:

1. the anatomical location and size of each gland and plexus (BMC)

2. the forces around them – from other glands or tissue within the body (BMC)

3. the spatial lines/pulls that emanate from the area or help to stimulate it (LMA)

4. the fascial pathways and spatial intention of the mover (BF)

5. vocalization and vibration in the area using spatial awareness (BF and BMC)

6. looking at how early motor development patterns relate to glandular and nervous system functioning (BMC and BF).

Physiology of the Nervous Systems and Glands

In standard physiology, the full set of endocrine glands is often referred to as the endocrine system but can also be called the "hormonal system" or "glandular system." As a whole, this system serves as a behavioral regulator. Focusing on embodiment of the glands and the entire endocrine system has numerous roles. One is experiencing new biological resources, similar to discovering the sensation of movement of the lungs in order to breathe more fully. Another is to regulate the moods and feelings that arise from the different hormonal

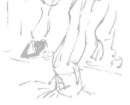

Chapter 3A

activity of each gland. A third is to access the chakras by grounding the subtle experience within the physical body.

The endocrine system is equally powerful and even more so as the elements work together. The BMC community has been referring to and embodying the neuroendocrine system as a way to gain insight about behavioral and mood changes, as well as strong energetic shifts. These explorations began at the School for Body-Mind Centering in the 1970s, inspired in large part by the writing of Alice Bailey. Readings by Dr Temple Fay were also distributed (Alzaga et al 2006).

Neuroendocrinology investigates reciprocal influences of neural connections (local and specific) with the impact of hormones (widespread and systemic). The neuroendocrine system's ability to control behavior stems from the fact that this control has a choice of coming through the endocrine system to shift moods, or through the nervous system to act more discreetly (in one part of the body). This covers the gamut of behavioral choices – those that are basically unconscious (hormonal) and those that are deliberate and conscious (governed by different parts of the nervous system). In DE it is found useful to bring cortical awareness into glandular physiological responses in order to regain "grounding" or "centeredness."

Pituitary: The Neuroendocrine Hub/Junction

You may have heard of the pituitary gland being referred to as the "master gland." The reason it is called the master gland is that it directs the release of hormones from other endocrine glands. The pituitary is a conduit for directives from a specific part of the brain, the hypothalamus, which links the

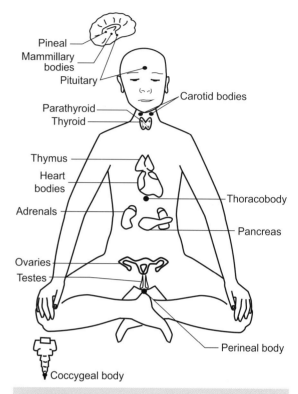

Figure 3A.1
The endocrine system as taught in Dynamic Embodiment[SM] and Body-Mind Centering[®]. Credit: based on original drawing by Amanda Latchmore.

nervous and endocrine systems. Also known as the hypophysis, the pituitary has two lobes, one dropping forward and the other behind. The anterior lobe is glandular and functions to direct other glands to release hormones through the bloodstream. The posterior lobe is neural – acting through the electrical pathways of the nervous system to help regulate the output of diverse hormones through various influences. The anterior pituitary is the central regulator of the endocrine system, coordinating signals from the hypothalamus in the brain (centrally) and endocrine glands (peripherally).

Labels on Figure 3A.1: Pineal, Mammillary bodies, Pituitary, Carotid bodies, Parathyroid, Thyroid, Thymus, Heart bodies, Adrenals, Thoracobody, Pancreas, Ovaries, Testes, Perineal body, Coccygeal body.

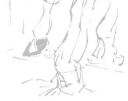

Deep to Superficial, Central to Periphery, Core to Distal

Deep in the brain is the hypothalamus, a neuroendocrine region that produces hormones that signal, through nerve or endocrine tissue, whether to release or inhibit hormones, working closely with the pituitary gland to regulate stress (adrenals), basal metabolism (thyroid), growth (thymus plus all neuroendocrine cells), reproduction (gonads), and, for cisgender women, lactation.

The hypothalamus works closely with neuroendocrine cells, which modulate cell growth and proliferation. The hypothalamic hormones regulate pituitary hormone release, among other triggers of physiological functions such as water/salt balance, and release of vasopressin and oxytocin, enabling the brain to respond rapidly to physiological shifts. These include making the hormones that guide the "releasing-hormones" for corticotrophin, dopamine, growth hormone, gonadotrophin, and thyrotrophin.

According to Hinson et al (2010), the anterior pituitary is composed of five different cell types, each of which secretes a different hormone (see Chapter 3B). The somatotroph is its main kind of secretory cell. Between 10 and 30 percent of the other secretory cells are lactotrophs. This part of the pituitary is associated with the accumulation of excessive subcutaneous fat, and other conditions such as hypogonadotropic hypogonadism and growth retardation.

Underlying Principles and Guidelines for Your Practice

DE provides many pathways for learning how to follow physical sensations. To access the internal body if there are no strong sensations already, it is important to have guidance from anatomy or physiology. In this chapter, each gland is described in terms of its location, its function, the potential metaphors or meaning of this bodily tissue, and where its impact resonates, as well as which chakra it relates to. It is not necessarily easy to learn how to embody the glands guided solely by the written word. Therefore, drawings, images, and guided somatic activities are provided to assist finding awareness. Whether working with your glands and chakras on your own for self-care, teaching a class, or doing a healing session with a client, work with at least three glands and/or chakras at a time. Learn more about the fascial lines/spatial pulls that emanate from the area or help to stimulate. Be alert to your own spatial intention as you move. If you desire, discover the benefits of vocalization and vibration. Explore how to use sound to expand internal space and to feel that space, proprioceptively. Consider how your habits impact your practice. Discover more about features of early motor development patterns and how they relate to glandular and nervous system functioning in childhood and at any other stage throughout the lifespan.

To embody the chakras is to experience the power of the combined sensations derived from the experience of how the neural and endocrine systems (see Fig. 2.5) combine to form the powerful neuroendocrine system. In DE, you take time to experience each system separately, before attuning with their combined sensations. The nervous system is discussed in Chapter 6 in the context of neurodevelopmental movement. In this chapter, you are introduced to each gland and invited to "feel into" it.

Why Embody the Neuroendocrine System?

In case you are wondering why to activate the glands or the chakras through embodiment of the neuroendocrine system, and why to do

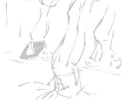
so within the Sun Salutation, here are several potential motivators:

1. It is exciting to understand the subtle energetic body, as well as to feel it as a bodily source for soul or spirit level consciousness.

2. Just as the suggestion of using props (e.g. pillows) for restoration while practicing movement, or "going easy on yourself," is helpful, so is having more inner bodily resources for engaging in self-care.

3. Embodied investigation shifts the practice of yoga from being an imagined experience of glandular balancing to being a tangible physicalized exploration resulting in self-discovery.

4. If you are a kinesthetic, sensate learner, you can shift a purely physical workout to a physical workout that is linked to moods and emotions.

5. In an age when, most likely, at least one person you know is struggling with thyroid, adrenal, or reproductive glandular imbalances, it is useful for one's health to have information about the physical, emotional, and spiritual impact of attuning with the hormones and glands.

Activating the Glands: Sacred Space, Sacred Feelings

How exactly does one activate glands using the anatomical–spatial method of DE? One inroad involves adapting methodologies from BMC for organ awareness for use with the glands. In BMC, two organ embodiment tools are compression and tensile stretching. DE finds that these same tools help stimulate the energy flow of an endocrine gland. Space Harmony principles from Laban/Bartenieff studies further support embodiment of the glands.

Here are three types of organ activation from BMC that involve using spatially defined actions that DE employs to stimulate or calm a gland:

1. Preparation: "Take out the slack." With muscles, "taking out the slack" involves moving the two ends of a muscle, the tendons, pulling them away from each other. With glands, the surrounding fascia or muscles positioned over the gland can be put into a taut state by moving the far ends of that structure (muscle or fascial sheath) apart. Think of pulling an elastic band into its resting length or a tad beyond it. During this process you are learning to find the tensile forces of the tissue.

2. Activation by Pressure: Putting weight into a body area compresses it. That compression increases sensation. Learn how each asana has a body part/area that takes pressure in order to balance. When one is standing, the body parts that are compressed are the feet. When one is lying down, whether prone (on the belly) or supine (on the back), the body generally relaxes. Once one or more body parts are lifted up, the body weight redistributes, causing compression into the supporting area. This area is often referred to as a fulcrum, which serves as support for moving parts. When the fulcrum is near or on a gland, somatic awareness registers this pressure as a stimulus to the gland. Please explore body positions that put extra gravitational pressure on any area along the spine that feels comfortable. These positions will most likely be related to glandu-

lar stimuli since the glands are situated all along the spine. This type of exploration is called "compressional support."

3. Activation by Tension: Experience how to go beyond the resting length of a body area by making or "drawing" an arc by arching the spine. This process increases the tension on the top surface of the body – the one lifting up. The height of the arch can become a point of suspension between two ends that are in high tension. If the suspension is in the area of a specific gland and you allow sensation to pour through that area using awareness of the area deep to the stretched fascia or muscle, this creates a tensile structure – a tensegrity. This tensile positioning is called "suspensional support."

Suspend to Stimulate

DE also uses the spatial concept of "suspension as support" or "suspensional support." This concept, along with "compression as support" or "compressional support," is applied to activating volume and vitality in the organs in both BMC and DE. DE also uses it with glands.

What does BMC mean by "suspensional support"? Bridges are suspension-based: they suspend from highly tuned wires pulling across long expanses. By finding tether points to anchor the body, and then positioning the body part that needs activation at the apex of the tension point, usually with an arching of that body area, one can form a tensile force that brings "energy" to that high point, the top of the arch. In the human body, this involves making a shape with the body that expands in space with tether or anchor points employing "counter-tensions" – pulls in opposite directions. These also exemplify tensegrity.

Using the Laban/Bartenieff system for spatial specificity and the Body-Mind Centering® system for anatomical specificity, DE combines the awareness of the anatomical placement of the glands and the sensations of its existence with the use of spatial tensions that occur when

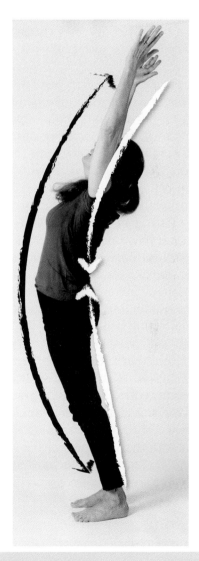

Figure 3A.2
Compressional support underlying suspensional support. Photo by Serge Cashman.

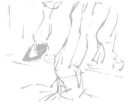

creating counter-pulls between the two ends of a muscle or on the fascia. This is a type of bio-tensegrity. These movements become a natural inroad to stimulating the glands – activating or calming the energy needed for hormone balancing. The stimulation of the glands can be further elucidated through Space Harmony practices from LMA; however, it is simpler and more traditional to engage in the practice of yoga and can be done specifically with the Sun Salutation.

While practicing the Sun Salutation, both compression and suspension are applied not just to the organs but also to the endocrine glands. This process enlivens a three-dimensional experience of the glandular system. The activation process can be pictured as creating a soft, elastic, crystalline form with the body.

Working within the already existent yogic practice of the Sun Salutation is a wonderful first step. This is because the Sun Salutation uses fairly simple spatial actions: up, up and back, down, back and low, up and down, engaging many different body parts at the same time. The action is predominantly within the sagittal plane, also known as the plane of the wheel – a narrow form that goes forward, up, down, and back. Generally there are no spirals, no big twists, and no off-vertical movement. This fits with its purpose – greeting the rising of the sun along the horizon line. The narrow wheel shape of the sagittal plane also correlates with the alignment of the glands in the body – up and down, forward and back, with only a little side to side.

Neuroendocrine Awareness Dynamic Embodiment^SM^-Style

DE asks you to become alert to the awareness that comes from the nervous system as well as that of the glands. Listening to the information

that rises up or settles down from the endocrine system can result in developing emotional/behavioral sensitivity that helps you attune better to yourself and others. The endocrine system can be stimulated or relaxed by finding the spaciousness around any specific gland. As described earlier – DE Practitioners (DEPs) believe it is the intersection of strong gland centers with strong nerve plexuses (where many nerve fibers arise) that is the seat of each chakra. This parallels the nervous system but is distinct in that hormones are released systemically into the entire bloodstream and therefore impact the whole body. From a somatic perspective, the glands regulate cycles and these cycles can both impact movement and be influenced by movement. Examples are:

1. The circadian cycle, relating to the cycle of day and night, now known to be governed by the melatonin released by the pineal gland

2. The rush of energy that comes from the release of "adrenaline" stimulating a short cycle burst of energy (of course this can become chronic – see below and in Chapter 7)

3. The rhythm of your own metabolic rate – how fast or slow you function – as regulated by the hormones of the thyroid gland.

The impact of the systemic nature of the glandular system is that its effect is on the whole body, often instantly. Glandular secretion sets different rhythms or cycles of energy flowing through the whole body. These rushes of energy can come in slow waves over the day or month, or can be instant. They can cause one to feel "out of control" or chaotic. Or they can provide the "just right" mood or energy level for one's chosen activity.

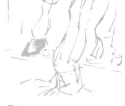

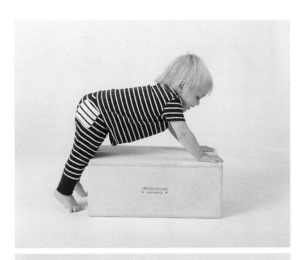

Figure 3A.3

"Thymus reaching" of the arms with whole-body glandular support. You can see this from the aliveness throughout the body. Photo by Serge Cashman.

A familiar example: think about when something scares you. At that moment, adrenaline rushes and impacts the entire body, causing an increase of blood flow to the arms and legs – for fight or flight. Freeze is another common response of the sympathetic nervous system, discussed later. It takes time for this rush to dissipate.

Locate and Move

In DE, whatever your reason for embodiment – health, relaxation, trauma recovery, vitality – it is important to locate the gland and then the fascial and related muscle tissues in the area around a gland. Once the muscles are located, tension is employed by pulling from their polar opposite locations. Once they are found, the pulling is like stretching out a hammock and tying it to two distant trees – the gland can then feel supported and will relax as it hangs and swings. The anchoring into the tree is maintained by its tautness.

From BMC, locate and "somatize." To somatize is to imagine feeling sensation and/or embodying a movement. Spend time doing this with each gland using sound, touch, and movement, and notice the differences in the rhythms of the sounds, touch, or movement that are resonant with each distinct gland. A key aspect of activating glands is to locate them along the spine, either high or low in the torso or head, and to then open the space around them up by "taking out the slack." While "taking out the slack" awakens tissue, Laban Space Harmony teaches how to find the subtle counter-pulls that stretch the system out into big space, referred to as a "large kinesphere." Kinesphere refers to the space different body parts can occupy and move through without taking a step. Occupying a large kinesphere is being as expansive as possible without taking a step. Bartenieff studied and devised exercises and explorations to practice identifying "where in space you want to go" and called it Spatial Intent. Bartenieff exercises also teach you to feel both fascial interconnections and superficial to deep muscular "kinetic chains."

Glandular stimulation responds to movement – specifically, movement that has a clear awareness of counter-pulls in and through the muscles or fascia, and out to specific spatial endpoints. DE practices Space Harmony and the use of specific counter-tensional pulls (counter-pulls) to actually stimulate the gland, using tensegrity (spatial pulls that create support for posture and whole-body movement). DE blends concepts of space from all three systems: BMC, LMA, and BF. You are guided to activate different tensegrities in the body while moving through the Sun Salutation: for instance, reaching the arms high while also standing with grounding, or reaching one leg back (and low) while the rest of the body projects forward, or forward and up (e.g. with one's gaze or arms). This process includes acknowledging

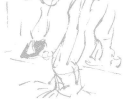

and feeling the sagittal nature of Sun Saluta-tion. The movement is narrow, moving mostly forward and back with up and down aspects – like a bow and arrow – as often depicted by Sagittarius. In order to find recuperation and inhabit our full three-dimensionality, activities are offered throughout these pages to ensure "spatial recuperations" – such as a spinal twist or two that takes you out of the sagittal plane.

Grounding: Emotional and Behavioral Connections

DE, like BMC, includes an understanding that the release of hormones may trigger unex-pected shifts in mood and therefore behav-ior. In BMC there is acknowledgment of a phenomenon referred to as "the chaos of the glands." One may experience chaotic feelings when the surges of hormonal activity stimulate big mood swings. In embodying the glands, it is possible to stimulate the hormones and have different mood swings. To avoid this, work with "grounding the glands" in three ways:

1. opening up the flow between the glands;

2. embedding the exploration in structure – movement that activates a balanced use of the musculo-skeletal system; and

3. working with ritual – in this case stimu-lating the glands through familiar move-ment to create a comparative framework to help one notice how one feels from one day to the next.

This supports the understanding that there is plenty one can take control of in working with the glands – for instance, responsibility for posture (careful skeletal positioning), use of breath and meditation, and other lifestyle choices. There is also much to learn from the sciences – from anatomy, somatic awareness,

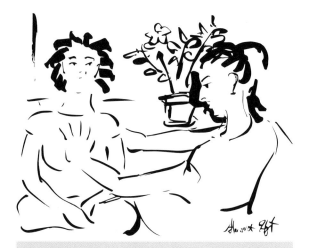

Figure 3A.4
Open hands and heart help us connect, by Stewart Hoyt.

and integrative medicine (e.g. hormonal bal-ancing through brain-activating movement). And one can integrate broader social somatic understanding such as the impact of cultural and intergenerational influences on moods, behaviors, and glandular/hormonal triggers.

Anatomical Information to Foster Greater Interoception

This approach focuses on embodiment of the glands through sensation. Recall that when perceiving the organs or glands you use a sense called interoception – perception of the internal body. Having anatomical information describ-ing each gland's location helps with embodi-ment and finding the spatial pulls between areas around the glands. To reiterate, in order to feel the glands, it is helpful to know their anatomy – to be able to "find them" and to activate them either through "suspending from them" by establish-ing a tensile structure, or "through compres-sion" by pouring one's body weight into them.

The glands that secrete hormones affect our moods and behaviors; this impacts

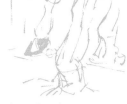

behavior – our expression. From a somatic movement perspective, by tracking moods, one can get to know the hormones. Becoming aware of our bodily posture and the dynamics of our movement also reveals insights about endocrine balance and imbalances. The goal of glandular embodiment is to gain ease while moving or holding a posture, or to balance the gland itself. This is done by integrating anatomical embodiment information as functional tips for the practice of the Sun Salutation.

More information can be gleaned from paying attention to the use of space. For instance, what types of forces do you succumb to during the day? The most common is the force of gravity pulling down, compressing joints and causing tiredness. However, sometimes, besides sinking, you can shape into positions of retreat or enclosing, which can represent shying away from intensity or attack or taking time for yourself. Other times you can be ready to move out into space – "the world" – to act or assertively defend taking on positions of advancing or spreading or ascending. These actions (called Shaping in the LMA/ BF work) are most personally expressive when they happen in the torso, but they can also occur in the limbs. Once you understand your bodily interaction with three-dimensional space, you can also use this spatial awareness to "open up the glands." And, if you know which glands support what moods or behaviors, you can be conscientious about which glands to stimulate. This chapter serves as a guide to coming to understand the different glands and how they *may* interact within you. Each person is different.

The biochemistry and molecular biology of the glandular system is complex and highly individualized. Hence this is just a map, not the actual world. You are exploring with guidelines, and you may discover new territory.

You can explore embodying the glands to overcome physical or emotional challenges (see Chapter 7) or simply to enhance the ease or meaningfulness of your Sun Salutation practice. Students report that practicing with "glandular support" helps them derive all the positive benefits of Sun Salutation plus an almost effortless unfolding of the movement. The integration of glandular support leads to new experiences of alignment, flexibility, and energy.

Grounding: Body Connectivity from BF

DEPs use many BMC resources, such as the neurodevelopmental patterns to be described in Chapter 6, and safeguards, such as attending to the gland above and below it ("working in threes"), to ensure a flow between the glands. DEPs also take time to experience and share how "glandular support" reinvigorates human movement efficiency as explained through BF. Using the connections to early motor coordination and neurodevelopmental practices from BF, the practice of the Sun Salutation opens up even more resources. One key avenue for experiencing the flow of glandular stimuli and staying grounded is to use the six bodily connections that Bartenieff identified as neurologically significant.

As described in Chapter 1 (see Fig. 1.4B, repeated here), the most common Bartenieff body organization connections are:

1. head–tail

2. and 3. scapula–fingers (of each arm; see Figs 5.4 and 5.5)

4. and 5. sit bone–heel connection (of each leg)

6. scapula–sacral connection.

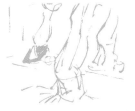

For instance, by feeling how the sit bones connect to the heels you engage your hamstrings, and your balance is more solid. When you then add in the power of the root chakra and the coccygeal body, that grounding intensifies.

The goal here is to explore each phase of the Sun Salutation as both a physical (musculoskeletal) and a chakral (neuroendocrine) experience. In DE, you experience the combination of the skeletal support by understanding embodied anatomy of BMC and the efficiency of body mechanics from BF. This is then supported by the energetic quality of the glands which often allow the body to feel lighter, more expansive and, if approached carefully, more grounded at the same time. For many, this approach heightens the spiritual nature of the practice.

For grounding, begin with the skeletal system – the weight and clarity of shape of the bones help contain endocrine chaos and can give "spatial intention" to help clarify action in the world. This is about knowing where you want to go or what you want to achieve. Having a clear intention clarifies the action. Your embodiment of the Sun Salutation with awareness of the skeletal alignment, the glandular energies (related to chakras), and neuro-developmental coordination allows for balanced glandular exploration. "The container" of the Sun Salutation ritual and the profoundly "hard-wired" neurodevelopmental movement from childhood becomes an anchor that works to center and ground. This is especially needed if your glandular or Kundalini experience can tend toward being chaotic. The ritualized practice of the Sun Salute helps you track your physical and emotional experience over time. The familiarity and structure of it also help to engage in glandular stimulation within a "container." All in all, this makes for gentle realignment and balancing.

The Specific Glands and Bodies

Chart 3A.1 lists the glands and the bodies, which include some only known within the Body-Mind Centering®-derived somatic systems. Bodies are gland-like structures along the spine that have no known secretion but through BMC somatic research feel as if they have glandular attributes. This somatic research process is substantiated in the sections teaching about the history of the pineal and heart bodies, which are now referred to as the pineal gland and heart glands, respectively.

Each gland has its own role within the rhythms of life – leading to different dynamics of movement and resonance. These align with different cycles in life: for instance, moment-by-moment sugar levels, the perception of daytime/night-time awareness, daily baseline metabolism, or monthly cycles, and the various impacts on reproduction, growth, and aging. This energetic awareness, when applied to movement or postures, can bring insights to the body-mind connection since each gland has a purpose that is also quite metaphoric/

Chart 3A.1	
Thirteen Endocrine Centers Along the Spine	
1	Coccygeal body (balanced by the perineal)
2	Gonads – ovaries/testes
3–5	Adrenals, pancreas, thoracobody
6–7	Heart bodies and thymus
8–10	Thyroid and parathyroids, and carotid bodies
11–12	Pituitary and mammillary bodies
13	Pineal gland

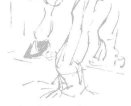

archetypal. For instance, the pineal regulates sleep (think of Rip Van Winkle), and the gonadal release of testosterone and estrogen regulate sex, evident in most films these days. And on a purely physical level, glandular support makes movement freer and easier. In the case of the Sun Salutation, each asana flows into the next when concentrating on the experience of a particular gland or two.

Locating Each Gland and Body and Understanding Its Purpose

Now let's learn more about each of the glands. The chart starts with the glands at our *base*, at the bottom of the pelvis (the pelvic floor), and moves up the spine to the top and back of the head. The choice to begin from the base of the spine first grounds us on a physical level while moving higher up into domains of the body that have been defined as spiritual. The first glands are related to basic survival and embodiment, "being on this planet," and when awakening a gland moving up the spine, the awareness can be likened to moving onto a more "spiritual level." By sensitizing to the pelvis first, feel 'weightedness' before moving toward the head.

What is a Body?

From a BMC and DE perspective, there are both glands and "bodies" within the endocrine system. Glands are made of endocrine tissue that is known to secrete hormones. "Bodies" are tissues that are not known to secrete hormones. Bodies such as the carotid and mammillary bodies are known in anatomy books but do not have a known endocrine function. From a BMC perspective, these two sets of bodies are endocrine-like in their movement quality or exude a similar quality

of "energy." While studying organ health with Yogi Ramaiah, Bainbridge Cohen also was studying the work of Alice Bailey (1947). When exploring the energy centers she sensed that the chakral energy could be glandular. Not all bodies identified in BMC as hormonal have research using scientific methods, but the pineal and heart were both identified by Bainbridge Cohen as endocrine, first confirmed by somatic specialists in BMC lineages as endocrine-like, and some years later found by science to actually secrete hormones. In this lifetime the BMC community experienced the definition of the "heart bodies" shift from having a "felt" endocrine center to being based on more western scientific knowledge of functioning regarding the atria, atrioventricular node, and aortic arch in connection with the release of hormone-related substances. Similarly, functions of the thymus were discovered somatically first.

> ### Martha's Personal Story: Somatic and Western Scientific Discovery of the Heart Bodies
>
> Over the course of the 40 years that I have been studying and working with the concepts and principles of Body-Mind Centering® I have seen what the BMC community refer to as "bodies" be renamed as glands. In the summer of 1976, a group of people studying BMC dedicated an entire month to investigating the experience of the glands. At the time there was no known function of the pineal gland – at least in accessible anatomical texts. By the early 1980s research revealed that the pineal releases melatonin – now a familiar hormone that has even become a central ingredient to the "jet-lag reduction" industry.

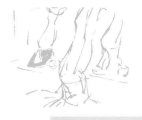

Chapter 3A

Another example involved the heart bodies. Yoga has identified the heart chakra. In the 1970s and 1980s it was certainly known that the heart has an electrical component, but there was no evidence that the region secreted hormones. In 1986, I came upon an article while teaching "Balancing the Endocrine System" in Toronto, Ontario, in Canada and shared it with the School for Body-Mind Centering. The article reported research showing that hormones are released from the aortic arch. Additional practitioners were sharing information and experiences.

Later research demonstrated release from the heart's atria. It is still rare for these areas to be referred to as the "heart gland." However, atrial natriuretic peptide (ANP) is now known to be a strong natriuretic and vasorelaxant hormone, released from the heart region as well as at other sites, including the brain.

Sensory Cues

Return now to the base of the spine and identify all the glands and bodies that can be contacted in DE (and other somatic systems based in Body-Mind Centering®). These are the glands/bodies and related themes that emerge from their hormonal function (if known), and/or from the felt experience of BMC-influenced somatic practitioners.

In BMC, the use of somatization involves guided language for "going into each gland" to establish its location and then find sensation. What can be sensed is the gland itself or the full-bodied experience of the hormone traveling through the bloodstream and the related rhythm or energy that this hormone creates. The systemic (whole-body) shift of energy that courses through the bloodstream can be referred to as a "hormonal surge." The specific shift that occurs due to a particular hormonal surge is referred to as a "shift in mind-states." This shift can happen in other body systems as well – by paying attention to muscles, organs, nerves, circulating fluid rhythms, or bones.

In DE, one can engage in this investigation sensorily – using proprioceptive/interoceptive awareness. A further goal is to learn how to begin to feel the sensations of each gland and to make the link to how these sensations inform our behavior. For instance, you can investigate whether the gland and its hormonal rhythm are depleted, in excess, or balanced.

Adrenals as Example

When you feel tired day after day, you may be experiencing adrenal fatigue. Or when there is a rush of angry or fearful feelings and a desire to run or attack something, adrenaline and cortisol (the hormones of the adrenals) are usually coursing through the bloodstream. These active or overactive adrenalized states can result in anxiety, panic, or aggressive moods or "mind-states." When depleted, sluggish attitudes and movement may be evident. From somatic awareness, one can also feel these shifts of state that affect behavior. As all somatic approaches do, DE asks you to slow down to feel inside (Eddy 2016, Kourlas 2021). There is a request to notice correlated moods – "Do I feel overactive energy in my mid-section just under the floating ribs near the beginning of my lower back, just above my kidneys? Is it buzzing?" Or "When I put my attention in the area of the adrenals, do I feel a wave of exhaustion? Or does the area feel easy, breathing and full of reserved quiet energy?" These are respective sensations of the adrenal gland in different states: activated, depleted, and balanced.

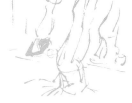

Snapshot: Glands and Physiological Function

Coccygeal body – unknown glandular function, possible neuroendocrine cells

Reproductive glands/gonads (ovaries and testes) – regulating sexual development and reproduction/fertility cycles in men and women

Adrenal glands – medulla: fight, flight, freeze response; cortex: sodium and sugar levels

Pancreas (part digestive organ/part glandular) – regulating sugar/glucose in body

Thoracobody – unknown body, postulated to help with breath

Heart bodies (now heart glands) – blood flow through the heart, blood pressure regulation

Thymus gland – adolescent growth, fighting off toxins, immune response

Thyroid gland – metabolic speed, regulating temperature

Parathyroid glands – regulation of calcium levels

Carotid body – not considered glandular, no known hormone; chemoreceptor, carbon dioxide and oxygen levels

Pituitary gland – master gland; the gland that stimulates other glands

Mammillary bodies – not considered glandular, no known hormone; function is consolidating memory Body-Mind Centering® – leads limbic system

Pineal gland (formerly bodies) – circadian rhythm/sleep cycle

Impact on Moods and How to Observe Them

Below is another "snapshot" of how each of the glands impacts shifts in human behavior experienced by the somatic research of the School for Body-Mind Centering. The shifts are changes in qualities of being, "mind-states" – a change in mood or energy such as feeling sluggish, alert, full of love, fearful, playful, creative, powerful, expressive, grounded. These shifts can be observed using LMA by looking at changes in movement quality. For instance, sluggishness is often accompanied by heaviness in the body, dropping into gravity. Alertness can be seen as increased acuity to timing and the environment, "being awake" and well oriented. Fearfulness is aligned with being adrenalized and can show up as quickness while also exuding strength. Playfulness could be fluctuating shifts of energy – allowing for changes such as sudden and light movements, to more free-flowing action. "Groundedness" can be observed in a weighted presence, as in feeling strong and self-aware. People will vary in how they express themselves (and their creativity), and these individual subtleties can be observed and named as well.

In performing the Sun Salutation with awareness of the glands, the idea is to become more aware of your own moods. By paying attention to mood changes you can also speculate what hormones are impacting your behavior. You may then choose to focus on bringing attention to that gland during your practice. You can then track any potential shifts in your moods or behavior. Generally aligning the glands while moving calms the glands down and integrates them with the other parts of the body – the bones, muscles, and organs. Focusing on activating one particular gland can be used to "wake it up."

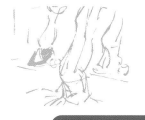

> **Snapshot: Glands and Metaphors in Life Relationship Beyond the Body**
>
> **Coccygeal body** – grounding, cosmic rootedness
>
> **Reproductive glands** – survival of the species
>
> **Adrenal glands** – survival of the person or family
>
> **Pancreas** – relating to others
>
> **Thoracobody** – relating to feeling full or empty
>
> **Heart bodies** – caring about others, love
>
> **Thymus gland** – immunological self-defense and protection
>
> **Thyroid gland** – creative expression of all types
>
> **Parathyroid gland** – balancing our muscles for action
>
> **Carotid body** – quieting the mind and empowering the voice through quiet space
>
> **Pituitary gland** – vision and envisioning
>
> **Mammillary bodies** – connection to memory, including smell, as well as to the limbic system, our emotional center; guardian of the perceptions
>
> **Pineal gland** – hearing, and connecting to night and day

Glandular Complexes

The pituitary, as the "master gland," is involved with various hormonal interconnections between those glands that serve a single function. These are referred to as complexes. There is an initiator gland (the pituitary) and its hormones interact to connect the other glands to complete a task. For instance, the pituitary–thyroidal–gonadal complex works together for reproduction. Regarding the specific hormones, the pituitary gland produces luteinizing hormone (LH) and follicle-stimulating hormone (FSH), and the gonads produce estrogen and testosterone. In simpler terms, in conceiving a baby, the pituitary sends hormonal messages to the thyroid and ovaries fairly simultaneously and they activate hormones that relate to the phases of follicle stimulation and the dropping of an egg. This coordination is critical in fertility. Similarly, the pituitary works with the thyroid and adrenals to deal with stress. The pituitary triggers the production of thyroid-stimulating hormone (TSH), which in turn impacts the production of adrenaline. This is another reason to "Work in Threes" when embodying the glands.

Bringing Stability/Grounding

When working with the glands, some say people are working with potential chaos. This happens most often when one is not involved in a movement regimen, has eaten poorly and is feeling "off," whether emotionally or physically upset. When any one endocrine gland releases hormones, they stream into the blood and then affect a person's complete mood instantaneously. The widespread carriage of the hormone by the bloodstream results in a change to the whole being. This is known as a systemic response. A systemic response is good when a surge of adrenaline for survival is needed. It is also true for the excellent functioning of the thymus to fight off an infection. When there is chronic imbalance or when too many short-term surges happen, both the body and related behavior can be "off base." We can act in ways that are more driven by our hormones than by our desires and strategic thoughts.

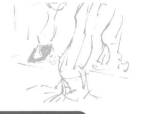

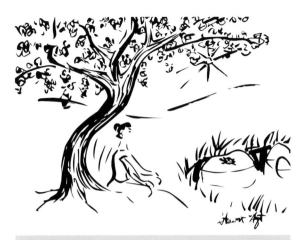

Figure 3A.5
Activating interoception through grounding and centering, by Stewart Hoyt.

In order to "ground" the experience one can turn to the nervous system to access positive thoughts and/or a meditative state of mind. This involves activating the "high brain", the cortex or "cortical brain." One type of cortical engagement is the use of imagery or language. If selected carefully, these images can calm down the sympathetic nervous system action that is often affiliated with, for instance, adrenal intensity. You can also use affirmations. These cortical disciplines help return to choice making versus simply being glandular reactive.

Another strategy for calming glandular energy is to feel the containment provided by the muscles and bones. BMC connects specific joints to glands and uses pressure through them to feel more grounded.

Activity: The Droplet Experience

A glandular meditation that reviews the location and energetic impact of each gland.

Goal of experience: Tuning in to each of the glands and where the energy resonates.

History: This "droplet experience" is adapted from guided somatizations led by Bonnie Bainbridge Cohen, first experienced by Martha Eddy in the 1980s.

Activity: Locate yourself in a comfortable space, ideally lying on your back so that the image of a feather dropping into a pool of water can be supported by your own image of gravity moving through your body from front to back.

 Begin with the descent of a feather in the lowest part of your torso just in front of the coccyx. Allow this feather, this droplet, to produce concentric circles as if touching water. Notice where the energy ripples from your coccygeal bodies.

 Moving up just a couple inches along the midline of your body, imagine a droplet that is the weight of a feather falling about 2 inches below the navel. This is a reflex point for the gonads, at the level of the ovaries or vas deferens as an anchor point. Once again notice any ripples of concentric circles as if this droplet has ever so lightly contacted water and its waves travel outward, in this case through your body. You can imagine allowing that energy to move out, down towards the ankles.

 Coming up higher to the navel, once again imagine a droplet creating concentric circles radiating out and notice the energy moving around the region of the lumbar spine, through the sacroiliac joints, and even down into the knees via the thigh bones.

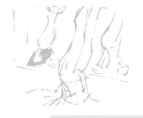
Moving up a little higher to the solar plexus, the soft tissue between the ribs, knowing that the pancreas is nestled in there, allow a droplet to disperse until that spot ripples outward. This time feel the ripples through the entire rib cage, then down through the abdomen such that you feel equal energy all the way to the toes and up through outstretched arms. In other words, the solar plexus radiates circles of wave-like action through the whole body, alive in the distal parts of the periphery of the body.

 Please go just above this area where the last little bone of the breastbone, the xiphoid process of the sternum, hinges like a tail. Just behind the xiphoid process in the soft tissue of the organ cavity, notice a sensation that is similar to that of other bodies of the glandular system. Allow the energy to ripple out, allow it to move again through the ribs and really to all apparatus of the breath, the diaphragm, the crura, which are the tendons of the diaphragm, down into the tail region and upward all the way to the head, through the breathing mechanism of the nose, trachea, and bronchi.

Moving up to the center section of the sternum, on either side of the sternum locate two reflex points for the heart bodies. Then come into the center of the sternum where this energy converges from the two different points. Feel the heart bodies concentrated and then, with either a very light pebble or lovely feather, make contact with your imaginary pool at this level of the body. See those concentric circles moving out through the upper body, in particular out to the wrists, embracing everything along the way.

Moving up to the top bone of the sternum, which is called the manubrium, know that just behind it is the thymus, at the midpoint of the manubrium. Invite the droplet,

whether water or feather or something else. Feel the radiation, the positive radiating forces and the circulating through the entire body with a special focus now on the area that radiates out to the edges of the elbows, to the tips, the olecranon processes.

 Moving now into the throat region, here there are three different sets of bodies making up seven different bodies: first the thyroid, an H-shaped gland just behind the Adam's apple. Come into the isthmus of the thyroid gland (the crossbar of the H) and allow that droplet experience to happen here. Feel how it radiates out: where it does so strongly, where perhaps it is a little weaker, and enjoy how it radiates out through the shoulders to the elbows. Feel the breath shift. Notice your voice perhaps jiggle if you need to adjust your posture; notice if your spine is lengthening and your organs are deepening, and their contact with the earth. How do your legs feel? Might you want to jiggle your toes?

Now, to find the parathyroid glands, go to the corners of the H, four different spots where each of the parathyroid glands is nestled. Even though they operate separately, feel the radiation in concentric circles from all four, or you can play with each one separately, feeling the relationship once again to the axial skeleton, knowing that these become the support to each arm and leg when a limb reaches out and expands into space.

Move up to the third area of the throat related to glandular energy. Locate the carotid bodies with no known hormonal function but active in registering carbon dioxide levels. They are under the jaw in the width of the throat, in the crevice where the carotid arteries split/bifurcate. Come now into the midline at the level of the hyoid bone. At the midpoint of the hyoid bone

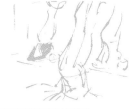

find the droplet and see where it goes, registering any symmetry or asymmetry in the rippling. Notice what wants to happen to bring in more balance – follow the energy flow within your body.

 Moving now up to the head glands, bring your attention to the third eye area between the eyebrows. Imagine a droplet near the pituitary gland, feather-light, radiating out, circling the eyes, feeling the counter pulled to the tail.

 Next, move ever so slightly up to the top of the bridge of the nose between the ears to where the mammillary bodies drop down from the fornix of the limbic system off the hypothalamus; feel the midpoint between the ears in the top area of the nose and find the droplet at the level of the olfactory nerve, really at the level of the temple.

Perhaps this droplet is a little heavier to go deeper into the skull. See, feel, or imagine what is there. How does it radiate out? Does it relate to your nose?

Finally, move to the pineal gland further up this slight diagonal from the third eye, through the mammillary bodies, just another centimeter back with the trajectory up to the crown of the head. It is located closer to the cross-section of the temples. Allow for a droplet into the depth of the skull and just notice if you feel the resonance into the crown of your skull. Then what do you feel? Is anything vibrating? It registers vibration of sound, waves, and particles. How does this resonate down through your entire body?

Notice how your entire body feels now. Move gently and pay attention to any parts of the experience that seemed important.

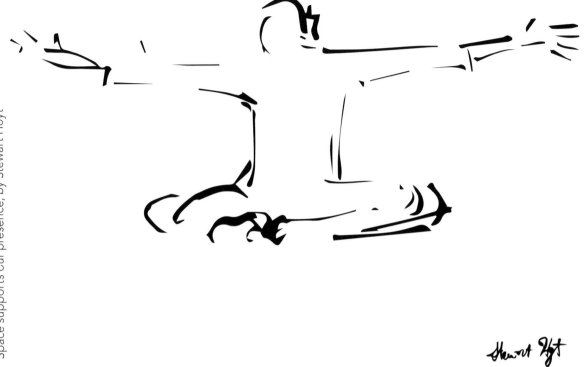

3B Diving Deeper Into Glands

Experiencing Each Gland: Locate/Breathe/Sound/ Energize

By now you have read that Bonnie Bainbridge Cohen (BBC), founder of Body-Mind Center-ing® (BMC®), was interested in organs, glands, chakras, and energy centers, along with more traditional explorations of anatomy and kinesiology. She was motivated to learn as much as possible and was guided by what she learned about organ healing from Yogi Ramaiah, and from her own investigation of the book *Esoteric Healing*, by Alice Bailey. Bailey (1947) describes how energy centers have three main purposes – to vitalize the physical body, to bring about the development of self-consciousness in humans (meaning self-awareness, not overly concerned

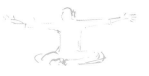
about others' opinions), and to transmit spiritual energy so that every person can become a spiritual being. The role of spirituality and mental as well as physical health is being explored widely in this century. Bainbridge Cohen has been a leader in this process for 60 years.

Before reading more about the history, location (anatomy), and function (physiology) of each gland and body, this is a reminder to invite you to pause and embody along the way. There are various avenues to stimulate, awaken, and balance a specific gland: by locating it, by breathing into the region, by making sound that vibrates the area, and by using touch, movement, or visualization to energize it. In summary, an easy and powerful way to connect with and stimulate the glands is to remember: "Locate/Breathe/Sound/Energize"

- **Locate it:** learn the anatomical placement

- **Breathe:** breathe into the area and feel it expand (Dynamic Embodiment^SM, DE^SM, calls this "volumizing")

- **Sound:** vibrate it with your vocalizations

- **Energize:** direct the tip of your finger to the location or a combined location of paired glands, or somatize by imagining the gland in order to then feel its energy.

Deepening into Locate, Breathe, Sound, Energize

- **Locate:** locate the gland anatomically, then picture and feel (somatize) the description of the bodily structure (the gland or body)

- **Breathe:** breathe into the location and don't let it deflate during the exhalation

– you can do this by hissing through your teeth to create internal pressure. BMC does this with organs and it is quite palpable since they are much bigger three-dimensional structures inside our bodies. As you exhale, feel the area keep its tensegrity

- **Sound:** vibrate the area with your sound or the sound of others. Allow it to penetrate it. Play with pitch – lower sounds for lower body glands and higher sounds (within one's range) for glands in the chest, neck, or head

- **Energize:** access to the energy of a gland is through vibration activating the area. Methods include touching the area with your fingertip, using sound, or imagining or engaging in gentle movement. Use a light touch with the tip of your finger on the energy point related to a gland. Spend time in stillness further cultivating this energy, expanding it by feeling it.

Enjoy trying out some of these embodiment cues while reading the next section.

The Glands, Chakras, and Body-Mind Centering®/ Dynamic Embodiment^SM Connections

The following section is a guide that shares information about 13 glandular structures commonly explored in BMC/DE. It includes the related chakra, and whatever is known so far about its physical shape, location, hormone, function, BMC mind-state and/or DE quality, anatomical history, and BMC somatic history of each. The detailed information is meant to guide you in your cognitive understanding and your physical embodiment using the "Locate, Breathe, Sound, and/or Energize" approach.

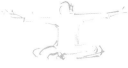

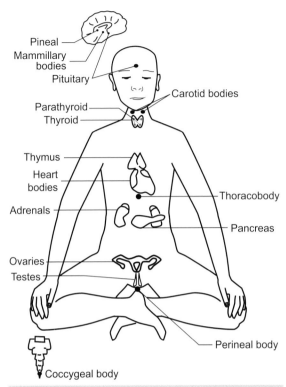

Figure 3B.1
The endocrine system as taught in Body-Mind Centering® and Dynamic Embodiment℠. Based on original drawing by Amanda Latchmore.

Coccygeal Body or Bodies Supported by the Perineal Body (Chakra 1)

Physical Description

The coccygeal body (CB), also known as Luschka's body or the coccygeal glomus, is not a familiar structure to scientists or lay people. The "coccygeal body" is rarely depicted in anatomical drawings. However, cadaver research has shown that humans have one to nine small pea-sized bodies. Generally, there is one large glomus surrounded by other smaller nodules that are irregularly oval in shape. They can be several millimeters in diameter, composed of epithelioid and smooth muscle cells and heavily infused with nerve innervation. Each glomus is serving to shunt blood from an artery to a vein avoiding capillaries, and is also referred to as an arteriovenous anastomosis. In this manuscript, our focus is on the root chakra which also includes the perineal body (PB), a more familiar anatomical structure, which in this book is a keystone to the glandular activity in the region. It is the central fibrous skeleton of the perineum (which has a pyramid shape in men and is wedge-shaped in women) and is the place where the connective tissues of muscles and septa join. The PB, also called the central tendon of the perineum, is located where the anal region and the urogenital triangle meet.

Location

The CB is generally thought to be a glomus at the base of the spine, anterior to the tip of the tailbone (the coccyx) in the back diamond of the pelvic floor, which is created by the muscles between the coccyx, pubis, and sit bones. The CB can be referred to as the intra-coccygeal body, as it can be located inside the coccyx bones themselves, within the fatty tissue around the bone, and/or in the surrounding ligaments – specifically the superficial and deep ano-coccygeal ligaments.

Hormone

There is no known hormone, sparking speculation about glandular function (Conti et al 2000).

Function

The coccygeal is usually called a body, not a gland, as it is not known to secrete a hormone.

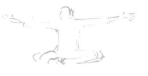
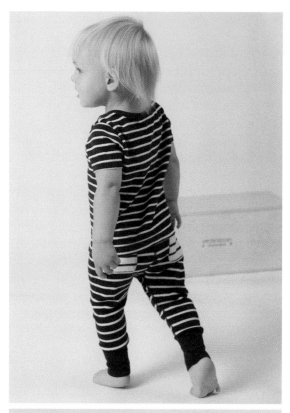

Figure 3B.2
Coccygeal thrust from tail to head. Photo by
Serge Cashman.

However, a research study (Conti et al) in 2000, referring to the "coccygeal gland," found that it may create blood cells (hematopoietic function) and might have a modulatory effect on the immune system, given the sympathetic nerve innervation. The blood flow may be critical to carrying hormones or neurotransmitters. It has been postulated that if the bodies do have an endocrine function, they use what are referred to as "nor-androgenic hormones" that regulate the sympathetic nervous system (relating to fight/flight). This relationship could in turn support immune system functioning (Davison & Michalak 2017). Hence

this possible function might also be a reason for searching for neuroendocrine cells at this base, which is so full of both the sympathetic and parasympathetic innervation. The PB supports the integrity of the diaphragms of the body and most importantly is the beginning point of development for the entire middle body (the muscles and bone and more). It spawns not only the mesoderm but also the containers for our periphery: for instance, the extra-embryonic container.

Body-Mind Centering® Mind-State/ Dynamic Embodiment℠ Quality

It has been hypothesized since the 1960s that there is a glandular-like energetic quality in this region and that it relates to survival of the self and the species through the capacity for self-love and the love instinct. When lacking, it could lead to being deeply self-critical (Bainbridge Cohen & Mills 1980, Bainbridge Cohen 2020, Hartley 1995). When embodying the CB, one notes that one quality is of deep stillness and rootedness. The CB, together with the PB, creates grounded strength. The PB provides a deep support for all parts of the body from the development of the middle body and its impact through the central axis of the body (gut, nervous system, and more). The PB resonates outward to the periphery, the body boundary of our personal kinesphere, and even extends off the body. Hence the connected CB/PB center is a cycle from root to cosmos and back again.

Anatomical History

The adult CB was first described by the anatomist Luschka circa 1860. In 1942 Hollingshead identified it as "glomus cells" – large round cells with a large nucleus in the center. Studies from 2002 and 2005 indicate that a larger structure is

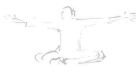

surrounded by smaller ones. A 2017 study confirmed the existence, number, and location of up to nine CBs. The PB may have held a stronger endocrine function earlier in our human history (Davison & Michalak 2017).

Bonnie Bainbridge Cohen (BBC) History

The interpretation of the CB as a gland in the BMC community is derived from somatic exploration guided by two facts: knowing the power of the root chakra from Bainbridge Cohen's reading of the author Alice Bailey, and physically feeling the "consciousness of glands" stirring in the rear pelvic floor area. As the School for Body-Mind Centering curriculum has expanded to include embryology, the PB has been included in an understanding of the root chakra. According to Bainbridge Cohen (2021), in comparison with the CBs, the PB is "different in consciousness as a ground for holding." If working together, the two sets of bodies "help to ground the Kundalini energy."

Reproductive Glands – Gonads – Ovaries and Testes (Chakra 2)

Physical Description

These are a pair of hormone-releasing glands, which are critical to reproduction as well as related to sexual desire and vitality of the reproductive organs. The location and functions vary for biological men and biological women.

Location

In a cisgender (gender matches biology determined at birth) female the ovaries are about 2 inches below the navel, and slightly to the left and right of midline, surrounding the uterus and connected to the uterus by the fallopian tubes. In a cisgender male the testes are the glands; they are inside the scrotum that hangs down from the pubic region behind the penis.

Functions

In cisgender females they stimulate the release of the egg as part of the fertility and menstrual cycles and guide menopause as well as the development of secondary sexual characteristics – development of breasts and pubic hair. In cisgender males they impact sperm development and movement, as well as sexual desire and the development of secondary sexual characteristics – beard, chest hair, drop in voice, and pubic hair.

Hormones

Estrogen, progesterone, testosterone, and androstenedione are produced in different levels in males and females. Estrogen and progesterone are produced in larger amounts in cisgender females, and testosterone and androstenedione are more dominant in cisgender males. However, there are great variations in levels of production of these hormones across the continuum of gender.

Body-Mind Centering® Mind-State/ Dynamic Embodiment℠ Quality

The focus is on preservation of family; the movement quality is a binary of left and right sides, of strength and downward pulse into the earth. It is epitomized by the chanting within many Native American dances.

Anatomical History

There have long been empirical observations of cyclical behavioral changes that seemed

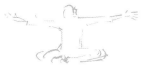
biological. It was not until the mid-1850s, though, that the scientist Claude Bernard discovered that glands secreted substances that influenced other organs. In 1906, secretions, called estruc, from the ovaries were shown to produce cyclic sexual activity in non-human females. The term "estrogen" was formed by adding "gen" from the word "*Gennan,*" which means to produce. Estrogen was isolated as a hormone in 1929.

BBC History

Given that traditional anatomy and science, as well as chakral references, pre-date the development of BMC, these glands have no separate BMC history. However, within the BMC community at least three practitioners teach about the embryonic development of the genitalia and related glands and/or clitoral parallel of the penis in terms of erectile function (Bindler, Eddy, Lyons) and related mind-states. These serve to break up a binary definition of gender. From a DE perspective, the influential work of Judith Kestenberg identifies movement qualities of both an inner (more vaginal) and an outer (more penile) genital rhythm as central to human physical and psychological development (Kestenberg Amighi et al 1999, Eddy 1993). The inner genital movement involves swaying, while the outer genital rhythm can be seen in projectile-like movement – jumping, spraying. According to the Kestenberg Movement Profile these two rhythms are integrated in all adults, of whatever gender, into a combined "U curve" rhythm.

Adrenal Glands (Chakra 3)

Physical Description

The adrenal glands are a pair of right and left walnut-sized glands. There are two parts in each gland – the lower part (the medulla) and the upper area (the cortex). The medulla has three sections or zones – zona fasciculata, zona glomerulosa, and zona reticularis.

Location

Each gland sits over the top of one kidney. Adrenal describes proximity to the kidney, *ad* for toward, and *renal* for kidney.

Function

The adrenal glands serve to provide a strong surge of energy when the body is under stress. Hence, they are considered a key to personal and familial survival. Self-preservation is evident in the fight, flight, or freeze response. Familial preservation is evidenced in the classic example of a mother lifting a car to save her child. Personal survival also requires a strong immunology. The adrenals also secrete glucocorticoids and catecholamines that regulate immune cell activity, cytokines, and the proliferation of bacteria. The implication here is that the health of the adrenals also impacts one's immune response.

Hormones

Epinephrine (same as adrenaline), norepinephrine, cortisol, aldosterone, and androgenic steroids are secreted. Epinephrine is the hormone that became the medication Adrenaline and is therefore popularly referred to as such. It is quite similar to norepinephrine. Cortisol is a glucocorticoid hormone produced by the zona fasciculata that plays several important roles in the body. It helps control the body's use of fats, proteins, and carbohydrates; suppresses inflammation; regulates blood pressure; increases blood sugar; and can also decrease bone formation (Deak 2008). Aldosterone is a mineral-based corticoid hormone that is created in the outermost layer by the zona glomerulosa. It helps in the regulation of blood pressure and the balance of sodium and potassium by sending signals to the kidneys. Sodium gets absorbed into the bloodstream and potassium is released to the urine. DHEA and androgenic steroids are the substrate for what will become estrogen and androgens in the gonads. They are created in the zona reticularis.

Body-Mind Centering® Mind-State/Dynamic Embodiment℠ Quality

Mind-state involves huge surges of power for self-protection and survival; the movement quality is that of strong and sudden impulses. The sympathetic state induced also allows for a calm, strong state of clarity if well regulated.

History

Chemists Jōkichi Takamine and Keizo Uenaka discovered adrenaline in 1900. Takamine also was able to isolate the pure hormone from the adrenal glands of animals. *Epi* and *nephros* are similar root words to *ad* and *renal* – also meaning "above kidney." While these hormones have been identified for over a century, cortisol and androgenic steroids are relatively new to the scene. The fight/flight response was named in the 1920s and the freeze response was named in 1977. It is interesting to note that Adrenaline is the brand name of a pharmaceutical that was created to replicate epinephrine.

BBC History

BMC's glandular embodiment began in the 1970s. Its approach predates many theories of trauma recovery. One focus is how to relieve

and support the impact of the adrenals from repeated fight, flight, and freeze responses. Embodiment and movement practices of BMC have influenced somatic psychology as well as other somatic movement approaches to trauma recovery, such as Dynamic Embodiment.

The Pancreas (Chakra 3)

Physical Description

The pancreas is a digestive organ and also a gland because it secretes a hormone. Within the digestive organ there are little bodies called the islets of Langerhans that secrete insulin. These pancreatic islets constitute 1–2 percent of the pancreas volume and receive 10–15 percent of its blood flow. The pancreas is a bit fish-shaped – with a big head and a body that ends in a slender tail.

Location

The head of the pancreas sits in the solar plexus region at the apex of the abdomen – where ribs

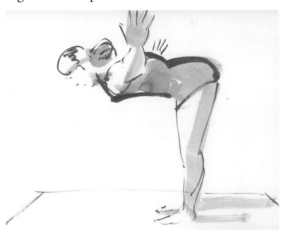

Figure 3B.3
Radiating out from the pancreas/solar plexus, by Stewart Hoyt.

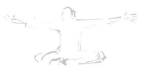

6–10 converge in an upside-down V shape at the front of the chest. The rest of the pancreas extends back and slightly up into the left back area of the ribcage.

Function

The hormonal component of the pancreas regulates blood sugar levels and energy production in the body. Endocrine cells of the pancreas are comprised primarily of two types – α and β cells. Diabetes is a metabolic disorder characterized by hyperglycemia (high sugar levels) and has recently been found to be impacted by eating habits and the level of incretin, a hormone released from the gut.

Hormones

Insulin is the most well-known hormone of the pancreas. It helps glucose, the most basic bodily fuel, find its way into the body's cells. Somatostatin is another hormone produced by the delta cells of the islets of Langerhans within the pancreas. This hormone serves to block the secretion of both insulin and glucagon from adjacent cells. Insulin, glucagon, and somatostatin work together to control the nutrient levels going in and out of the bloodstream. Amylin is also important in helping insulin function and controlling appetite.

Body-Mind Centering® Mind-State/ Dynamic Embodiment℠ Quality

Relationship is a key theme since the pancreas sits at the base of the diaphragm and therefore at the bottom of the ribcage – the container for the lungs and heart. It is perceived as a transitional gland moving from survival of the species to relationships with other people. The movement quality is one of spaciousness and integration – it expresses bodily force or exuberance when it is most extended, reaching out far into space.

History

Much has been learned about the pancreas because of diabetes. When pancreatic hormone levels are severely out of balance diabetes mellitus occurs. Type 1 diabetes (T1DM) is a serious disease during which the pancreas stops producing insulin; it affects many children and adolescents. People with type 2 diabetes (T2DM) have poor responses to insulin, which can progress to not making enough insulin. Amylin was discovered in 1987.

Body-Mind Centering®/Dynamic Embodiment℠ History

The pancreas has been known as a gland, so it was explored amongst all the other glands to find its contribution to human consciousness. DE, combining both BMC and Graf-Burnham Body Systems, explores the sweetness of life as well as overall digestive health such as the regulation of eating, calling on feeling full. This relates to the DE principle of "being as big as you are" (including in the stomach). Hence it has been used in helping with managing bulimia and other eating imbalances.

Thoracobody (Chakra 4)

Physical Description

This body is unknown to science and is included in this lexicon due to a felt sense that these bodies are vital to breathing and the diaphragm, as well as the endocrine system.

Location

The thoracobody is hypothesized to sit just behind the xiphoid process, the lowest bone of the sternum. This is a juncture which creates

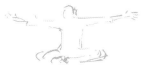

the shape of a triangle at the apex of the solar plexus, where the ribs attach to the sternum (also known as the breastbone). The xiphoid process articulates with the body of the sternum, moving, like the tailbone/coccyx, forward and backward in small movements.

Function

As the xiphoid process moves forward and backward that leverage helps move the sternum and ribcage. The body may give support to this action and breath, especially as it moves in a counter-pull from the xiphoid process, creating spaciousness (Bainbridge Cohen & Mills 1980).

Hormones

None is known; there is a possible relationship to carbon dioxide.

Body-Mind Centering® Mind-State/ Dynamic Embodiment℠ Quality

The thoracobody aligns the entire endocrine system by being the heart of breathing and being, emptiness and fullness, openness, and defenselessness. The movement quality in BMC and DE experience involves the movement of the xiphoid process toward and away from the thoracobody impacting movement or lack of movement in the diaphragm (Bainbridge Cohen 2020). While the movement of the xiphoid process acts as a skeletal pump for the ribs, allowing the thoracobody to move away from the xiphoid bone, the diaphragm expands, helping to create the vacuum for the filling of the lungs. During exhalation, the xiphoid and thoracobody move back together as the diaphragm domes upward. On the other hand, if the xiphoid bone and thoracobody constantly move in the same direction,

as if a single unit, this can inhibit the action of the diaphragm in either direction. Explore ungluing this togetherness. Having additional energetic support for this critical life function has a great logic to it. The thoracobody sits nestled in the solar plexus region, which is often referred to as a nexus of powerful energy, supports breath, and radiates up and down to help orchestrate the entire endocrine system. If you discover other sensations and meanings, please share your experience with the authors!

Anatomical History

Searches for a body or a glomus in the thoracic region resulted in no "normal" findings. Only one study revealed that six cases worldwide exist of benign glomus tumors of the mediastinum. These tumors are more often found in fingers and other limbs (Kanakis et al 2015).

BBC History

Bonnie Bainbridge Cohen had a "problem," and she always perceives a problem as a difficulty to learn from. This challenge involved her 10th rib being separated from the cartilage. One of her students, who was also a massage therapist, would work with her regularly. During a massage, she felt a glandular awareness in the nearby area of the lower sternum. She discovered a small depression in the thoraco area and spent time bringing consciousness to it by asking questions of her own somatic experience such as, "What is the type of consciousness here?" Later she saw a drawing that correlated with her experience – it was a drawing of the solar plexus with a triangle on the upper apex and she correlated this with what she felt, locating what she named the "thoracobody" there (Bainbridge Cohen 2020). Perhaps a hormone will be discovered in the future. It may

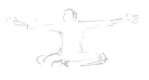

be linked to Bainbridge Cohen's awareness of the pervasiveness of carbon dioxide in every cell, the neuroendocrine functioning being in every cell, and the role of the thoracobody with external and internal respiration.

Heart Bodies/Heart Glands (Chakra 4)

Physical Description

Postulated to exist in and around the heart are what are called the heart bodies (BMC), also referred to as the heart gland and/or the aortic bodies.

Location

They are found on either side of the sternum at the level of the 4th rib, and in the heart (aortic arch and atrioventricular node). The phenotype has a predominance of endocrine cells.

Function

There are two types of bodies with physiological functions to be considered when working with the heart. The aortic bodies are chemoreceptors with a connection to the vagus nerve. The aortic bodies are similar to the carotid body, as they work to monitor changes in oxygen and carbon dioxide levels (PaO_2, $PaCO_2$, and pH in the arterial blood). The heart gland is a name sometimes given to tissue in each section of the heart muscle that releases hormones. The hormones released from the atrial region (ANP, BNP, and CNP – see below) assist in the functioning of the circulatory system with a direct impact on blood pressure.

Hormones

Atrial natriuretic peptide (ANP) is also referred to as atrial natriuretic factor (ANF). It is a strong natriuretic and vasorelaxant hormone released from the atrial region of the heart, as well as at other sites, including the brain (Goetze et al 2020). Natriuresis is the excretion of sodium by the kidneys; therefore a natriuretic peptide is a peptide that induces natriuresis. There are three natriuretic peptides: ANP, BNP and CNP. BNP is brain natriuretic peptide, and CNP is C-type natriuretic peptide. The release of these peptides by the heart is stimulated by atrioventricular and neurohumoral action, which can occur in response to increased pressure in the area, or other factors affiliated with heart failure. The main physiological actions of natriuretic peptides is to reduce arterial pressure by decreasing blood volume and systemic vascular resistance – reducing the stress on the heart. These heart glands help keep the heart pressure normalized, establishing just enough volume – "being as big are you are in the heart."

The aortic bodies, as chemoreceptors, give feedback about oxygen and carbon dioxide's partial pressure as well as pH, as established by the carbon levels. An additional set of bodies includes the para-aortic bodies, which create catecholamines, specifically chromaffins, which monitor blood acidity but also respond directly to stress through regulating the breath.

Body-Mind Centering® Mind-State/Dynamic Embodiment℠ Quality

The mind-state is the expression of love, group consciousness, and sympathy. The DE movement qualities include widening from the heart out to the sides of the body and also feeling the depth of the heart out through the fingertips and eyes. The DE perspective is that the heart glands help keep the heart pressure normalized, establishing enough, but not too much,

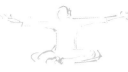

volume to allow the heart to "be as big as it is designed to be" – supporting big-heartedness.

History

Investigations looking for natriuretic properties of a polypeptide carried out between 1971 and 1983 located the first hormonal response in the heart area with a substance called ANF, now known as ANP. Another polypeptide isolated from the brain in 1988, BNP, was subsequently shown to be a second hormone produced by heart atria in different mammals. The third, CNP, also is mostly in the brain but produced in the heart, and its function is unknown.

BBC/Dynamic Embodiment[SM] History

The term "heart bodies" was not known in science until 1986; however, in BMC Bonnie Bainbridge Cohen explored the heart region, guided by the writing of Alice Bailey, and discovered a sensation of bodies with a glandular quality as early as 1977. This continues to be explored with strong embryological investigation that relates to subtle concepts like discerning the central as well as right and left energy points from the felt experience of the specific anatomical structures. DE distinguishes between the atrial hormonal function of working with volume, and the aortic bodies' chromaffin neuroendocrine function of monitoring the blood's level of acidity, checking for respiratory acidosis as measurable with $PaCO_2$ evaluation (35–45 mmHG).

Thymus Gland (Chakra 4)

Physical Description

The thymus gland has two separate lobes connected by a central medulla and a peripheral cortex, made of lymphocytes and reticular cells. The reticular cells form a mesh that is filled with lymphocytes.

Location

The thymus lies behind the highest bone in the sternum – the manubrium.

Function

The thymus provides a dual function – along with its glandular function, it is also central to the lymphatic part of the immunological system. The thymus works with the spleen, adenoids, and tonsils. The thymus is a receptor for puberty growth hormone or human growth hormone but not its producer. Originally only known for adolescent growth spurts, the thymus gland is now known to be critical in the immune system and the development of T-cells stimulated by diverse hormones.

Hormones

Thymopoietin, thymulin, and thymosin are produced by the thymus. Thymopoietin and thymulin assist in the differentiation of different types of T-cells. Thymosin interacts with the immune response (heightening the ability to fight off viruses) and stimulates pituitary hormones such as growth hormone. The pituitary hormones are thought to reside in the cytoplasm of the thymus epithelial cell. The thymus gland's epithelial cells also are believed to have receptors through which other hormones can regulate its function. The thymus gland may also make small amounts of some hormones that are mostly produced in other areas of the body, such as melatonin and insulin.

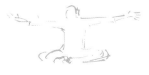

Body-Mind Centering® Mind-State/Dynamic Embodiment℠ Quality

The thymus relates to courage based in love, self-protection, self-defense, letting go before climax, and activating for health and energy. DE relates it to both a light and a strong presence of self. It is interesting to note that cold water stimulates the immune response. Much can be learned from Japanese culture – Misogi rituals, martial arts, and Kiai all help develop immunological strength.

History

Thymosin, identified in the early 1970s in response to the AIDS epidemic, is now known as an important hormone of the thymus, in that it stimulates the production of disease-fighting T-cells by developing its progenitor cells to T-cells. As written in 1979, "The question is no longer to decide whether thymic hormones exist, but rather to elucidate their biological significance and potential clinical applications" (Bach 1979, p. 277). One main action is the cleansing away of debris from fighting infection.

BBC History

During the early BMC years the thymus was considered by medical science to atrophy after age 12, when it reaches its largest size for most people. However, the BMC community experienced the thymus to be active throughout life. One BMC practitioner repeatedly found larger-sized tissue in her cadaver research. Further experience centered on how the gland was largest in body proportion at age two, and largest in size for adolescents, but more importantly on how it continued to be significant in adulthood.

Thyroid Gland (Chakra 5)

Physical Description

The thyroid is an H-shaped gland with each lobe approximately 4 to 6 cm in length and 1.3 to 1.8 cm in thickness. The isthmus (horizontal bridge) measures less than 4 to 5 mm.

Location

It is located behind the "Adam's apple," the laryngeal prominence of the thyroid cartilage, close to the vocal chamber (the larynx).

Function

This gland is central to the body's rhythm because of its impact on metabolic rate, also

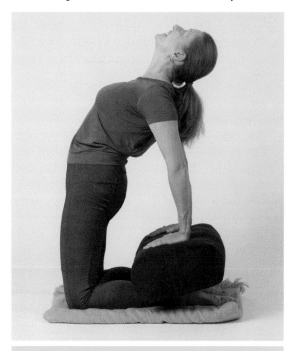

Figure 3B.4
Suspensional support of thymus and thyroid in camel. Photo by Serge Cashman.

known as the basal metabolic rate. This rate impacts heart and breath rate and body temperature. It sets a rhythm for how fast the different glands and even organs function.

Hormones

The thyroid makes two main hormones – triiodothyronine (T3) and thyroxine (T4). Adequate amounts of iodine (a chemical element that is an essential part of the diet) are needed for the thyroid to create these hormones. Another hormone produced in parafollicular cells or C-cells of the thyroid gland is called calcitonin, which serves to reduce calcium and phosphorus levels in the blood, impacting bone health. It works together with the parathyroid hormone. Calcitonin reduces calcium levels by the short-term inhibition of the osteoclasts (cells responsible for breaking down bone) and by decreasing the resorption of calcium in the kidneys. The secretion of calcitonin is also inhibited by somatostatin, released by the pancreas or by the C-cells in the thyroid gland.

Body-Mind Centering® Mind-State/ Dynamic Embodiment℠ Quality

The thyroid is the keystone of the endocrine system. It is linked with experiences of creative expression, artistry, conviction, and self-sensitivity. It supports the transition of relating to that which is upon the earth to relating to that which is of the heavens, the beginning of self-consciousness. Experiences can lead to atheism or, if overly strong and of the earth, the person can become like a crusading evangelist. The movement quality of a balanced thyroid is one of freedom – moving with diverse movement qualities, singing every range, and sounding like different animals, freely.

Anatomical History

The scientists who first published on the thyroid include Leonardo da Vinci (drawings), Andrea Vesalius (anatomical drawing and function), and Thomas Wharton (who named the gland).

BBC History

The thyroid was explored by Bonnie Bainbridge Cohen from 1973 to 1976 because it was known to be a gland and taught in 1977. Somatic explorations during this time revealed the thyroid's role in moving from group consciousness to personal expression.

Parathyroid Glands (Chakra 5)

Physical Description

These are small, round glands.

Location

They are located behind the distal corner of the H shape of the thyroid gland in the throat.

Function

The parathyroids monitor levels of calcium in the blood. They serve in calcium balancing and therefore in setting the rhythm of muscular contractions, including muscle cramps.

Hormone

The parathyroid glands produce parathyroid hormone (PTH), sometimes referred to as parathormone or parathyrin, which releases calcium into the bloodstream via actions in the bone, the kidneys, and the intestines, usually when the calcium levels are considered too

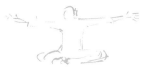

low. PTH raises the blood calcium level by breaking down the bone (where most of the body's calcium is stored) and causing calcium release; increasing absorption of calcium from food into the intestine, especially through its effects on vitamin D metabolism; and increasing the kidney's ability to hold on to calcium that would otherwise be lost in the urine.

Body-Mind Centering® Mind-State/ Dynamic Embodiment℠ Quality

The parathyroids relate to empathy and gentleness – softening the adrenals – expecting others to perceive you as you perceive yourself; they can also be used in manipulation. DE quality – as taught at the School for BMC, the activation of the parathyroid with a clear laryngeal sound can bring in a type of poised bow and arrow tautness and clarity – direct, light, and bound, with readiness for action.

History

The parathyroids have been known to exist since they were discovered in the neck of a rhinoceros in 1852 by Richard Owen. He encountered one and described it as "a small compact yellow glandular body attached to the thyroid at the point where the veins emerged." Starting in the 1920s they were found in humans and then by the 1960s their functions were more understood: specifically, in 1963, by a scientist named Virchow. The first complete description came from Dr Sandstroem of Sweden in 1980 when he identified two parathyroid bodies in his extensive autopsy work.

BBC History

The consciousness of the parathyroids was explored by Bonnie Bainbridge Cohen in

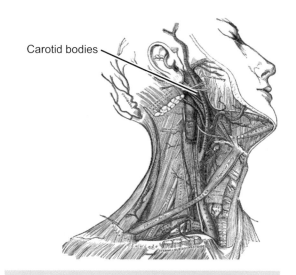

Figure 3B.5
Find the carotid bodies in the "neighborhood" of the carotid arteries, drawing from the book *Gray's Anatomy*, first published in 1858.

1973–1976 because they were known to be a gland. This material began to be taught as part of the BMC curriculum in 1977. The experience of whether the upper or lower or right or left parathyroid correlated with the actions of the right or left leg took time to refine.

Carotid Bodies (Chakra 5)

Physical Description

One carotid body sits nestled at the base of the sino-carotid nerve, within the bifurcation of each of the right and left carotid arteries. They are not typically referred to as endocrine glands. They are known to serve in reading the level of carbon dioxide in the bloodstream. The carotid bodies are not to be confused with the coccygeal body, which is also known as a glomus. The carotid is referred to as the glomus caroticum.

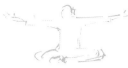

Location

They lie under the jaw, close to either side of the hyoid bone; the carotid pulse can easily be found there.

Function

The carotid body is a chemoreceptor, which registers the amount of oxygen (and thereby carbon dioxide) in the blood (internal oximeter).

Hormone

No known hormone is associated. Bainbridge Cohen (2020) discusses her experience that carbon dioxide itself, the one compound that every cell makes, feels neuroendocrine.

Body-Mind Centering® Mind-State/ Dynamic Embodiment℠ Quality

The carotid bodies are a base for the head glands which relate to perception and spiritual realization, and provide a counter-support to the pelvic glands. Carotid embodiment supports courage, honor, effortless expression of life force, and mastery. The carotid energy is expressed through silence, the pauses between words. In DE explorations, stillness and slow, earthy, methodical movement can also be supported by the carotid energy, as well as monotone phrasing or timelessness. DE investigates the relation of blood and breathing through the balance of the coccygeal, thoracobody, heart bodies, and the carotid.

BBC History

Bonnie Bainbridge Cohen explored the carotid region because of Alice Bailey's reference to a carotid gland. As with the thoracobody region, she felt there was a glandular consciousness there (Bainbridge Cohen 2020). Bailey's book (1947) included statements depicting the carotid gland as the mechanism through which what she called the Spiritual Triad, together with the soul and the personality, works. At present, the School for BMC is exploring the role of carbon dioxide in the neuroendocrine system. Based on BMC, DE is exploring the inter-relationship between the carotid and coccygeal bodies, together with the thoracobody, all in conjunction with the biochemistry of breath and its impact on the two branches of the autonomic nervous system.

Pituitary Gland (Chakra 6)

Physical Description

Also known as the anterior hypophysis and/ or "the Master Gland," the pituitary serves to regulate all other glands. In particular, it signals the thyroid to speed up or slow down and wake

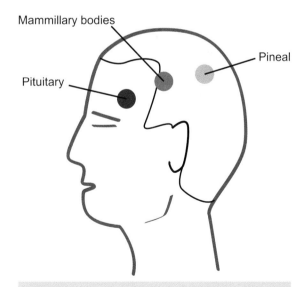

Mammillary bodies

Pineal

Pituitary

Figure 3B.6
Locate the pituitary, mammillary, and pineal.

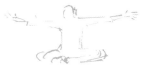
up the other glands. The pituitary–thyroid–adrenal complex is one such glandular relationship triggered by the pituitary.

Location

The pituitary is located in the center of the brain/skull – between the eyebrows and above the cavity of the nose (nasal cavity).

Function

As the master gland, the pituitary helps guide the release of hormones from other glands – most notably from the gonads, adrenals, and thyroid gland.

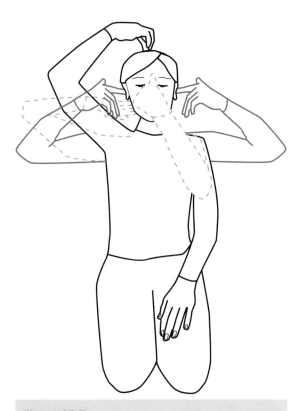

Figure 3B.7
Pituitary map. For description, refer to page 92.

Hormones

- Thyroid-stimulating hormone (TSH)

- Follicle-stimulating hormone (FSH)

- Luteinizing hormone (LH)

- Prolactin (PRL)

- Growth hormone (GH)

- Alpha melanocyte-stimulating hormone (α-MSH)

- Vasopressin

- Oxytocin.

All of the hormones of the pituitary are secreted in response to hormonal messages from the hypothalamus of the brain.

Body-Mind Centering® Mind-State/Dynamic Embodiment℠ Quality

The pituitary is linked with compassion, knowledge, integration of one's personality, love of humanity, devotion, seat of intelligence, conceptual memory, and linear thinking. At its extreme, it can be associated with compulsiveness, racism, sexism, and paranoia. DE movement quality is of openness within stillness or movement, lengthening of the tail with a long spine, and related clarity of hip joint action.

History

The pituitary was first found in the 1740s and was believed to be secreting an unknown substance. Harvey Cushing – neurosurgeon at Yale University during the early 1900s – led a shift from the nervous system being the major communicator of parts. His surgical prowess allowed him to find the pituitary – recognizing both lobes and noticing that there were different functions in each. Using early technology of the X-ray he learned that the pituitary had an impact on other areas of the body.

BBC History

Bonnie Bainbridge Cohen explored the pituitary from 1973 to 1976, teaching its embodiment in 1977. The "third eye" was familiar to her. She developed explorations of pituitary pathways that connect to the skin (and its "nectar of well-being"), as well as sequences from the neck glands through the pituitary to the pineal.

Mammillary Bodies (Chakra 7)

Description

These small bodies are nestled in the center depth of the brain (distinct from the mammary glands of the female breast system).

Location

One mammillary body hangs down from the fornix on each side of the limbic system (like small breasts, hence their name) to cranial

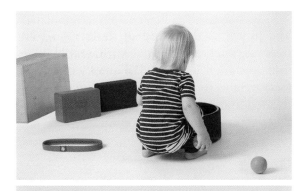

Figure 3B.8
Reach of the head from the mammillary. Photo by Serge Cashman.

nerve zero and to the olfactory nerve (that registers smell) in the posteroinferior area of the hypothalamus.

Function

As nuclei of the hypothalamus, the mammillary bodies function in memory recollection. Memory information originates within the hippocampus. Theta waves are known to activate neurons in the hippocampus which then transmit through the fornix to the mammillary bodies. The medial area may also relate to spatial memory *and in this way to* amnesia, as well as other behavioral themes such as emotion and reward, and goal-directed behaviors.

Hormone

This is not known.

Body-Mind Centering® Mind-State/ Dynamic Embodiment℠ Quality

Keystone of the neuroendocrine system and guardian of the perceptions, the mammillary body underlies insight, suspension between space and time, merged with the past. The movement quality of the mammillary relates to dynamic alignment – feeling suspended by the anti-gravity force on the top center of the skull, allowing uprightness with light yet free-flowing stability. All time, all space. No time, no space.

Anatomical History

There has been an awareness of the mammillary bodies since at least 1881 when BA Gudden published about their role in a German psychiatric journal. However, knowledge of the pathways to and from the mammillary bodies and their function is still advancing. Initially pathways were seen between the hippocampus (and onward to the thalamic nuclei and cingulate cortex) and the related mammillary body on each side. Now the tegmental segments of Gudden are also thought to be involved, broadening our understanding of what structures retain and circulate episodic memory (Vann & Nelson 2015). Given the importance of memory in general, and the role of episodic memory in trauma recovery, this finding is definitely worthy of further investigation.

BBC History

Bonnie Bainbridge Cohen investigated how the mammillaries support consciousness (1973–1977). At the onset she explored the line between the pineal and pituitary and felt "the Guardian of the Perceptions" there, bringing about clarity. After 1977 she saw an article with a photo of the Temple of Luxor superimposed on the mammillaries and recognized this as the location, the seat of this clarity. Years later at Esalen, she was moved by her colleague, world-famous neuro-endocrinologist Candace Pert's, description of how she discovered peptide T through research into the opiate receptors, led by the experience of her patients with AIDS. Bainbridge Cohen (2020) links natural opiates to these bodies, cranial nerve zero, and the pituitary.

Pineal Gland (Chakra 7)

Physical Description

This tiny pea-like structure often has calcifications that help it to appear more distinctively on X-rays.

Location

It is located along body midline, above the midbrain, in the depth of the brain, aligned up and back from the pituitary gland, near the entrance of the canal between the 3rd and 4th ventricles (canal of Sylvius). The pineal area has been called the crown chakra and its energy is felt to project up and back out of the skull at the region of the fornix (soft skull).

Function

It serves as a light receptor, helps to govern the sexual cycle, and is linked to skin pigmentation. The pineal glands have impact on immune modulation, restraining tumor growth and interaction with oxygen free radicals, and on calcium dependent metabolic processes (Chronobiology.com nd).

Hormone

Melatonin, formulated from tryptophan, is released to help regulate the sleep cycle. It is designed to perceive night and day to help in maintaining the circadian rhythm. Another function of melatonin is that it also regulates the absorption of melanin, which is related to skin pigment.

Body-Mind Centering® Mind-State/ Dynamic Embodiment℠ Quality

The pineal is the gland of darkness, all-in-oneness, integration of the spirit, seat of intuition, and high will. The DE quality of intense focus relates to remote state – space and flow. Related movement can often be directional and deeply responsive to sound.

History

The epiphysis (pineal) was not known to be a gland until melatonin was identified in 1958 (Wurtman 1985). In 1981 the release of melatonin was discovered by Alfred Lewy (2003)

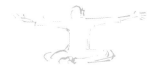

and found to be related to light (Chronobiology nd). The Society of Endocrinology reports of melatonin that, "although it appears not to be essential for human physiology, it is known to have a range of different effects when taken as a medication" (Society for Endocrinology nd). There are many social implications of the glandular action of the pineal in relationship to melanin–pigment tone that can be investigated (Azikiwe 2017).

BBC History

At the School for BMC in the 1970s the pineal was referred to as a body within the endocrine system, since it was experienced as having glandular consciousness. Since the body was known in anatomy books, Bonnie Bainbridge Cohen chose to investigate how it supports our consciousness circa 1973–1977. She knew from spiritual studies that the pineal area has been called the crown chakra and its energy is felt to project up and back out of the skull at the region of the fornix (soft skull). She personally called it the gland of darkness, relating it to the birthing crown and feeling that it could be that humans exit through this crown as well. When she presented the pineal experience at a think tank at Esalen (organized by Don Hanlon Johnson) there were several physicians and one endocrinologist in attendance, amongst others. Bainbridge Cohen presented her experience of the pineal as a gland and the endocrinologist announced that melatonin had just recently been identified and that it was secreted at night. This was a deep corroboration of lived experience with scientific inquiry.

Working in Threes

When working with the glands, always consider at least three at a time; it is best to not work in isolation. The practice of working with the full complement of the gland in threes can present two choices:

1. pick the glands above and below that are in closest proximity, or

2. pick any two glands in the chakral area above and below your focused gland. This could be the root and crown chakra area glands to help bring in the whole spine. (Learn more about the chakral connection in the next chapter.)

Working with at least three glands at a time ensures balancing of the glands and greater connectivity throughout the body. This is useful for feeling the open channel or flow of energy between the glands, and it may also support experiencing the inter-relationships of the glands to other body areas such as the organs, fascia, or the muscles. The glands are all connected and work together. This process also applies to the chakras.

The tip of the finger action can lead into another hands-on approach to balancing a gland: vibration. When working with vibration it is especially important to remember the Principle of Threes: bring attention to each gland above and below the desired gland. Vibrating can be the most likely way to awaken the gland – you can vibrate with gentle movement or sound.

Examples of glandular threes include:

- Thyroid – with parathyroid "above" and thymus below

- Adrenals – with pancreas above and gonads below

- Heart glands – with thymus above and thoracobody below

- Thymus – with thyroid/parathyroids above and heart glands below.

As described in locate, breathe, sound, and energize, you can open these glandular connections up in various ways: by creating spatial patterns – visualizing lines, pathways, and crystalline forms – or by vibrating them to create spaciousness using sound and/or touch. You can also simply somatize, physically feeling each of the glands, above and below the chosen gland. "Working in threes" is ultimately about balance and holism, counter to our culture's tendency to focus on one thing and sometimes to become so focused that overexertion and burnout occur.

Working in threes can also be protective when working with blocked energy. There is often a primary focus on one gland to open up blocked areas. Since it may involve moving stagnant energy, it is important to open a pathway for that flow to move out of the body. It helps for the circulatory system to be alive, to satisfactorily move the hormonal overflow. Begin by locating glands further up and down the spine from the gland you are focusing on – either a small amount, as in "Working in Threes" described above, or at either end of the whole spine. Use an image of breathing between the selected gland in the direction of the gland or glands below it and above it. You can be quite kinesiological with your breath – understanding the anatomy of the breath from the skull (nose and mouth) through the throat (trachea) into the chest (lungs and pleura) and finally through the diaphragm and its tendons (crura) into the pelvic bowl and pelvic floor. In other words, breathe with attention to the air moving through the nostril or mouth for the head glands, moving through the trachea for the throat glands, sensing air going in and out of the different lobes of the lungs to become more aware of the chest glands, feeling the movement of the diaphragm to stimulate the central torso glands, and finally the resonance of the crura that move into the bowl of the pelvis to feel the lowest glands. Remember to include the movement of the thoracobody to integrate the entire endocrine system.

Why Working in Threes?

To illustrate the power of this work, I'll (Shakti) give an example. When I taught my practicum class at the end of my somatic movement therapy training, Martha arrived partway through class. She arrived when I was guiding the class into the pancreas after working on all of the glands below. She dove right into the work and began to feel dizzy. This reminded her of a story which she shared with the rest of us later. When she was 18, in her first class with Bonnie, she arrived at a workshop after searching all over the building through a warren of rooms. Everyone was working with the pancreas. She joined in. The rest had worked their way up from the coccygeal bodies. She fainted. She was not grounded.

Linda Tumbarello, Body-Mind Centering® practitioner and teacher, and DEP, has had a similar experience, leading me to understand that it is best to have activated adrenal embodiment before pancreas. Then the adrenals can support the pancreas. Pancreas can reach up higher and with less effort with the support of the adrenals.

Ultimately, there are lines of energy for the flow of the endocrine system. By awakening the neighbors – the nearby glands – both the glands and the hormones they secrete can become more balanced. Also, include working forward and back as well as expanding right and left, along with the luxurious opening to a flow up and down.

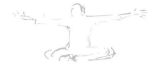

Bonnie Bainbridge Cohen (2020) explains how to ground, in order to counteract the possibility of fainting: start with contacting the coccygeal–perineal bodies for deep rooting. Then go to the gonads, which help take energy down through the ankles towards the feet; finding the adrenals, bring the connection into the knees through the femur, and also expand through navel radiation upward to the head and arms. In this way the adrenals are the first of the lower glands to bring the energy up through the head. The pancreas with its energy out through the tips of everything (feet, hands, head, and tail) completes the cycle. However, if you start at the periphery with just the fingers or toes there is no central axis. This can happen when beginning with the pancreas. Energy needs to go down through the feet first to be grounded. Contact the lower glands to ground.

Having some guideposts of glandular anatomy and physiology is a first step to embodiment. Being aware of how both the glands and the hormone interact impacts consciousness and energy. In order to gain more physical access to increasing or decreasing glandular tone it is helpful to use spatial expansion and vocalization, as well as compression and grounding, respectively.

Specifics about Dynamic Embodiment^SM and the Sun Salutation – Focus on Spatial Tension and Glandular Stimulation/Balancing

Bartenieff's vocal work in the dimensions and planes helps expansion. Integration with the BMC concepts of compression and suspension as well as Laban's Space Harmony allows for more dynamic balancing. The LMA principle that *visible movement expresses to the external world what is experienced inside* forms the basis of an excellent somatic investigation.

The DE approach to the Sun Salutation is meant to be easeful and also seeks to balance the endocrine glands, the hormonal system. It does this through activating breath, increasing embodied knowledge of all layers of anatomy, the use of the voice, and a keen experience of how to organize the body in space (spatial dynamics). "Spatial dynamics" include becoming aware of how each human chooses to move through space and how to use "the support of space." Space has personality, as evidenced in different landscapes, architecture, or crystalline forms. DE teaches how to activate spatial pulls much like what happens in constructing a bridge. By learning about how the body occupies space and practicing activities for doing so more efficiently and fully, movement can "flow" more.

Sourcing the experiential anatomy of BMC together with the concepts of shaping in space, DE explores how attention to the organs and the glands can "volumize" the asanas within the Sun Salutation. Similarly, by combining the importance of "body organization" and "connectedness" from Bartenieff together with Bainbridge Cohen's theories of how the nervous and glandular systems develop in response to infant movements, DE provides pathways for analyzing each transition for somatic movement from one asana to another. These resources provide support for the muscles and bones to feel lighter, freer, and more alive. Finally, by also including the Laban Space Harmony work together with applying a BMC organ principle to the glands, each explorer gains a DE inroad for understanding how the glands and hormones are being activated. This final exploration unleashes hormonal energies that have long been thought to relate to the

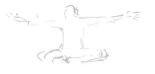

chakras within the framework of crystalline forms, the sacred solids. Early thinkers found that imagining the sacred solids within the body relates strongly to the chakras.

Said another way, when people embody shapes that match with the crystalline form of one of the solids while also focusing on aligning the chakras by feeling neuroendocrine sensations, they generally move with more energy and ease. They may even move into transcendent states.

It is important to recognize that other factors may intensify transcendent states: for instance, tuning into electro-magnetic fields, or taking care to enlist supportive biochemistry through what you eat, drink, or otherwise imbibe.

An example of an additional factor comes from Burnham Body Systems, which has parallels with BMC and is embraced by DE. Eva Graf, a teacher of Dr Linda Burnham, spoke of crystals in the joints of the body. Burnham correlates this statement with the work of Maurice Vogel, who identified that a type of liquid crystal exists as part of our connective tissue, which coats the top and bottom of joints. Dr Burnham (2020) reports that one can recognize the crystalline nature of the "lyotrophic mesophase" that exists in fascia and coalesces at the end of joints. The work of Vogel brings the esoteric aspects of yoga into a perspective that embraces physics as well as anatomy. Since "we are primarily crystalline beings we know that chakral energy precipitates down through all levels of life. This energy has to be stepped down (grounded in the physical body) in order for people to harness it, to use it in the third level of manifestation. It is possible to enter into one's wholeness through this work. I could potentially see anyone through the lens of this wholeness, each person aligned with the greater universe" (Burnham 2020).

If we also consider theories such as the possible existence of the lyotrophic mesophase within fascia at the end of our bones (at the joints), the esoteric aspects of yoga can become grounded in physics as well as anatomy. This book mostly focuses on anatomy, but when dealing with chakras many other levels of experience are awakened. Exploring tetrahedral, octahedral, cubic, icosahedral, and dodecahedral forces in our and around our bodies and activated by our movement can be life-changing.

To bring these ideas all together, DE invites you to explore the activation of glands and related neuroendocrine centers by:

1. feeling the spatial counter-pulls around them, creating tensegrity to stimulate the area

2. fully occupying three-dimensional space (with breath, sound, or visualization)

3. picturing the sacred geometry and related colors within and around the body (or body parts)

4. enhancing musculo-skeletal posture to support spaciousness

5. aligning the chakras and glands for vitality, improving glandular functioning and shifts in consciousness.

Grounding the Glands: Body Connectivity from Bartenieff Fundamentals

Dynamic Embodiment Practitioners (DEPs) use many BMC resources – such as the neuro-developmental patterns described in Chapter 6 and safeguards such as attending to the gland above and below it – to ensure a flow between the glands. DEPs also take time to experience and share how "glandular support" reinvigorates human movement efficiency as explained through Bartenieff Fundamentals. Using the connections to developmental movement coordination and neuromotor practices from BF, the practice of the Sun Salutation has even more resources. One key avenue for experiencing the flow of glandular stimuli and staying grounded is to use the six bodily connections that Irmgard Bartenieff identified as neurologically significant.

The most common Bartenieff body organization connections are: (1) the head–tail; (2 and 3) the scapula–fingertips of each arm; (4 and 5) the sit bone–heel connection on each leg; and (6) the scapula–sacral connection. For instance, by feeling how the sit bones connect to the heels you engage your hamstrings and your balance is more solid. When you then add in the power of the root chakra and the coccygeal body, that grounding intensifies.

The goal is to explore each phase of the Sun Salutation as both a physical (musculoskeletal) and a chakral (neuroendocrine) experience. In DE, you experience the combination of the skeletal support by understanding embodied anatomy and the efficiency of body mechanics. This is then supported by the energetic support of the glands, which often allow the body to feel lighter, more expansive, and if approached carefully at the same time, more grounded. For some, this approach heightens the spiritual nature of the practice.

For grounding, begin with the skeletal system – the weight and clarity of shape of the bones help contain endocrine chaos and can give "spatial intention" to help clarify action in the world. This is about knowing where you want to go or what you want to achieve. Having a clear intention clarifies the action. Your embodiment of the Sun Salutation with awareness of the skeletal alignment, the glandular energies (related to chakras), and neurodevelopmental coordination allows for safe glandular exploration. "The container" of the Sun Salutation ritual and the profoundly "hard-wired" neurodevelopmental movement from childhood become an anchor that works to center and ground. This is especially needed if your glandular experience can tend toward being chaotic. Having the movement ritual of the Sun Salute helps you track your physical and emotional experience. It also helps to move glandular stimulation within a "container." All in all this makes for gentle realignment and balancing.

Accessing Each Gland – A Guided Somatization with Shakti

Now let's take some time to locate each of the glands in your own body and try an initial sensing of their qualities.

Bring yourself to a seated position, cross-legged on the floor. Use a cushion to support your pelvis.

Take three full breaths to center yourself. Now tune in to notice how you are feeling – your heart state, your emotions, your brain, your thinking, and your physical body. This reflects energy level –
being awake/tired, spacey/alert, desirous/listless.

Coccygeal Body

Let's begin at the base of the spine. Start by locating the tip of your spine or coccyx physically. You may want to use your hands to locate it. Begin by touching your sacrum. Reach behind your back. Walk your fingers down the spine of the sacrum until you reach its end, the tailbone. This is your coccyx. Sense into the bone, knowing that on the other side of it is the **Coccygeal Body**. This body, which the Body-Mind Centering®

world experiences as having endocrine function, rests on the anterior side of the coccyx. Use your superpowers, the power of the focus of your own mind, to rest your awareness in this location for a few breaths. Simply be there. you might discern an energy or quality; you might not (yet). This comes with practice. For now, simply enjoy being in the area with your awareness.

Gonads

It's time to move upwards. Climb up the spine with your awareness, coming to your belly. Bring your hands around to rest on your belly, locate your belly button, and move about 2 inches down and 2 inches out. These are the energy points for the **Gonads** (male and female).

If you are biologically female: rest a few fingers here lightly for a few breaths. Notice what you notice. Then to locate your ovaries, move your fingers a little further out and down. This is going to be different for each human. Some women know exactly where their ovaries are. At the monthly cycle, some women can feel which ovary is releasing eggs. Just go to where it "seems right," where your fingers fall. Often one ovary is a little higher, horizontally, than the other. Again, use your superpowers to fall into this area, inviting your awareness to BE in your ovaries, to sense their size (like a pecan in its shell). After a few breaths, notice if you can feel a quality of energy. Often, women feel this as a sort of sweet, high-vibration energy. Remember, the glands are electrical; they have an energy, different from the chakras, as it is more physically embodied. With the adrenals you might feel this energy connecting down to your knees, resonating through your lower back and sacroiliac area (adrenal–gonadal complex).

If you are biologically male: rest a few fingers in a similar location below and either side of the navel by a few inches. Stay there lightly for a few breaths. Now notice what you notice. Then you can locate your reflex points for your testes by moving your fingers a little further out and down. This is the ligamentous point or source of the vas deferens, the tube that supplies semen; the source is at the top of the tube. The tubes arch above the bladder and it is important to breathe there. Know that this area as a tube that sources semen is a powerful site. This is going to be different for each human. Just go to where it "seems right," where your fingers fall. After a few breaths, notice if you can feel a quality of energy. Remember, the glands are electrical; they have an energy, it is different from the chakras, as it is more physically embodied.

Adrenal Glands

From here, move your awareness up the spine and find the bottom of your ribcage, using your hands to palpate the sides and front of your body. Trace the bones with your fingers around to your back. Rest your hands here for a few moments, knowing that your two kidneys rest with about half covered by the ribcage, and half beneath it. They are kidney-shaped, 2½–3 inches in height, and are located forward and on either side of the spine. Rest your hands, should they reach here comfortably, to cover the kidney area at your back. Simply be in this area for a few breaths. Now imagine two caps, like two little hats, resting, one on top of each kidney. These are your **Adrenal Glands**. Bring your awareness here. Simply embody the area, your adrenals, for a few breaths.

Pancreas

Now bring your awareness to the front of the body, to your solar plexus. Rest on your hand here. A little bit behind your hand is the head of your **Pancreas**. It then extends back and to your left, in a diagonal line. Tuning into it can help you feel the depth of your torso, from front to back. Breathe here for a few breaths, sensing into the location and energy of this organ with glandular function.

Thoracobody

Now move a hand to your sternum, sliding it down to where the ribs attach on both sides. Slide a few fingers under this notch, your xiphoid process (it may be tender, so be gentle) and sense up and behind the bone. This is where your thoracobody is located. Breathe in and out of this area, sensing for glandular energy. When you inhale, move the bone and body away from one another; when you exhale, they naturally come back together. You may feel space here, or might sense the two being "glued" together. Be curious and investigate as you breathe into your thoracobody.

Heart Bodies

Now move your awareness upwards to your heart. Rest your hand on your sternum. And should you be able to reach it, place the other on your back. Now rest both your hands in your lap, while you continue to sense into the area. Behind your sternum, and in front of your spine, lies your heart. It is resting within the pillowing protection of your lungs. Immediately surrounding it is the pericardium. It actually lies a little left of center, so move your front hand so that the base is on top, and your fingertips are below your left nipple. Take a few breaths to feel your own heart, in between your sternum and spine.

Then sense a little more lightly for its endocrine function in the aortic arch. This was discovered by Bainbridge Cohen in the 1970s and named the **Heart Bodies**. More recently science has confirmed that there is indeed endocrine function at the heart.

Thymus

Now move your awareness up your spine, and your hands to above your heart in the middle of your sternum. Here lies your **Thymus**. The thymus is quite large in babies, actually preventing them from being able to bring their hands together at first! But slowly it shrinks during aging (to the shape of a small H under the top bone of the breastbone/sternum). Sense into this area for a few breaths. Allow it to help you feel the breadth of your chest and your pectoral muscles, extending into your shoulders and down your arms into your fingertips. Try bringing your hands into anjali mudra, paying attention to your thymus, then feel the body for the connection from thymus to shoulder to arm to elbow. And then out to your hand to open your arms wide from your body. Feel the heart–thymus, arm–hand connection. There is a major meridian here, going from heart to hand, in Chinese medicine.

Take a moment to pause and feel the larger picture of your whole "glandular spine." Sense for a few moments into the connection of your thymus to your heart bodies, to your pancreas, to your adrenals, to your ovaries, to your coccygeal body. Then come back up to the thymus. Allow this sensing to help you in feeling your height, your length, and your spaciousness within. There is room in between each of the glands. Notice how adding organ and gland awareness into spinal awareness is different than feeling solely the bones of the spine. You might sense more softness, curves, circles, three-dimensional fill of torso, weight, and volume.

Thyroid

Let's continue. From your thymus, move up your spine to your throat. Breathe in and

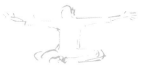

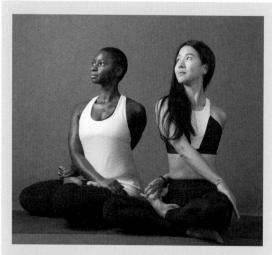

Figure 3B.9
Contralateral twist for parathyroidal activation.
Photo by Serge Cashman.

out. Feel the air coming in at the back of your mouth into your neck. Then bring one hand to your Adam's apple. This is the bump formed by the soft cartilage around the larynx; feel this area with a few fingers as you breathe in and out. This is where your **Thyroid** is. To open up this area, slowly move your thyroid and elbows counter to one another (like in Indian and Balinese dance).

Parathyroids

From this space of embodying the thyroid, bring your fingers to feel at the sides of the Adam's apple, as this is where your four **Parathyroids** are. Breathe in and out here a few times, into the space of your parathyroids. Breathe in, and exhale with an "Ah" sound. Both the thyroid and parathyroid support the voice. Use your voice to help you resonate your glands.

Carotid Bodies

Moving to up under the jaw, experience the soft tissue and the exocrine glands – the salivary and lymphatic glands that swell during an infection. In the front, under the mouth, you may feel more bony sensation under these tissues. If so, you have located your hyoid bone – a curved C-shaped bone in front of the neck. It is the base of the tongue. You can gently hold the two sides of the hyoid and then protrude your tongue.

You may feel a tug on this bone. Behind the hyoid and up and under either side of the jaw in the soft tissue you will find the **Carotid Bodies**.

From your thyroid, move into the whole of your neck, into the back of your throat (which you can feel filling with air as you do Ujjayi Breath) and into your mouth. Feel its three-dimensionality by sensing its height, width and depth. Bring your tongue to the roof of your mouth, feeling the upper palette. Sense the bone above it. Release your tongue.

Pituitary Gland

Move your awareness up through the bone and into the pituitary gland that is just above it, within your brain. Bring your finger to each ear, to your ear canal – sense in between these two points to find the **Pituitary Gland** in the center, just above where you had your tongue touching at the roof of your mouth. Sense into the gland. Just be here for a few breaths.

To fine-tune the location of your pituitary gland (see Fig. 3B.7 for pituitary map), move one finger to rest in between your eyebrows, and a little above, and the other finger to rest on your occiput in back. Release those finger touches, and bring one finger to rest at the top of your head, at the fontanel. Rest your awareness in between these three sets of finger touches.

You may be able to sense these upper glands quickly; don't be surprised by, or discount, your ability to feel shifts in sensation right away. You may hear tones rising in your ears, and/or feel the quality of your head space changing, as your awareness moves inward into your brain, and upwards with each gland.

Mammillary Bodies

From your pituitary location, sense upwards. Just a little bit up and back is each of the **Mammillary Bodies** (see Fig. 3B.8). There is an energy reflex point that you can touch here; bring your hands to both ears, to touch the upper point of the front wall of each ear canal.

Pineal Gland

Just above and a little behind this is your **Pineal Gland**. Bring a finger to touch the very top of your head, the place where your bones came together as a baby, your fontanel; this is the reflex point for the pineal gland.

Take a few moments here, to breathe in and out, with awareness focused on these three glands: pituitary, mammillary, pineal. Simply be here.

You are likely feeling spacious, heightened in vibration, and mentally acute. Maintain this spaciousness by feeling your width beyond your skin. Activate your peripheral vision to help you feel out to both sides; extend this beyond your eyes, as a sort of full-body peripheral vision, as you briefly check in with the other glands.

You are grounding by retracing your path: sense from the brain glands, to the connection to your thyroid/parathyroid. Now sense from thyroid to thymus. Maintain your sense of width and fullness, as you continue to center and move downwards to the heart/heart bodies, then thoracobody and pancreas. Take in a breath. Then connect to adrenals, ovaries and coccygeal body.

You've done it. You've visited, embodied, and therefore activated your endocrine system. Take a moment to notice what you notice. Then feel this glandular support of your center line and spine and sushumna. You may sense your more fully activated self. You may have access to a different type of awareness of self, of your body's health, and your body's aliveness.

Effects students, colleagues, and friends have noticed over the years include feeling more alert, feeling more circular/less linear, having a stronger sense of their anatomy, experiencing gentleness, having an experience of the divine feminine energy, and feeling refreshed.

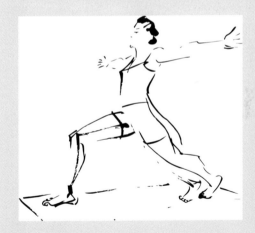

Figure 3B.10
Opening up to claim space – a tensile and glandular experience, by Stewart Hoyt.

93

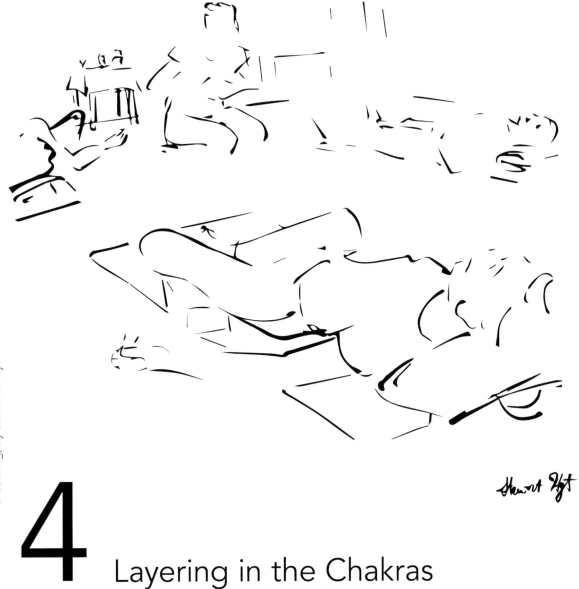

Breathing, by Stewart Hoyt

4

Layering in the Chakras

Guided Chakra Experience

Tuning into your chakras can be an expansive experience. Integrating chakra awareness and exploration with experiential anatomy grounds the exploration, making it easier for you to keep it with you, remember it, not get too spacey, and stay emotionally even keeled. Layering the chakras onto your awareness of the glands in this chapter grounds an energetic experience

in anatomy. Embodying anatomy happens through knowing anatomical locations, having either a picture or a sensation of the area and its function. Movement and touch as well as sound are great ways to bring sensation to an area.

The Sun Salutation is a structure for integrating this information. In Chapter 3 the endocrine glands were introduced in depth. Here the chakras, color, and sound are visited, In Chapter 5 Bartenieff Fundamentals cues will

Chapter 4

Chart 4.1					
The Chakras					
Note that chakras 2–6 have a front and back					
Chakras by Number	**Location**	**Sanskrit**	**Sound**	**Crystalline (Blair & Laban/ Bartenieff)**	**Yantra**
1st Chakra	Root	Muladhara	Lam	Cube	Square
2nd Chakra	Sacral	Svadhisthana	Vam	Icosahedron	Crescent moon
3rd Chakra	Solar	Manipura	Ram	Tetrahedron	Red triangle
4th Chakra	Heart	Anahata	Yam	Octahedron	Star of David
5th Chakra	Throat	Visuddha	Ham	Octahedron	Smokey gray egg within white orb
6th Chakra	Third eye	Ajna	Ksham	Dodecahedron	5 rays of violet light
7th Chakra	Crown	Sahasrara	Ohm	Dodecahedron	Rainbow petaled lotus

be added, and lastly in Chapter 6 developmental information will be layered in.

There are seven major chakras, all emanating from the body and moving out through the energy field. You can think of them as spherical, within the body, with a cone shape emanating from the body out, frontally as well as through the back body. The narrow end is at the body; the chakra grows in diameter as it moves outward (see Fig. 2.1). The chakras act as transforming stations: energy/chi/qi/prana comes into your crown from source/God/ Goddess/the universe and from the crown down, and each chakra transforms the energy down in vibration. So as you move from crown to foot, the chakras go down in pitch, color, density, and wavelength – from high pitch to low, sparse to dense, high wavelength to short.

Next is an experience, guiding you to move through them from the bottom of the spine upwards to the head. You may notice these shifts in vibration or density, just from reading

this material. As you proceed through these practices awareness of these aspects grows.

Here are some things to watch for:

- Energy in your body vibrating at a higher pitch
- Tones in your ears rising
- Seeing colors in your mind's eye
- Emotion or sensation in chakral area changing
- Changes in smell.

Guided Chakra Experience

 Root/Muladhara chakra: located at the base of your spine, at the pelvic floor. You can think of your pelvic floor as a diamond-shaped hammock suspended from these four bones: the two sit, pubic, and tail bones. At the base of your tailbone, on the anterior side, is your coccygeal body. This body is thought to have endocrine function, and helps free up movement in the hips and legs, all the way down to the toes, bringing in lightness and agility. It supports your connection to the earth with a "groundedness based on self love and the will towards personal survival" (Hartley 1995, p. 215). It supports the root chakra and the connection to the head's glands. Here is where your root chakra resides. It is red in color, emanating from the center of your pelvic floor. The Indian yantra symbol for the root chakra is a yellow square, perhaps the most stable shape. And this is a place where stability is needed – a healthy root chakra can indicate a healthy relationship to home, food, and finances. The element for this chakra is earth. Here you can chant the bija mantra lam, to help you access, tone, and clear the area.

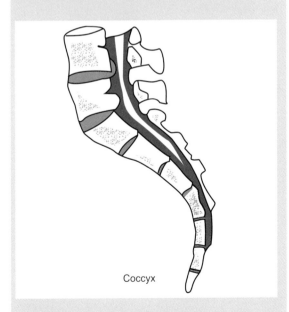

Coccyx

Figure 4.1
Locate the coccygeal body on the anterior side of the tailbone.

 2nd/Svadhisthana: located below your belly button. Also known as the hara or power center in Asian disciplines, this chakra is connected to your gonads (ovaries in those born female/vas deferens in those born male). Sense into this area a few inches below your navel. Bring two fingers down from your belly button; draw them 2 inches below, and a few inches apart from one another. This is roughly the placement for your ovaries or your vas deferens. Use your intuition, the smartness that is in your hands, to discern a more exact location in your body, i.e. one ovary is usually lower/higher than the other. Take a moment to pause with a light finger touch here; you might feel a light energy. Sense the connection from these points to your ankles, heels, forelegs, and sacrum. Making this connection, sense for the possibility of feeling your pelvis and lower body grounded and supported.

This 2nd chakra, unlike the root that is facing the earth, is at your front and back (see Fig. 2.1). You can visualize this as two cones (like orange traffic cones), with the narrow end at your physical body, widening as your chakra reaches out beyond your skin and into your energetic field. You can mist in the color orange to help balance this chakra, seeing it bathe and fill your belly space. You can chant the bija mantra vam to help you embody this area both energetically and physically. The element is water, less dense than the earth element below at the root. This water indicates the flow of this area – and the sensual and creative energy of the 2nd chakra. This creative zone supports the creative expression at your throat chakra; grounding the gonad helps ground the throat glands too (Hartley 1995). The Indian symbol is a crescent moon resting on its outer curve,

facing upwards. A healthy second chakra indicates a balanced relationship to your sensuality, sexuality, and creativity.

 3rd/Manipura: located at your solar plexus, at your center line just below the ribcage. Sitting right here is the white head of your pancreas – an organ that has endocrine function. Your pancreas then travels at a diagonal through your torso to your left side in back. Sensing into it helps give you a sense of the depth of your torso. It relates to the six ends of your limbs – hands, feet, tail, and head. "It gives energetic support to these six extremities, and maintains spatial tension between them" (Hartley 1995). It also supports social instinct, awareness of others, which supports love of others as its energy rises into the heart chakra. In Chinese medicine a sun is often visualized here with its yellow rays emanating out through the whole body, bathing it in yellow immune system-supporting light.

Along with visualizing yellow for this chakra, you can chant the bija mantra ram to help you feel and balance this area. The sun and the ram have a strong bolstering effect – supporting healthy confidence and sense of identity and self. "The health of this chakra supports the development of healthy love expressed at the fourth chakra" (Hartley 1995). In Egyptian culture, Ra is the word for sun. The element here is fire. When our self-esteem is stronger, via a balanced chakra, our will is supported in using the fire element of the chakra to act. The Indian symbol is a red triangle, pointing upwards to the heart.

 4th/Anahata: located at your heart. The heart itself has endocrine function, through the heart bodies, which are stimulated by homologous yield and push of the arms (Bainbridge Cohen & Mills 1980). You can take a moment here to put both hands on your heart and sense into the endocrine function (the energy points are on the right and left sides, of the sternum at the level of the nipples). From here play with pressing the palms of the hands together and then reaching out with both arms to embrace. These physical movements are supported by the heart bodies, as is reaching out through hands and eyes, and forearms and wrists in general. Then bridge into the heart chakra expansive energy. The Indian symbol here is a powder blue star of David. This star is two inter-linking triangles, one pointing upwards and one downwards. As it is the central of the seven major chakras, one triangle is pointing at the upper three chakras, the other to the lower three. The element is air. You can visualize the color green bathing this chakra, helping to bring it into balance as you chant the bija mantra yam. A healthy heart chakra indicates a balanced ability to receive and give love, and an ability to feel compassion.

 5th/Visuddha: here at the throat move into the more subtle elements; here it is ether – the element of space that holds the other four: air, fire, water, and earth. Connect with the endocrine system here by finding the area of the Adam's apple (prominent in most men and some women): press its side, try swallowing, and you will feel it pressing into your fingers. This is your thyroid. It supports your elbows and humerus. Try moving them opposite to one another; this will help free up the thyroid area. The parathyroids are also here, two on each side and at the back of your thyroid, supporting movement of the ribs, and movement between the ribs and scapula. Tuning into these glands helps you bridge to accessing your throat chakra. Like the 2nd chakra this is a major center for creativity as well as communication. Here is where you express your ideas and knowledge through the power and vehicle of your own voice. The parathyroids support gentle qualities of the voice; they "integrate vocal expression with finely articulated movements of the hands" (Hartley 1995, p. 219). Take a moment to feel your breath here. As you breathe in and out, feel the breath moving into and out of your throat. Imagine the feeling of a yawn, or actually yawn right now. Feel the openness in your throat? Try to maintain that. When balanced, your throat chakra connects to your higher wisdom from the upper chakras, as well as the love and wisdom of your heart, assisting you in expressing your message in a balanced and connected way. The Indian symbol is a white egg shape with a silvery egg shape within that. Bathing it in the color blue, while chanting the bija mantra ham, helps you to access it and to clear it and bring it into optimal health.

 6th/Ajna: the 6th or third eye chakra is located a little above and in between your eyebrows, seating at the same location as your pituitary gland. See the centuries-old painting in Chapter 2 (Fig. 2.2). In back, it emanates out at your occiput. To access it move upwards from your throat chakra into the cavity of your mouth. Take a moment here to somatically feel the fullness of your mouth – sense its width, its depth from front to back, and its height. Then bring your tongue to the top of your mouth, touch the roof, and press a bit. You are touching a small chakra here, *lalana*. Sense for the bone above. This bone is supporting and protecting your brain. Release your tongue, but keep your awareness at the roof; sense up through the bone to your brain above. Resting right here is your pituitary gland; this is also the location of your third eye or ajna chakra 6. This gland supports the visual function of the eyes and the imagination, intelligence, and conceptual thought (Bainbridge Cohen &

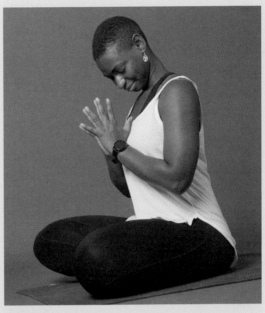

Figure 4.2
Third eye/pituitary. Photo by Serge Cashman.

Mills 1980). Be aware of the position of your neck and head. The head pulls forward from stress and tension, effectively closing this chakra. This pulling forward also happens specifically from overuse of this gland (visual functions like reading, writing). Also, if your head tilts upwards, this chakra gets too open, making you spacey (Finger 2005). To counter these tendencies, practice anchoring the pituitary to your tail. Sense the connection going down through your spine. This is a way to help you sense the realness of embodying the pituitary. You can further explore this connection by sensing how the pituitary underlies reach and pull from the tail. The Indian symbol is five purple rays of light emanating out in all directions. You can visualize this purple light moving from a central point outwards while chanting inwardly the bija mantra ksham, to clear and balance this chakra. Here is where you connect with your highest wisdom aligned with your soul's knowledge and source. The pituitary specifically supports altruistic love and compassion.

 7th/Sahasrara: located at your crown, just where the bones of your skull came together when you were a baby – your fontanel. The mammillary and pineal glands are our bridge to the crown chakra. From your pituitary, move upwards and back a bit, sensing these two small, round bodies, the mammillaries, that are at the midline of the body. Centering in them helps the head to reach into the space above it. This centering "can produce pleasurable feelings of spaciousness, timelessness, and an openness of the sense perceptions similar to those experienced in some types of meditative practices." Begin to move your awareness up a little higher, diagonally and back from the mammillary, to locate your pineal gland, above the midbrain. Centering here "can evoke a sense of the depth of time, of ancient history and eternity, past and future brought together in the present" (Hartley 1995).

Now, at the top of the endocrine chain, take a moment to sense back down your spine, your sushumna, and begin to see it as the stem of a flower. This stem is riding up through your body, with the various chakras along the way, and rising up through mammillary and pineal, and now to top of your skull, see your 7th chakra beginning to blossom. Its yantra is the Indian symbol of a thousand-petaled lotus. You can visualize this lotus blossoming upwards from the stem of your central line or spine, petals unfurling over your shining skull, as you chant the bija mantra ohm. A balanced and healthy crown chakra has you easefully connected with Source or God/Goddess, the cosmos and universe.

Grounding

Take a moment now, to bring your hands together in namaste (anjali mudra) at the top of your head, resting on your crown chakra. Then slide your hands down your face, gently encouraging the energy to connect to the other chakras and glands, and ground, as you slowly sweep your hands from face to throat, to heart, to solar plexus, to belly, to pubic bone, to hip fold. Slowly lengthen your legs, and bend and unbend your knees. Do some ankle circles and stretch as you please. Take a moment to feel the effects of this practice on your thinking, your heart/your emotions, and your physical body.

When you open your eyes, cast them to a 45-degree angle, looking at the floor/earth. This will help you ground.

Here are some things to watch for: in doing these practices your awareness grows. Often there are shifts happening that go unnoticed. This can be because the territory is new and it is not always easy to see the "landscape apart from the animals." You may notice:

- Tones in the ears that rise as you move up from the root to the crown chakra

- Your voice pitch changing from low to high

- A feeling of energy shifting from strong, low vibration to a higher, faster-paced wavelength vibration

- Images in your mind, perhaps even colors.

More about Bija Mantras

The bija mantras are the "seed" sounds, the sounds that the Rishis heard when they meditated on these zones of the body those thousands of years ago. The sound, or mantra, for each chakra is a Sanskrit word. Sanskrit, like Latin and Hebrew, is one of the languages that are sacred, the words having specific energetic vibration and meaning. Each of the chakra sounds is representative, like the yantra. These are the sounds that help to balance this chakra, this vibration. Become a scientist as you explore – try each sound yourself, and notice if that syllable (la for lam at the 1st chakra, for example) activates your pelvic floor, or not. Try using *la* at the 2nd chakra and see if it feels any different there, or does *va* really work better there? See for yourself; make it real. And that is the exciting thing about working with the chakras: they are real – as the confluence of the nerve plexus and the glands. Working with them is a great way to explore the "unseen" and find its palpable reality in your life.

When you try the mantras, explore with the vowel sound first, then add the "m" onto it, like an aum, turning it into a hum. Relax your lips so that you can feel the buzzing there. Intend for the sound to be filling and resonating your chakral area. It is an internal energetic massage.

More on Sound

Sound, like the colors of the chakras, changes in vibration when moving up the spine, from dense to light, from slow and deep-wavelength to high-pitched and fast. As you chant the bija mantras you are moving energy through your body. Stagnant areas will begin to disperse. There is potential here for the practitioner to experience a dramatic shift in chi flow with this practice. Allow time for rest and integration afterwards.

Sound affects us. A lot of the dots are not yet connected by science. Sound affects matter: it can change our brain waves, and tuning forks, Tibetan bowls, and/or your own voice can calm or activate your neuroendocrine system. Suren Shrestha, engineer and sound healer, illuminates this idea further, speaking to the power of intention: "When we use sound coupled with intention, which is the most important aspect of healing, we can direct sound vibration to raise the body's vibrational frequency" (Shrestha 2013). With chakra meditation we are exploring how sound, color, and yantra help balance and clear our chakras, therefore raising that frequency. There are some examples of how researchers and artists have made connections between sound and how it affects matter.

Cymatics is the name for a sound field of study, coined by Swiss physician and scientist Hans Jenney in the 1960s. It translates as modal vibrational phenomena. He continued development of a field that goes back to the 1600s, of putting sand or other fine particles on vibrating plates. The particles respond to frequencies by forming predictable symmetrical shapes similar to those found in nature. A certain frequency gives you the design seen on a turtle's shell (see Figs 4.3 and 4.4), another frequency gives us the pattern of a leopard's fur, and yet another the shape of a horse crab's body. German researcher and photographer Alexander Lauterwasser has continued this work with sand and water. See Figure 4.5 for the shape of a seven-petaled flower (like a datura), and Figure 4.6 for a spiral, as seen in nature in shells and cacti and more. The sound frequency of ohm gives us a mandala-like shape of a circle within a circle (how ohm is depicted in ancient Hindu paintings) (Lauterwasser 2011). "Once one's eye is open to the cymatic phenomenon, you can see it everywhere" (J. Volk 2015, personal communication). And how do you, the reader, feel or otherwise experience these images somatically?

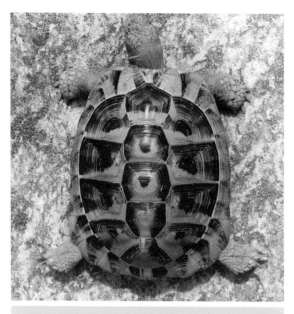

Figure 4.3
Turtle: an example of harmonic patterns in nature, this photo from book *Water Sound Images: The Creative Music of the Universe* by Alexander Lauterwasser, permission given by Jeff Volk for Alexander Lauterwasser.

Figure 4.4
1088 Hertz: Chladni sound figure at specific frequency; there are hundreds of such figures exhibiting the patterns of animals, this photo from book *Water Sound Images: The Creative Music of the Universe* by Alexander Lauterwasser, permission given by Jeff Volk for Alexander Lauterwasser.

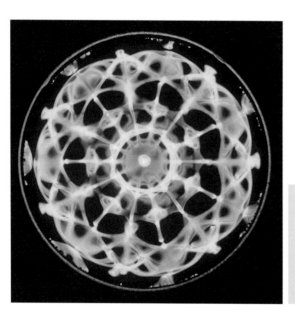

Figure 4.5
Seven-element structure: "standing wave", as found in seven-petaled flowers, seashells, this photo from book *Water Sound Images: The Creative Music of the Universe* by Alexander Lauterwasser, permission given by Jeff Volk for Alexander Lauterwasser.

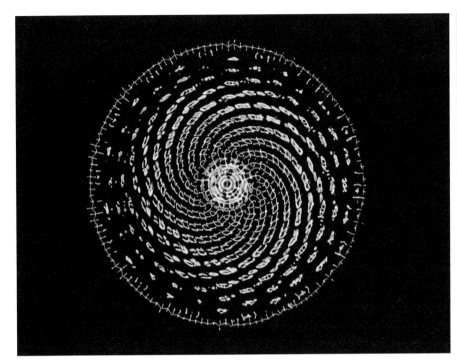

Figure 4.6
Water–Sound–Image with 14 spiral arms formed in a water bowl of 20 cm diameter. Frequency/ 102.528 Hertz: we can see this pattern in shells, cactus and other forms in nature, this photo from book *Water Sound Images: The Creative Music of the Universe* by Alexander Lauterwasser, permission given by Jeff Volk for Alexander Lauterwass.

Hungarian artist Gabriel Kelemen continues this work today with his research, drawings, and three-dimensional forms. Figure 4.8 encapsulates some of his work with spines, cellular nephrology, and evolution. He postulates that the energy vortexes that come out from the center of the earth at the equator shape everything that is born and develops on earth. This drawing shows us some of that impact from low to high frequencies affecting body size – large bodies with lower heart rates being affected by low frequencies, smaller bodies on the right being influenced by higher frequencies. The light spectrum and piano keys further illustrate this range (J Volk 2021, personal communication; Kelemen 2015). You can use these examples of sound affecting matter as inspiration, seeds for investigation. Does

sounding into your chakras and glands send wavelengths through your body, therefore changing the arrangements of particles?

Fabien Maman, acupuncturist and concert pianist, named by *Webster's Dictionary* as the father of sound healing, did experiments in the 1960s, where he played sound frequencies via tuning forks to blood cell samples, while Kirlian photographs were taken. The photographs show the cells becoming more vibrant and healthy in appearance, glowing with light, and literally changing shape (Maman 2008). Maman, when teaching and lecturing, tells of how his research and work with clients over the years have shown him that acupuncture treatments will be more effective and last longer when done with tuning forks instead of needles, and even better with the addition of color in the form of colored

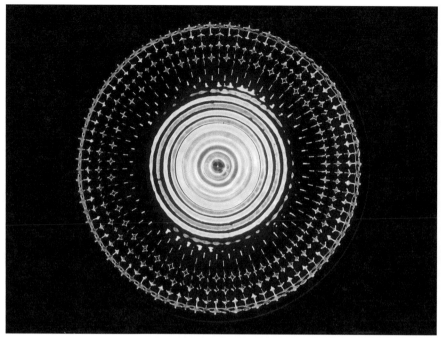

Figure 4.7
Multi-element/
"standing wave" 91.8
Hertz, by Alexander
Lauterwasser, this
photo from book
*Water Sound Images:
The Creative Music of
the Universe* by
Alexander Lauterwas-
ser, permission given
by Jeff Volk for
Alexander
Lauterwasser.

light and fabric (F Maman 2011, personal communication). When sounding into the body does it cause our cells to become more vibrant?

Maman's work inspired Dr Masaru Emoto to build his body of work as published in the series of books titled *Messages From Water* that first came out in 1999. His hypothesis in his experiments was to show the effect of prayer, intention, and the written word on the ability of water to form ice crystals when frozen. The word *love* written on a piece of paper wrapped around a test tube of water gives us beautiful lace snowflakes. The word *hate* resulted in molecules of water that are having trouble forming (M. Emoto 2004, personal communication, September 17). German scientists more recently have found that water does indeed have a memory. When a flower was placed in water each of the individual molecules of water was changed, with an imprint of

the flower detectable. They believe that water holds memory of all the places it has been, thus having the ability to connect us to those places if drinking it (Brown 2018). Our bodies are 70 percent water. Could this imprinting extend to our thinking, visualization, and sounding? Do our thoughts affect the structure of our cells?

Dr John Beaulieu, when teaching, tells of his experiences in New York University's anechoic chamber. This chamber removes all outside sound, making it so quiet that a person can hear their own heart, blood moving, and even the nervous system. He tells of the day when he was in a state of agitation because of an argument with a transit worker over his metro ticket. In the chamber he could hear a high-pitched buzzing in his ears, coming from his nervous system. He had the idea to go down to the street to the guitar shop and purchase some tuning forks. Back in the chamber, when

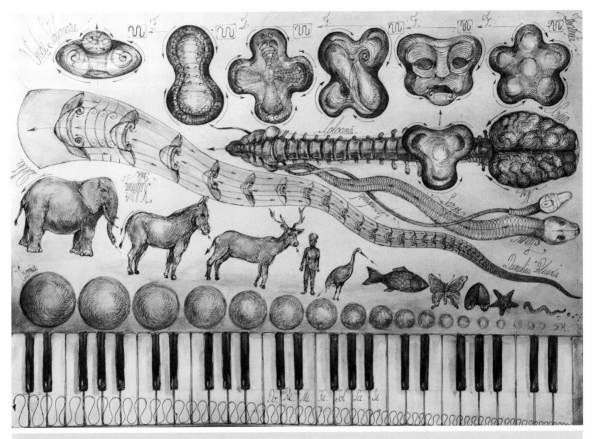

Figure 4.8
The dimensional spectrum relationship, by Gabriel Kelemen, The Universality of the vortex-sphere archetype, 2015. Permission given by Iulia and Gabriel Kelemen.

he played them close to his ears, the pleasing sound of the notes of a perfect fifth, the buzzing in his ears immediately quieted (J. Beaulieu 2011, personal communication). Thus began decades of research into the beneficial effect of sound on the human body.

Rather than drawing scientific conclusions from these bodies of work, use them as inspiration, and ask these questions doing your own personal bodily research, including when teaching others. This somatic process was modeled when Bainbridge Cohen, in the 1970s, together with her students and colleagues, investigated whether the heart had glands. They felt the answer was yes, and later science came out with the studies to prove it.

To further inspire, here is a quote from Jonathan Goldman: "Most people think of sound as energy that just goes into your ears and into your brain, and this, of course, is true. Sound does affect our brain and is able to entrain, or change, our brain wave activity, our heart rate, and our respiration.

"This by itself is extraordinary, since it means that you can induce different states of consciousness through sound. But sound

Chapter 4

affects more than that. Sound is capable of rearranging molecular sound. Think of what this means. There's virtually nothing that cannot be changed or fixed or shifted with sound" (Goldman, in Geissenger et al 2002, p. 19).

Color

Color is a lost art. It was known by healers to be effective before the rise of allopathic medicine at the beginning of the last century (Judith 1987). "If sound waves affect the physical arrangement of subtle energy, it would follow that color, being such a high octave of material manifestation, could influence matter in much the same way" (Judith 1987). The world of energy healing presumes that disease begins in the auric field, in the more subtle realms, before manifesting in the body. Healers today continue to use color to treat ailments ranging from fatigue and inflammation to sore muscles to issues with the eyes – using light and fabric. Dr Jacob Lieberman has noticed that when people dislike a color, then are asked where their physical issues are (neck pain, bladder pain, stomach issues), there is a high correlation between these colors and the part of the body associated with that color

by the eastern chakras (Lieberman 2018). Perhaps let Maman's experiences with color and acupuncture inspire you in your investigations of color with the chakras, including experimenting with the color of the clothes you wear. Can you explore visualizing color moving into a chakra and noticing if it affects your well-being?

Color Therapy

I (Shakti) had the experience 20 years ago, at a dance event, of not feeling well. I was considering going to bed early, after dinner, and missing out on the evening dance. I felt nauseous, tired, and a bit out of it. My friend Tom then asked me, "Want to try an experiment?" I was game. He guided me to sit still, and hold the glass of water that I had sitting nearby. He asked me to imagine a color, whatever color would be healing for me. I immediately pictured yellow. He suggested I see it coming out through my hands into the glass, filling the water. I did this, and then I drank it. Within a few minutes all of my symptoms abated. I have been holding this example as inspiration since, for my self-healing, with my clients, and with my students.

Honoring Ancestral Wisdom

Herbalist and herbal teacher Richard Mandelbaum, founding partner, director, and teacher at the ArborVitae School of Traditional Herbalism in New York City, has said that he often values the herbal recipes and healing stories that are passed down through families more than he values science. They are often the ones that are tried and prove true over time, that work and help us. When he brought a group of us on a herbal tour of Prospect Park, he was

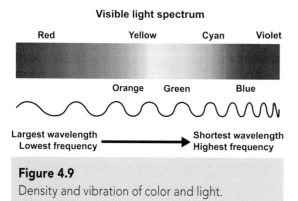

Figure 4.9
Density and vibration of color and light.

curious about what we had learned from our grandmothers. I was surprised, and impressed, as he runs a respected clinical herbal school in Manhattan. He inspired me to value my intuition and what I have learned and observed in myself, and from my community, and to not let our scientifically oriented western culture override that.

Going Deeper with Vocalization: Bartenieff Approach to Spatial Expansion with Sound

Practicing yoga can feel different depending on one's cultural lens. This is true for working with the chakras and vocalization too.

Bartenieff (1980) sourced some of her work with voice from Hindu and Buddhist meditation practices. She also taught an approach to Breath Support and related vocalization with the following guidance:

1. to support sagittal dimensional movement (and related planar and diagonal movement), introduce the "oooo" sound for breath and shape support

2. to support vertical dimensional movement (and related planar and diagonal movements), introduce the "aaah" sound

3. to support horizontal dimensional movement (and related planar and diagonal movements), introduce the "eeee" sound.

Using the resonance of her suggested sounds in different chambers of the body – low (pelvis), middle (chest), and high (head), Bartenieff often worked with the following sounds progressing from the lowest chakra to the highest. Various Laban/Bartenieff faculty

(Bradley & Parker 2020) recall this specifically as the following:

- Ooooo (the "u" sound in boot) in the pelvis (1st chakra)

- Oh (the long "o" sound in boat) in the belly/dan tien/hara/gut (2nd–3rd chakra)

- Ah (the "a" sound in talk, or the sound sometimes made when finally understanding something) in the chest/heart (upper torso) (3rd–4th chakra)

- Ai (the long "a" sound in hay) in the throat (ehhh) (5th chakra)

- Ee (the long "e" sound in meet) in the head/third eye (6th chakra)

Dynamic Embodiment[SM] (DE[SM]) brings in silence or listening to a bell for the 7th chakra.

The oh and ai sounds combine two pure dimensions: "oh" = "ah" and "oo" – vertical and sagittal (forward and back); "ai" = "ee" and "ah" – horizontal and vertical. Whether working with one pure dimension or a combination of two or three, this is the beginning of space harmony through sound, which uses the counter-pulls of bio-tensegrity. Vocalizing using careful shaping of the mouth and selecting pitches that vibrate in specific glandular regions becomes even more powerful in areas where the gland is near a nerve plexus – a chakra.

The spatial choices made also reflect enculturation of gender identities, of race and ethnicity, along with family dynamics. Denise Cavassa (2020), a seasoned Laban/Bartenieff trained Movement Analyst, adds a broader perspective about cultural variation in how vowel sounds are used with movement: "I also

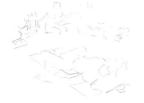

see that Bartenieff's sounds resonate (no pun intended) with her cultural experience and language – the same way that movement expression and interpretation does across cultures. For example, European movement histories have traditionally expressed along the dimensional cross (the 3 cardinal dimensions – the vertical, horizontal and sagittal dimensions), as well as a notion of rising from the ground; whereas cultures whose music was/is more centered around connecting to the earth and the drum as a primary rhythmic indicator have more transverse expressions [three-dimensional movement like an infinity symbol moving along a diagonal]. The meanings behind the movements are also related to how the body organically expresses sound (sighs, expressions of joy, etc.) within the socially-accepted modes for movement and non-verbal communication.

A recent example was a conversation with scientists who [included] a female West African, a female German, and a male German. They were together during lunch when a funny story was being told. When we got to the punchline and everyone laughed, the West African woman opened her arms and hands as she laughed; the German woman closed her arms to her chest and clasped her hands; and the German man patted the table with his hand and then extended it in an arching-upward motion… Tying in with this topic, the Germans both expressed, "Oh!" just before laughing and the West African woman said, "Eh!" Meanwhile, all parties were equally surprised and delighted with the punchline, yet their verbal and movement expressions were completely different."

Personal movement style and tone of voice has a long history in its development. What the movement means to ourselves and others also varies from culture to culture. However, almost every culture uses sound to resonate the body, and movement,

especially dance, continues to be a profound healing resource. Each can be explored with awareness of how space is being used or integrated. Adding in glandular sensations and chakral awareness has many potential outcomes.

Martha's Personal Story: How Sound and Movement Relate

I'd love to share a favorite lesson that had a memorable impact on a class I taught for a fellow CMA, Sarah Jane Burton, at the University of Toronto with her Opera students. I had them:

1. explore breath support while sounding and being aware of related shaping in the planes (one by one through all three)

2. move in the dimension and planes with the sound support (one by one through all three)

3. continue to move without the sound support but feeling the breath support (one by one through all three)

4. move freely through any desired dimensions/planes/diagonals with matched breath-sound support.

Their movement and sounds were astounding and one of their responses stayed with me forever: "Moving without sounding felt like going through a tunnel." She implied that bringing back the sound with the movement is like bringing back the light of day. It was glorious to be surrounded by such richness of sound and movement, and to see the liveliness of their interaction with such skilled vocalists/actors/movers. There was quite a bit more to the lesson. I often include this type of experience in yoga classes, somatic education classes for Dynamic Embodiment and in BodyMind Dancing classes.

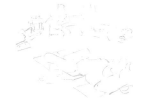

Spaciousness – Sacred Forms and Moving Inside of Imaginary Crystalline Space

Another way to work with the chakras is to stimulate the inner core through expansion, creating resonant spaces in the body. One image is to think of a large hall, perhaps a house of worship, and how that large space resonates sound. Similarly each musical instrument is shaped in space with different sizes and shapes of cavities to create their unique sounds. In DE one can choose to make highly symmetrical body shapes related to the "sacred crystalline forms," as first mentioned in Chapter 1 (see Fig. 1.2). Any of these five equally sided forms can be imagined either inside the chakras or outside of the entire body as additional inroads to experiencing each chakra's energy. It is because of the harmonic symmetry that the forms are considered to be sacred. These ideas were explored by Rudolf Steiner and many people who were involved with the Masonic traditions. Lawrence Blair experienced this sacredness and brought the crystals and envisioning colors together with working with the chakras themselves. Hence, space, color, and sound together can be a support for inner or outer movement.

Each of the sacred crystals can be found in nature, in geometry, and in movement.

DE movement activities include:

1. Practicing visualizing each polyhedron inside of each chakra region (see the inspiration in Lawrence Blair's list below)

2. Moving "inside the polyhedral shapes," using your imagination to picture your body in one of these sacred shapes. Explore moving as if inside a beautiful perfectly symmetrical home to explore their energies within and outside of the body

3. The visualization or movement can be modulated to be "stimulating" or "toned-down" for the needed balancing effect for either the chakra or related glands.

While not many yoga teachers work with the polyhedra together with the chakras, it is important to note that different groups may correlate them with different chakras. Sourcing Blair (1976), DE uses the following correlations between chakras and spatial forms. (See Chart 4.1, as well as Fig. 1.2 showing the sacred forms in Chapter 1, in order to better envision the location and inter-relationships.)

"The Root chakra is governed by activating imagery or movement from within the cube – 6 exactly equal sides

The Generative chakra is governed by the icosahedron – movement from any of the 12 points that make up the 20 triangular sides

The Solar Plexus is governed by the tetrahedron – 4 equal triangular sides – a pyramid

The Heart and Throat chakra share the octahedron – 8 equal triangular sides – two pyramids joined at their widest point

The Crown chakra is stimulated by the dodecahedron – the most round of the crystalline forms has 12 sides formed from 20 exactly proportioned "5 pointed" pentagonal sides (20 points)." (Blair 1976, pp. 124–136)

Working in Threes Through Chakras

When you are targeting a specific chakra for balancing, add in a chakra from below and one from above. This opens the pathways for the energy you have generated or cleared to move

into the rest of the chakra system, allowing for overall balancing. To be safe you could always ground through the root, and connect with the sky through your crown, at the start of any chakra balancing session. Or, if working with the heart, for example, you can add in the 3rd chakra below, and the throat chakra above.

A nice way to close your session is to touch a few fingers to the chakras below and above, and simply rest, knowing that these hand placements do the balancing work for you. Your two hands move the energy in between them, opening the flow up and down the chakral line. The authors know of a few situations where only one chakra was balanced, so fainting occurred. This is real: energy gets moved and it can cause overwhelm, dizziness, and nausea. So work slowly and gently, and always ground through your root.

Chakra Meditation Tips

As a practitioner or teacher, when doing or guiding a chakra meditation, telescope your awareness out into the whole room, or the group, when you are ready to take in more information. You will begin to observe the practice of an individual or a group affecting the whole space that you are in. Over time you will make your own connections, which may include:

- feeling the energy of a group or room brightening as energy clears

- a higher vibration or pitch in your ears as you move up into the high chakras

- a low tone in your voice and body as you and the group ground; a feeling of depth or earthiness with this

- stuckness or cloudiness in the space when someone is working with blocked energy

- joy or giddiness when the heart chakra grows bigger.

Chakras In and Out of Balance

You can keep these qualities in mind to get a sense of where you or a student may need balancing. These balances and imbalances can present emotionally and physically. Looking at the third eye, or ajna chakra, as an example: consider how many people are thinking a lot and reading a lot. This can cause a literal jutting forward of the head/chin, even a furrowing at the forehead. The forward head can be balanced by bringing awareness more into the center of the body, by embodying the energy and physicality of the pituitary and ajna chakra. With awareness in the center or back of the head, the chin and nose often drop, the back of the neck lengthens, and the weight of head and skull rearranges in a more aligned fashion over the centerline. Now the thoughts and thinking processes can be more easily informed by your deeper wisdom; you are less "cut off" from your body, and likely less spacey. The emotions and lower chakral centers can be more informed by this center as well, so likely calmer and more even.

Chart 4.2

Chakras In and Out of Balance

Chakra Number	Balanced	Out of Balance
1	Areas of money and home are easeful; have a sense of trust in being taken care of; secure, grounded	Areas of money and home are challenged, ungrounded; anxious
2	Easefully sensuous, expressive, access to creativity, emotions are able to be experienced – evolution can happen	Repressed sensually, emotions held in this area
3	Confident, connected with life purpose; good digestion; easy leadership	Low self-esteem; digestion difficulties; unsure of life direction
4	Loving, able to give and receive; feel compassion, empathy for others; erect posture	Difficulty in giving and/or receiving; numb self to feeling (close chakra) or drown in sadness (stuck) (Goldman 1994, p. 143); collapsed chest area
5	Can speak with ease; when balanced with surrounding chakras ideas are connected to heart and mind/wisdom	Difficulty speaking and expressing ideas
6	Have access to inner wisdom, intuition	Disconnected from wisdom beyond the ego, "stuck in the head"
7	Easeful connection with nature, source, cosmos	Disconnected from sense of being a part of something bigger

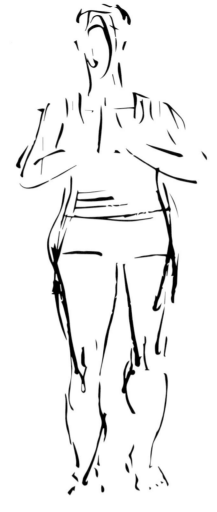

5 The Sun Salutation – Entering the Practice

The Practice, the Sun Salutation as Ritual

Daily practice of movement can be performed to connect with what is sacred in life. Practicing the Sun Salutation can be that special time to reconnect with your body and nature. Consciously feeling your breath as you move, and tuning in with awareness to the earth and other natural energies around you, are two ways to encourage this connection. Reaching the arms upwards can be reaching to connect with the sky, and acknowledging the sun, moon, and stars in the cosmos above, as you ground through your legs and feet attuning to your connection with the earth below. The sacred for you could include honoring animals. Some of the poses refer to animals, such as the cobra or dog, inspiring you to embody their movements or archetypal energies. The sacred

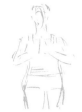

Chapter 5

connection of this practice could also be connected with community: connecting with the other hearts in the class, whether in person or online. This practice is a moment to pause from the other aspects of your life and simply be present with your body, as a moving meditation. When done regularly it becomes a ritual.

Rituals give us stability and continuity in our lives; they can foster a sense of peace and contentment. In addition this particular ritual has the potential to slow time down and give you not only greater health through increased embodiment, strength, and flexibility but also a deeper relationship with your experience of nature and the universe.

From the "somatic" vantage point of Dynamic Embodiment[SM] (DE[SM]), a ritual provides not only structure but also freedom to deviate by following movement experiences that you find satisfying. This could result in such adaptations as changing the specific form of the Sun Salutation or varying the timing of the practice. What is wonderful about ritualizing a practice is how it frees the mind, making more brain space available for self-reflection and learning. When doing something familiar the body has time to notice what is happening and also compare and contrast the status of how it felt on a different day or some time ago.

Preparation for Doing the Sun Salutation

Setting an intention can intensify mindfulness while practicing the Sun Salutation. These are themes that can help you set objectives or simply create a focused state of mind.

Key themes and inter-relationships:

- Moving through the Sun Salutation as restful experience

- Moving through the Sun Salutation to energize

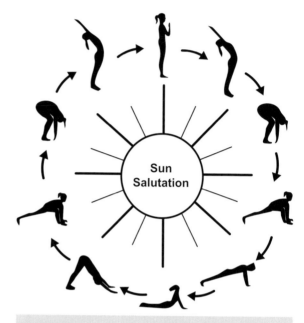

Figure 5.1
The Sun Salutation.

- Following your body wisdom – being true to yourself and your body (holding on to your personal authority)

- Accommodating/adjusting a given task to be loving toward your body

- Using props to enhance awareness – prioritize your comfort and pleasure

- Bringing in the feminine, through embodiment of the organs/contents/volume, three-dimensionality, and Laban's spaciousness vs being mostly linear and muscular

- Experiencing the glands in synergy – glands can support each other and you

- Relating conscious movement to understanding early childhood and how these developmental connections are serving throughout life. (See Chapter 6 for tips.)

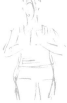

The Sun Salutation can also be a healing journey. To address spiritual, physical, and emotional balance and ease pain, take time to notice which of these processes strikes you in this moment. Which would you like to be working with? Consider these healing tools and inter-relationships:

- Breath, as organizer, which refuels the adrenals

- Gentleness, to calm the mind and be self-loving

- Flow, which means moving with ease from one pose to another; this quiet centering supports ease on the joints

- Embodiment, which starts with locating a part of the body and can involve safe and caring touch or picturing/visualizing of movement, allowing your mind to enter into the body to perceive its messages.

- Touch, which increases sensation. The somatosensory and motor cortices light up in correspondence with the part of the body being touched (Doidge 2007). Hence movement facilitated by touch (movement repatterning) helps increase capacity for consciousness while moving.

Integrating Glandular and Chakra Awareness into your Practice

Let's begin the Sun Salutation with glandular and developmental awareness cues: for those of you who have done this practice for a long time, there will be some new nuggets, and even a new lens through which to understand your practice. For those of you new to the Sun Salutation, this is a nice way to begin: these cues give you a strong scaffolding through which to enter the form.

Bringing glandular awareness into your practice brings in gentleness. You will find that this gentleness brings in ease throughout the body; and you will be surprised by the results on all levels – from transitions being more graceful, to finding more comfort in your body and actually being able to go deeper into the poses. Practicing this way has the short- and long-term benefits of balancing your endocrine system, and of you being in your body in a different, more three-dimensional way.

When you move through the Sun Salutation with developmental and glandular cues, you will be guided to feel your body in space in a new way. When you work with awareness of the glands you are able to contact a different aspect of energy flow that is established by spaciousness. Some of this comes from feeling your body move in two opposite directions to open up space for the glands. Other times it is through the pressure into the gland. When you work with developmental movement cues, you will experience your body in relationship to the floor, to the earth, in a manner that is grounding. Together, experience the benefits of compression and spaciousness throughout your body, in partnership with the floor and a feeling of how space supports you.

Work gently, at least at first. This is to get to know the movement and to experiment with the power of the glands and their energy. If you ease into the Sun Salutation you will be able to repeat it more and enjoy it more. In the next chapter you will learn more specific ideas from early infant movement practice that can (1) increase these compression and expansive connections through the body and, in turn, (2) support glandular activation. In Chapter 7 adaptive positions are provided for taking care of your body through improved posture and alignment, including ways to keep you moving after an injury or illness. Read it now if needed.

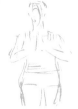

Chapter 5

Enjoy and titrate your experience – selecting just enough stimulus to keep your practice alive. You can choose to focus on keywords, specific poses, or anatomical concepts. Find below two guided experiences: (1) one with the glands as a focus and (2) one using a chakra and Bartenieff focus.

Note: Chart 5.1 follows this guided Sun Salutation experience; it may be helpful for you to look at this first, or use the two together.

Guided Sun Salutation

Start standing, feet hip width apart, arms at your sides, palms facing forward.

Take a moment to center and feel your feet touching the ground: make a connection to sky, connection to earth. With this action you can already feel the connection between the solar plexus and your feet by pushing off the floor upward into your diaphragm. This stimulates and integrates the pancreas.

Take three breaths in and out to center, and feel that connection and begin to activate all of the muscles from ankles to calves, quadriceps/hamstrings, as if plastic wrap was helping you engage/squeeze all the muscles from feet to waist. This is enhanced by moving the thoracobodies and supports rejuvenation of the adrenal glands.

From the waist upward, elongate your spine (feeling the mammillary bodies rise). This action is supported by the lower half of your body, which is actively engaged through the pancreas, while the upper half gently reaches for the sky, which is supported by clear breath entering the upper chest, and the upper breastbone moving with energy supported from the thymus.

 You are standing in **mountain pose**.

From mountain pose, bring hands into namaste (anjali mudra), and connect with your heart.

As you press your hands together feel the energy from behind the center of your breastbone, near your heart (including the heart bodies), into your wrists/palms. Allow the flow to power your connection but keep the musculature easy, relaxed. Add a nice breath in.

Then, slowly breathe out as you reach your arms up in front of you, at your center line, to over your head, remembering your thymus energy resonating in your upper breastbone. Feel it as a base for your shoulder girdle to reach from (supported by your center (adrenals) and feet (pancreas) as well, of course!).

 Arch gently back, into the spinal extension movement, repeating the **first backbend** of the practice maintaining pancreas, thymus, and adding mammillary activation.

Inhale, then exhale (from the thoracobody) and open arms wide as you fold forward from the hip joints in slow motion, perhaps bending at the knees, elongating at the spine, and reaching through the top of the head (using

 mammillary support-breathing, deeply smelling the air) as you come down into **uttanasana**, hanging, resting your adrenals on your thighs, as you breathe in and out. Bend and unbend the knees to help warm up the hamstrings. Rotate your thighs internally slightly to help open up the low back. Together these actions balance the adrenals. If you choose to feel a reach down into the floor with your heels as you straighten your knees by lifting your sit bones up, you can attune with thyroid energy.

While rising, inhale and reach forward with arms, hands, or fingertips placed on the ground or blocks in front of you (activating thymus, heart bodies, or pancreas). Lengthen your spine (all the head glands), feeling the breadth across your chest and the three-dimensionality of your torso, which can activate the thymus as long as you feel your breastbone (sternum) elongating and breathing.

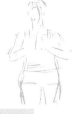

 Now exhale, as you reach your right foot back, with a counter-pull from your neck to include your parathyroid gland on that side, tips of toes pressed into the floor, now in **lunge.** Reach your right heel back as you reach your left knee forward, to increase your stretch or intensity of the pose. Relax your reach for a gentler pose. Note the nice stretch you are getting in your left psoas right now. The spine is long, chest wide, and shoulder blades are moving towards one another. It is the lengthening of one leg away from the body core that can help promote parathyroidal balancing. (Walking backwards with a big long stride is another option.)

Bring your hands flat on the floor, take a nice inhale in as you connect your wrists to your heart bodies, and reach your left foot (using right upper parathyroid support) back to join your right, coming into **downward dog** (feeling the push of your arms into your heart and the push of your feet into your pancreas). Your feet are hip width apart, your torso is long, and your legs are straight. Bend and straighten at the knees a few times to continue warming up the leg muscles, particularly your hamstrings with awareness of the adrenals. (Once warmed up, consider straightening both knees, and involving the thyroidal reach of both legs into the floor.) Breathe in and come up on your toes, sending your tailbone closer to the sky, which can activate the master gland, the pituitary. Now, keep your tailbone reaching for the sky in this way, maintaining your newfound length in your spine, as you slowly reach your heels back towards being flat on the floor (allowing for pituitary–thyroidal balancing).

Let your head hang. Bob your chin a few times to encourage a relaxed neck. You are upside down. If you actively reach your head to the ground, to stretch the muscles of the neck or

between the shoulder blades, you may feel mammillary activation, promoting perceptual alertness (including smell) and awareness of midline support for alignment.

Press your hands into the ground, checking to see if you can press each finger down with equal weight. Experience width across your palms. Breathe and connect into your heart region and heart bodies as you do this. Inhale, and glide your torso forward into plank pose; your torso is parallel to the ground. (You may add a reach of your head and even of your tail as you do this, stimulating the pituitary and the mammillary bodies.) Your arm strength is helping you to hover above the floor. Breathe in and out a few times here. Inhale and then, either holding your breath or exhaling, slowly lower knees, chest, and chin to touch the earth. The breath and folding of the body rejuvenate the adrenals. Inhale, and slide your heart and chest forward in between your hands into a gentle **cobra pose.** Palms are flat on the floor, chest is wide; reach your sternum forward as you relax your shoulders and move your shoulder blades closer together, all with thymus support. Exhale.

Inhale, and press your weight through your arms and hands into the ground as you send your hips up and back into **downward dog.** This time stay for five breaths, finding length in your spine as your tailbone reaches for the sky and your palms press into the ground. Heels reach for the floor. Downward dog combines balancing of four glands: the heart bodies by pushing back from the hands/wrists, the pancreas by pushing up to the sit bones and into the thoracic diaphragm from the two feet symmetrically. The interaction becomes a dance also including the thymus and thyroid, by feeling a simultaneous reach of two arms, and of both heels, into the floor, all the while also pushing from hands and feet toward your core.

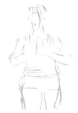

Chapter 5

Inhale. Lift your head up a bit and look forward (mammillary bodies); see the place on the mat where you are about to place your right foot. Exhale. Inhale. Now lift your right foot up off the ground (with parathyroid support), and sweep it forward, place your foot inside your left palm. Exhale. You are now in the opposite leg forward **lunge.** Pushing from the forward or back foot into the pelvic floor can activate the coccygeal body. Enjoy the enlivening of the pelvic floor as well. Enjoy the stretch. Bring in parathyroidal energy or imagery as you reach your right knee forward and your left heel back. Note the stretch in your left psoas. Keep the spine long and eyes forward.

Inhale, sending your left foot forward to join your right. Feel the push of your feet up into the solar plexus with aliveness through the pancreas as you unroll or use a flat back hinge at the ilio-femoral joint. Exhale. Inhale, and reach the top of your head forward using mammillary curiosity – sniffing or breathing fully; it will help you find more length in your spine.

 Exhale, and fold at your hips, finding your way back into **uttanasana.** Your neck is relaxed; your head is upside down. Breathe in and out as you press each toe into the ground. Feel the idea of condensing back to center here – an adrenal reprieve as we gather; whether in an elongated stretch state or a folded relaxed state, one connects with the glands, the muscles, the organs, the fluids.

Inhale, and reach your arms wide like wings, collar bones wide, as you upwards swan dive. This can be a quintessential thymus-leading activity. However you prefer to rise, come up to standing, and then to whatever extent you can, allow your upper arms to come up by your head, as fingertips touch above. Decide if you want to gently arch backwards into a backbend.

 Exhale, and come back to center, hands coming together into **anjali mudra** or prayer pose.

Fingertips touch. If you press your palms together you will stimulate the heart region. If you feel a strong push from your hands into the body core you can activate the heart bodies.

Let your eyes close. Take a few moments to feel the effects of this practice on your mind/your thinking, your heart/your emotions, your body, and your connection with Spirit. And anything else you might notice.

After absorbing the experience, it is time to do the other side. *One Sun Salutation is actually a set of two.* On this first Sun Salutation you reached forward and back into the lunge poses with your right foot. For the second, the only difference is when you move into lunge pose, step back with your left foot. And when you step forward again into lunge after your second downward dog, you reach forward with your left foot. These partnered versions also ensure balanced activity to each of the upper parathyroids and to the coccygeal/perineal bodies.

Welcome if this was your first Sun Salutation!

Whether new or experienced with this movement ritual, invite this guidance and knowledge to enrich your practice and your life.

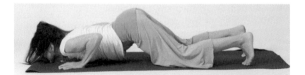

Figure 5.2
Knees – chest – chin, Ashtanga Namaskara, salute with the eight limbs. Photo by Serge Cashman.

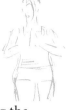

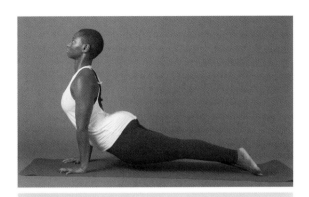

Figure 5.3
Reach through top of the head, mammillary; reach through the arms, thymus. Photo by Serge Cashman.

Next practice the Sun Salutation initiating the lunge with the other side, and focus on chakras and Bartenieff Fundamentals.

A circle of interaction between Bartenieff and Bainbridge Cohen led to the lines of connection depicted in Figures 5.4 and 5.5. Bartenieff planted the seed of the scapula–finger connections. Based on her exploration of the scapula–finger relationships introduced by Bartenieff, Bainbridge Cohen identified refined musculo-skeletal connections matching specific fingers to specific parts of the scapulae. Using these images can strengthen your Sun Salutation as you take weight into your hands or reach out into space with your arms.

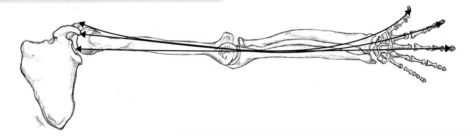

Figure 5.4
Fingers to scapula connections – front view. An interactive influence between Bartenieff's general idea that relating the fingers to the scapula would support movement efficiency was refined by Bainbridge Cohen to include specific correlations between each finger and each part of the scapula. These are taught in both the Laban/Bartenieff and the Body-Mind Centering® systems now. Drawing by Marghe Mills-Thysen, Certified Teacher of BMC and Feldenkrais Practitioner.

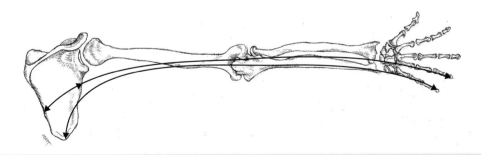

Figure 5.5
Fingers to back of scapula – back view (depicts index to acromion process, middle to socket, ring to blades of scapula and pinky to wing). Drawing by Marghe Mills-Thysen.

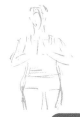
Guided Sun Salutation with Chakra and Bartenieff Fundamentals Cues

Standing – feel the heel–sit bone connection and find your breath support. Sense your pelvic floor; see and sense lines of energy, like roots, moving down through your legs to the earth. Breathe energy back from the earth up into your feet, legs, and hips. See red light filling your 1st chakral area.

Reach your arms up over your head, by lowering your shoulder blades toward your sacrum as you stretch your fingers up. Now arch back gently while feeling the connection between your tail and head. Breathe blue light into your throat and the back of your neck, activating your throat chakra.

Bending – feel your head–tail connection as you fold at the hip joint; reach from your tail up through your third eye and crown as you float downwards into a forward bend (bend your knees if that helps you get more range of motion at your hips). You may keep your spine expanded or condensed – long or curled in as you like.

Lunge back, this time reaching your left foot back – find your heel–sit bone connection with each leg to help with grounding. Breathe into the fullness of your torso, flooding your solar plexus and kidneys with yellow light for three breaths, activating your 3rd chakra.

Downward dog – feel your hand to shoulder blade (scapula) connection. You may focus on the pressure from each finger into different parts of the scapula.

For five breaths, breathe into your 2nd chakra at your belly, and exhale through your heart. You may find that this softens the torso.

Plank – make sure your arms are connected to your back – meaning your scapular muscles are engaged toward your spine and toward your sacrum; establish clear tensile support through the rest of your body. Do this by feeling the length from your head to your tail and from your sit bones to your heel, all lined up parallel to the ground. Then feel the tensile energy of the counter-pull from heels to head.

Fold knee–chest–chin – keep your shoulder blades connected to your sacrum by sliding them down your back as you fold into this position.

Upward dog/cobra – experience a rocking from feet to top of head. Breathe green light into your heart. Feel the fullness across your chest as you hug your elbows towards your sides.

Downward dog – feel your superficial muscles stretch as the deeper muscles engage in the core for core support.

Lunge forward, reaching your left foot forward – find the breath support for contracting the psoas to bring the leg forward. Allow your hands to expand outward to enhance your balance.

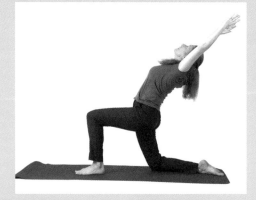

Figure 5.6
Lunge with parathyroid support for reach. Photo by Serge Cashman.

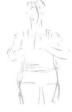

 Stepping into the folded low central stance, allow your upper body to shape into a curve to allow your knee to fit between your hands.

Coming up – feel all connections – heels to sit bones, tail to head with freedom in the hip socket, sacrum to scapula, and scapula to fingertips.

 Arch – continue all of the above into an arched spine.

Ending – allow your breath to expand your chest as you feel your hands compress into the heart region, keeping your shoulders released downward with the scapula to sacrum connection.

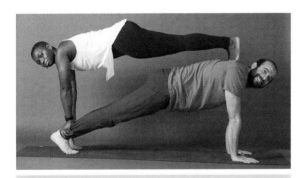

Figure 5.7
Playful spirit in integrative plank. Photo by Serge Cashman.

Some Key Variations/ Recommendations for the Sun Salutation

 • Please bend your knees as much as you need to feel comfortable at any time. This is to prioritize the ability to lengthen the spine. If your hamstrings are tight during downward dog, bending your knees can help you keep the spine fully elongated.

• You may always choose to move your arms out to the side in back bend and folding over (versus stretched up over your head and forward – sagittal).

• Play with your chin and mouth leading spinal flexion and extension versus the eyes – this gives the eyes a break. You can also initiate from the top of your head as another option. Each focus point will feel different on your neck and spine.

• If you are invigorated and your joints seem resilient, feel free to jump forward or back. Use this choice to jump with both legs symmetrically in and out of plank or downward dog once you are warmed up – jumping brings in vitality of muscles, focus, and strength.

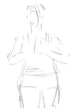

Chapter 5

Chart 5.1		
Reviewing the Ritual – Describing the Sun Salutation in Everyday Language with Body-Mind Centering® Concepts		
Engaging in the Sun Salutation Using some BMC Language		

	Mountain Tadasana	Allow the weight of the pelvis to drop into the flesh of the feet and then push up from the feet into the solar plexus (pancreas), creating space in the lower back and breath in the upper torso (thoracobody).
	Anjali Mudra	Bring the palms together (heart bodies).
	Backward Bend Thru – Urdhva Hastasana	Extend the spine into a small backbend as you arch back (with care to not pinch nerves or compress too much) with a choice of any variations on the use of the arms reaching sidewards, or forward and up (thymus).
	Process Forward Bend	Lengthening from the top of the head (mammillary bodies), bend forward; flex clearly at the ilio-femoral joint, also known as the acetabular–femoral joint or hip joint.
	Arrival Uttanasana	Flex the spine, release the head until inverted, folding over the thigh with the head near the legs (adrenal relaxation)… moving the hands towards the floor. It is okay to bend the knees.
	Right Lunge (Ardha-Alana) back	Keeping a clear contact with the stable leg, feel the push of each leg back up to your pelvis – up into the hip socket on that side (coccygeal) as you reach the other leg back (parathyroid support) into a long, low step.
	Downward Dog – Adho Mukha Svanasana	Second leg steps back. Then flex clearly from the hip joint with the sit bones and tail reaching up and back, while pressing from the hands towards the sacrum/hips. This makes a triangle between the two hands and sacrum; as that push becomes clear let it continue into a reach of the tail (stimulating the pituitary) so the tail uncurls and is also connected from the push of the hands into reaching fully, with the tail making a triangle of forces between the arms and tail.
	Plank	Keep level to the floor instead of arching upward and hold a posture on elbows or hands, feeling the legs reach backwards (thyroid).

(continued)

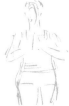

Chart 5.1 (*continued*)	
Reviewing the Ritual – Describing the Sun Salutation in Everyday Language with Body-Mind Centering® Concepts	
Engaging in the Sun Salutation Using some BMC Language	
Knee–Chest–Chin (see Fig. 5.2)	Begin to lead with the head with support of active engagement from the feet to the head – another important triangle – and then lower the chest and chin (stretch of thyroid while relaxing adrenals).
Cobra	Push from the tail (carotid) to move the thymus and breast bone further forward with the senses of the head active (head glands).
Upward Dog Urdhva Mukha Svanasana	Variations: straighten arms, keep legs active as you raise hips, pressing into tops of feet, hug elbows towards torso, rotate inner thighs to ceiling to protect low back, move sternum forward and up, maintain length in back of neck, be mindful to protect wrists. Blocks recommended.
Downward Dog	Repeat as above.
Right leg steps forward	Reverse action described above – this time reach the knee and foot through the swing of the legs.
Uttanasana (Forward Bend)	Flex the spine; release the head until inverted, folding over the thigh with the head near the legs (adrenal relaxation), moving the hands towards the floor. It is okay to bend the knees. Relax, breathe out, allow for adrenal renewal time.
Return to center (Urdhva Hastasana) and Backward Bend	Find grounding and integrity – the desire to be upright and face the world. Bring compassion into this moment as the arms are activated and repeat the deep spinal extension with thymus support.
Mountain Tadasana	Allow the weight of the pelvis to drop into the flesh of the feet and then push up from the feet into the solar plexus (pancreas), creating space in the lower back and breath in the upper torso.
Anjali Mudra	Bring the palms together (heart bodies). Rest for a moment. Be aware of the position of your feet on the floor, the state of your heart and your mind. Prepare to begin the other side, this time stepping from the left leg back into lunge, then the left leg forward into the second lunge, ending here in Anjali Mudra after you have done the second side.

Learn more about the gonads and pubic bone connection to support the lower back in cobra. See also low back section in Chapter 7.

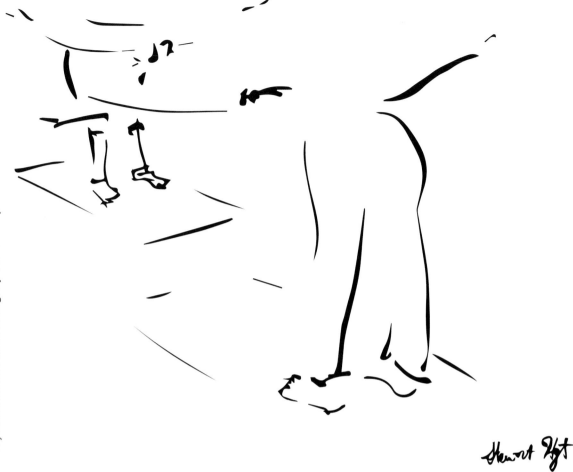

Thymus/heart bodies soaring, by Stewart Hoyt

6 Developmental Movement and the Sun Salutation

This chapter explains how the "developmental patterns" of early infancy relate to engaging with the glands in each pose. Dynamic Embodiment[SM] (DE[SM]) believes that the practice of the Sun Salutation is enriched by the developmental aspect of the DE knowledge. This DE focus on early childhood movement stems from the Body-Mind Centering® (BMC®) understanding of conception, embryology, birth and infant movements, and the Bartenieff idea that each of these patterns of movement can be seen in adult non-verbal and expressive behavior. BMC teaches us how deep postural support evolves from healthy digestive processes, sensitivity to symmetrical and asymmetrical patterns, and the power of infant, childhood, and adult maintenance of equal joint space – taking care to not compress any areas unnecessarily.

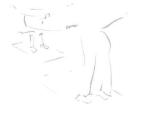

Chapter 6

Body-Mind Centering® Approach to Neuromotor Development

In BMC most of the developmental movement patterns are performed on our bellies or rolling, and then on the hands and knees until, if possible, on the feet. These movements are practiced in a specific order to reintroduce how most humans learned to come to standing or upright posture. BMC calls these identifiable and shared patterns that are common to most people *Basic Neurocellular Patterns* (BNP). These BNP form the baseline for lifting the head and, if possible, rolling, crawling, sitting, creeping on all fours, standing, and walking.

BMC and Bartenieff approaches to early childhood movement also consider how movement is a form of brain stimulation. All movement coordination emerges during the first year of life, calling on different combinations of brain activation. The entire nervous system, which is pervasive, ever-changing, and relational, engages through the alternation of paying attention to body cues, environmental cues, emotional desires, and mental goals. Each of these sensations results in motor responses that need to be experienced to become automatic. This begins early on through reflexive responses, and then through exploration and play becomes a toolbox of choices that allow for volitional actions.

Body-Mind Centering®'s Basic Neurocellular Patterns (BNP)

Vibration/Cellular Breathing/Sponging/Pulsation

Navel radiation

Mouthing

Prespinal

Spinal push from the head

Spinal push from the tail

Spinal reach from the head (Fig. 6.1)

Spinal reach from the tail (Fig. 6.2)

Push of two arms (homologous) (Fig. 6.3)

Push of two legs (homologous)

Reach of two arms (homologous)

Reach of two legs (homologous)

Push of one arm and then the other (homolateral)

Push of one leg and then the other (homolateral)

Reach of one arm and then the other (contralateral)

Reach of one leg and then the other (contralateral) (Fig. 6.4)

Prevertebrate and Vertebrate Patterns

In the list in the box the first movements are activations of energy, first starting in the whole body, that then begin to differentiate, in the embryo and then the fetus. These are considered prevertebrate patterns because they do not involve bones. Beginning with the spinal push of the head, bones are involved – in this case the cranium and spinal column.

Even before the School for Body-Mind Centering began to deeply investigate embryology, studies had already included prenatal movement, and even some embryological movements. Vibration, cellular breathing, sponging, and pulsation are actions that are part of embryological life. Breathing exists at the moment of conception and involves cellular

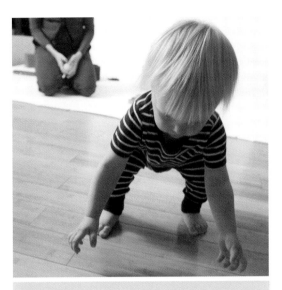

Figure 6.1
Spinal reach from the head. Photo by Serge Cashman.

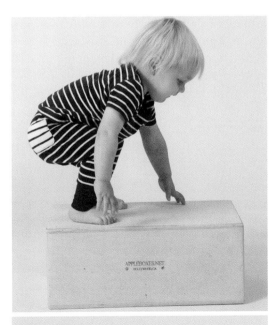

Figure 6.2
Spinal reach from the tail. Photo by Serge Cashman.

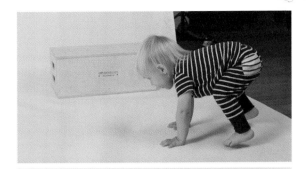

Figure 6.3
Push of two arms. Photo by Serge Cashman.

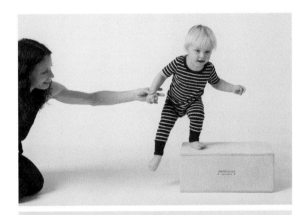

Figure 6.4
Reach of one leg. Photo by Serge Cashman.

breathing – the give and take of nutrients at the cell membrane. (Later in life, breath is taken in through the nose or mouth as "external respiration" – using all five lobes of the lungs as well as each of the diaphragms of the body (the crura); see Figure 7.3 for how these tendons can extend into the pelvic bowl. In fetal cellular breathing, the blood is supplied through the baby's navel to every cell; this was named navel radiation, distributing equal energy to each part of the body – the head, tail, arms, and legs. Mouthing is the coordination of movement to suck, also practiced *in utero*, that also activates the digestive tract (and its glandular

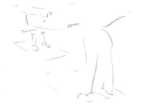

Chapter 6

function). The notochord and then the spinal cord are also soft tissue – the spine without the spinal column. Each of these body parts has movement qualities that are different from the types of movements humans have once bones and muscles are fully developed and interacting with gravity.

Yield & Push, Reach & Pull

One of the unique contributions of BMC is an analysis of how each baby movement just before birth and after birth is performed using actions that involve pushing and/or reaching. This differentiation of movement types is at the heart of the "BMC developmental consciousness." Bones are levers that push other bones. Muscles are pulleys that pull bones while expanding and contracting body parts.

History

Bonnie Bainbridge Cohen learned much about neurodevelopmental constructs when she studied in Europe with the physiotherapists Dr Karel and Berta Bobath, and from her childhood and young adult experiences with dance. Berta Bobath, physiotherapist, developed the "Bobath Concept," now known as NeuroDevelopmental Therapy. It was the Bobaths' work with reflexes, righting reactions and equilibrium responses, that Bainbridge Cohen studied and took further. Perhaps her training as a Laban Movement Analyst with Bartenieff helped her see directionality and initiation of movement more clearly in order to determine the difference between a push versus a reach & pull. She also recognized that, in order to push off a surface to travel, one must first connect with the surface. She calls this connection "yielding," as it usually involves releasing body weight into gravity while also feeling the support of the receiving surface. Similarly, she

identified how, in order to move through a large space, reaching and pulling is supported by a push. To move one's center of weight the reaching action must be followed by a pull that moves the full body to the new spot. Yield supports pushing while reaching is supported by pushing. Reaching is best followed by a pull in order to complete a weight transference. In 1991 Martha Eddy described this process in the following words:

Defining yield, push, reach, and pull (and grasp and absorb): "A push pattern is a movement that travels from one part of the body through the core of the body, usually deriving its impetus from interaction with (pushing away from) another surface (the floor, the uterine cervix, another person). For example, a spinal push from the head begins at the head and sequences tailward. Push patterns give the body a compressed feeling. This compression reinforces a bodily sense of self and provides as well an experience of support from the environment. This is entirely different from pushing something (or someone else) away.

A reach pattern is most efficient if it follows a clear experience of pushing. It travels from one part of the body outward into space, pulling along the rest of the body as a follow-through of the movement. For example, a spinal reach of the head initiates with the head and often leads to a change of level for the entire body, or at least an elongation out into space. Reach and pull patterns give the body an expansive feeling. They increase one's kinesphere and serve to make connections with the environment (including other people).

Some years later it became important to discuss what the baby was pushing away from and how it made enough contact in order to be able to then separate. What does it take to effectively push oneself away? It is important to give in at times, to yield, feel supported by gravity, weight sense, before activating a strong weight. This

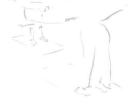

learned strength allows the ability to extend away from this contact. This statement is full of metaphors that are keystones in the developmental relational process. The pull is the culmination of the reach. The reach is an extension into space that takes you out into the environment, often destablizing your center of weight. The pull regathers you to land safely in the next place. Each of these four processes [yield to push to reach and pull] is critical to be able to apply effectively for different desired actions or in relationships. There are two important factors in understanding the role of yield and push, and reach and pull in development: (1) 'yield and push' underlies 'reach and pull,' and (2) when initiating with one limb, a well-executed push thrusts through the body homolaterally (compression through body tissues of one side of the body – right foot to right arm or left arm through to left leg), while a well-executed reach of one limb brings out a muscular cross-lateral connection (activating a diagonal kinetic chain)" (reprinted in Eddy 2015, pp. 23–24).

Once born, babies no longer float in the protection of the uterine fluid but deal more directly with gravity. Movement becomes relational through all the surfaces of the skin plus through all the tissues of the body, no longer buoyed up by liquid (except as a cellular memory, which of course has a huge level of potency). One can rest into these real or remembered environments (floors, furniture, and walls, or uterus or memory of it). As newborns and through infancy into adulthood we can then push off from our surroundings to move our bodies away. This push can support extending further out into the world when followed by reaching – often an expression of wanting something. Finally the reach can complete itself in a pull, as in reaching out for a hug, stepping forward and pulling oneself or the other person into this embrace (Eddy 2015).

In more recent years Bainbridge Cohen has incorporated other phases of a movement. Grasping and absorbing are also important. You may want to explore yield–push–reach–grasp–pull–absorb.

Your Experience

With practice you can take note of when you are:

- yielding – connecting with the earth or another supporting surface by releasing your weight fully: embodied resting

- pushing – feel the yield and then use it to push away, allowing yourself to be propelled in space, often in order to separate or move away

- reaching – extending out toward something, often with desire

- grasping – choosing to connect with something, holding it, and anchoring

- pulling – once anchored in some way to the space beyond the body's boundary, use it to move the body through space (to locomote, whether on our feet, our forelegs, or in a wheelchair)

- absorb – taking time to digest the experience, to notice where you have gotten to. Recognizing: recognizing that you have arrived.

With this knowledge you can discern if the chosen movement is the most efficient action for the task or expressive movement at hand. This principle of types of initiation of movement (yield & push, or grasp & reach & pull, then absorb) varies in how each person comes into relative uprightness in the first 24 months after conception. The patterns developed in childhood can often still be reflected in adulthood.

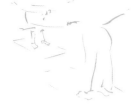

Chapter 6

For movement to be learned, to be a choice versus a reflex, takes practice. Once learned, practice also allows movement skills to become refined. Picture an infant transitioning into a toddler ... the walk is not yet steady or smooth. That level of coordination takes practice over time. This is true all life long. These patterns can feel optimal or suboptimal. The concept of movement repatterning or re-education in somatic movement supports gaining awareness of movement habits in order to make choices about how you move today, with an understanding that patterns are based on repeated practices from earlier phases of life (Eddy 2016). Your own current sensations of posture and movement are what are important to track in order to learn more about past and present.

Martha's Personal Story: Tuning into Glands Stimulated by "Baby Movements"

As part of studies within Body-Mind Centering®, Bonnie Bainbridge Cohen shared a system of interaction between glands and joints. The work was initially derived by Bonnie from her yoga experience and exploration of Alice Bailey's insights, and further researched deeply through BMC embodiment practices. Those of us studying or teaching with the School for BMC in the 1970s were part of the empirical research team who "felt into" a gland and explored how each related to specific bones and joints. We all shared what in the body was resonating for us. As a profoundly insightful person and perhaps because she is a Laban Movement Analyst, Bainbridge Cohen got specific – what is initiating each movement, the gland or the bone? And what did we feel as relationships between them? The developmental movement, full of neurocellular connectivity, was a key to these interconnections. A case in point in the 1980s was whether the reach

of the arms or the legs related more to the thyroid or to the thymus. It continues to be a dialogue and it includes the joints. Fellow students, clients, and faculty weigh in to verify somatic BMC investigations. The community settled on the experience that the thymus is related to reaching from the arms and the thyroid to the reach of the legs.

Bartenieff Fundamentals – Finding Comfortable Ways to Practice Baby Movement

Exploring these early childhood movement patterns can sometimes be impossible or uncomfortable to do. Modifications are always an option. Being more disability-sensitive and integrative of all senses versus being visually dominant can help. The Bartenieff Fundamentals teach how these patterns of bodily organization exist inside other movements. For instance, they can be done on the back surface of the body (a supine position) or in sitting or standing. Bartenieff Fundamentals provide language that matches the developmental progression of BMC's BNP, using more everyday words: breath, core–distal, head–tail, upper–lower, body halves, and diagonal or cross-lateral movement.

The Bartenieff aspect of the DE work further establishes the early childhood concept of interconnectivity, especially between the core of the body and each of the limbs, and its relevance for older children and adults. In exploring sound and movement from the navel center or body core through each of the six limbs, integrated awareness and action are practiced. The Laban/Bartenieff perspective furthers an understanding of the value of transposing in space the early neuromotor connections developed on the floor. The Sun Salutation's body organization occurs at many levels and directions in

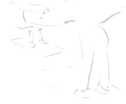

space, and moves through a developmental progression (see Chart 5.1 and related box).

DE also integrates Bartenieff Fundamentals in the following way: by learning how to derive musculoskeletal support from breath, proper weight shifts, and maintaining awareness of connections between key body parts – sit bones to heels, head to tail, shoulder blade to fingers, as learned in the context of neuromotor development as well. Neuroendocrine support and activation can be achieved by using all of the above concepts.

This DE approach recognizes that there is no one type of body or movement performance that is "normal" but that all bodies are different. The early infant motor development process exists for all people, including those with disabilities. All people develop differently. Much is to be learned from all types of bodies and abilities. There is no one normal way to develop or move. Each person is unique and so is the developmental process. The "conception to death" journey is individual and culturally influenced. DE honors this diversity and seeks to find language for this.

For everyone, movement efficiency is an outcome of practicing developmental movement at any stage in life based on whatever is possible. Early movement is shaped by breath patterns and informed by the *in utero* experience of being "grounded"/attached to our oxygen supply via our umbilicus as a life-giving support. DE embraces the idea that finding support for each movement enhances movement experience.

Practice, Practice, Practice

Without time to explore diverse activities in different contexts, it is also possible to not get enough practice to strengthen certain muscle groups or find healthy posture. This is true of babies when put in a seated posture before crawling, before the spine is well supported by the muscular development that comes from movement. If that is one's own infant experience, the spine may still need to be strengthened in later years, as a child, a teen, an adult, or an elder. The body can learn at any stage in life, although as life experience expands over time, there is a need to break down habits first, before finding and embedding new experiences through practice.

Practice is especially needed if one "skipped" a pattern (or two) as young children. A pattern can be skipped because of our genetics, birth experience, or siblings and having busy parents – for instance, they can be busy or overwhelmed, or just get excited and encourage us to learn how to walk before naturally ready. Spending time on the belly or all fours strengthens our abdominals and teaches us spatial tensegrity from the head to the tail. The related skills of compression and suspension are critical to transfer to uprightness as adults. Time on the floor also "integrates" various motor reflexes. If we are positioned upright too soon it is important to practice these movements later in life. The Sun Salutation provides time on the floor, including rising up and lowering down – what a ten-month-old spends time doing repeatedly. Another reason to practice developmental movement is when too much time was spent on devices, much like adults spending too much time in chairs. When not given enough time on the floor to explore gravity and strengthen in relationship to it, young children may not develop adequate abdominal strength and bodily integration to support healthy posture and efficient movement.

Variations, Yoga, and Connections to Animals

You can practice these BNPs with different imagery and dynamics. You may find that you

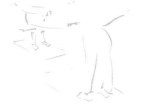

can ooze like amoebas, or wiggle or wriggle from the spine to awaken the core of the body. While in a prone position (face down toward the floor) one can discover the power of the symmetrical use of the arms or legs, crawl like lizards with a side-to-side emphasis, and come to sit and creep like babies or mammals. Similar to many yoga asanas, these movements echo our animal roots. For instance, the cobra includes a spinal reach of the head, like a snake. Upward dog can be evocative of a frog – with two arms pushing as the head reaches. Downward dog could be a base for beginning to crawl like a bear. There are many other examples. Fun for children!

Bringing in the Glands

For the purposes of practicing the Sun Salutation with the support of the glands, now focus on the patterns that involve the skeletal involvement of the body, beginning with the spinal push of the head.

What is the purpose of studying developmental movement and combining it with the Sun Salutation?

How babies are positioned in their mothers' wombs may impact how they fare at birth and how the first 14 months of each baby's *ex-utero* life proceeds. Likewise, the birth journey and the environment and relational influences on an infant all affect postural and kinesthetic development. These experiences can then impact the rest of one's development through the lifespan.

While each person is unique and has specific genetic imprints, humans are also socialized into certain movements, forming habits based on life experience. People often fall into the automaticity of these habits by constantly practicing the same movements in the same way. Developmental movement knowledge and practice can help bring consciousness to habits,

or change them to improve efficiency. There are three significant points to highlight here:

1. Practicing BMC's BNP of embryology and motor development, whether as an infant, a child, or an adult, is grounding because these movements involve getting reacquainted with the floor and experiencing support.

2. BMC's BNP also integrate with perceptual development and can be mind-brain opening.

3. The endocrine glands are stimulated by movement during infancy and continue to be activated by these specific coordination patterns from babyhood throughout the lifespan.

4. One can stimulate the correlated gland in various ways.

5. Neuroendocrine activation is found by using specific "tensile" or "compressional" relationships within the developmental movement patterns, which helps settle the body, potentially because they organize the "chaos of hormonal activity."

Next, the Sun Salutation is analyzed from a developmental, neuromotor perspective using DE's combination of BMC and Bartenieff Fundamentals (developmental organization) cueing. In BMC, the BNP are postulated to correlate with a specific gland. Glandular balancing involves becoming more aware of these musculo-skeletal actions from early infant movements. In order to integrate the support of the glands there is particular awareness of the LMA/DE concept of counter-tensions (counter-pulls) that create experiences of spaciousness and lightness. These have a direct impact on the skeletal system as well.

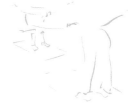

Focusing on the Joints and Glands

When one is being guided through yoga poses, especially from a DE approach, another key connection is often made – the connection between the glands and the chakras and each of the joints. The idea is that there is a type of resonation of energy from the glands outward to specific joints. BMC has created a sophisticated map of these interconnections by observing infants, exploring these movements and studying the progression of this perceptual motor development.

Infants and toddlers are using diverse levers (bones) and stances as they explore developmental movement. Engaging in life requires movement for relating to people, locomoting toward desires and curiosities, and balancing on smaller and smaller surfaces (from belly to the feet). When weight bearing, whether kneeling or standing, bones put pressure onto the joint. This pressure can come from compounded weightedness or through elongating into space. Meanwhile, the tendons pull on the joints. These sensations in the joints are first stimulated by specific developmental movement patterns, which also have a fulcrum of compression or tensile stretching into specific glands and joints. Once you embody the inter-relationship between glands, joints and movements, it becomes more clear that these are resources for bringing ease to each asana and heightening awareness of chakral energy.

Chart 6.1			
Understanding Gland–Chakral–Joint Relationships: What Joints Are Impacted?			
Chakra #	Location of Chakra	The Endocrine Glands/ Bodies Clustered by Chakras	Related Joints and Senses (from Body-Mind Centering®) – Dynamic Embodiment℠ Embraces this Hypothesis
1	Base of Spine	1: Coccygeal body	Hip joints – ilio-femoral = pelvic–femoral or acetabular–femoral joints
2	Lower	2: Gonads – ovaries/testes	Ankles, forelegs, arches of feet
3	Middle	3–5: Adrenals, pancreas, and thoracobodies	Lower back, pelvic, sacro-iliac, lower back and knees, fingers/hands and toes/feet, and sternal
4	Chest	6–7: Thoracobody, heart bodies, and thymus	Sternal, carpal, shoulders, wrists and elbows
5	Neck	8–10: Thyroid and parathyroid and carotid bodies	Neck, ribs, and hyoid bone
6	Head	11–12: Pituitary and mammillary bodies	Seeing and smelling/taste
7	Crown	13: Pineal gland	Hearing

(Source of Gland–Joint Relationships: B. Bainbridge Cohen, M. Mills (1980). Developmental movement therapy. Sebastopol, CA: Mills–Thysen.)

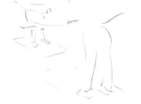

Chapter 6

Working with the glands or chakras also can support skeletal and joint functioning.

In yoga classes, ancient yoga practices are cited saying that the pose resonates energy outward to nearby joints. Body-Mind Centering® and its derivative programs like Dynamic Embodiment^SM have been exploring chakral/glandular relationships to specific joints and postulate the following relationships:

Joint Relationships from an Endocrine Gland Perspective

As Chart 6.1 outlines, the extended BMC community has explored, researched, and embodied glands and discovered supportive correlations between a gland, a movement, and joints. From this BMC perspective, an important resource is the movement most likely experienced as infants (or some variation on it) and the way each "developmental movement pattern" resonates with the glands and a related joint. The list in the box shows these relationships between developmental patterns and glands (Bainbridge Cohen 1992, 2003, 2018, 2021).

As described in the box, DE also works with the neuromotor coordination patterns as stimulants for the glands. In Chart 1.1 each Basic Neurocellular Pattern (BNP), as named by Bonnie Bainbridge Cohen, or Neuromotor Developmental Coordination (NDC), the term from DE, relates to glands and in turn to specific joints as well. To make this connection to glands and joints, focus on the following:

Movement coordination is learned through the brain, from varying how the body travels through space – wriggling as newborns, rolling and lizard crawling, coming to sitting (this is a level change, which involves traveling upward), quadrupedal creeping (typically called crawling), standing, and

Body-Mind Centering®'s Basic Neurocellular Developmental Patterns (BNPs) Correlated with Glands and Joints

Respiration – thoracobody

Navel radiation – adrenal

Spinal push from the head – pineal

Spinal push from the tail – carotid

Spinal reach from the head – mammillary

Spinal reach from the tail – pituitary

Push of two arms – heart bodies

Push of two legs – pancreas (islets of Langerhans)

Reach of two arms – thymus

Reach of two legs – thyroid

Push of one arm (and then the other) – gonads

Push of one leg (and then the other) – coccygeal

Reach of one arm (and then the other) – parathyroid

Reach of one leg (and then the other) – parathyroid

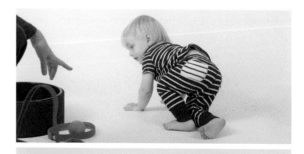

Figure 6.5
Hunter changing levels. Photo by Serge Cashman.

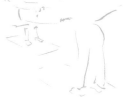

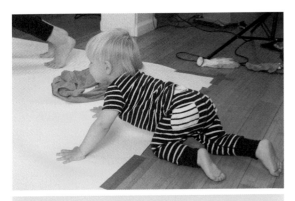

Figure 6.6
Crawling on all fours with active head–tail connection. Photo by Serge Cashman.

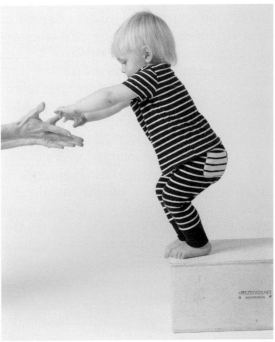

Figure 6.7
Symmetrical reach for mother's hands. Photo by Serge Cashman.

toddling. Each of these movements is coordinated with also having fulcrums into different areas of the body. This is where the pressure of gravity helps to stabilize movement. It is also why babies rock – stimulating the area. Once it has strengthened in place the internal body part can become a support for moving through space. BMC has correlated these specific movements with specific glands.

Bringing in the Gland–Joint Connection

Why does the DE system focus on the joints? Joints are where movement comes into play! Posture and movement may be improved by bringing awareness to the balanced use of the joints. This BMC principle is called "maintaining equal joint space." Laban's Space Harmony supports being spatially precise about movement choices. This precision helps clarify connections between joints and glands.

What is exciting about BMC's neuroendocrine movement awareness is the construct that both the brain and the glands are activated by the BNP.

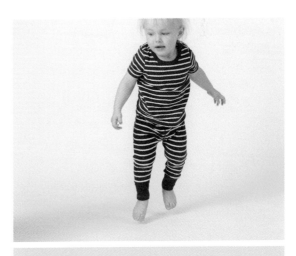

Figure 6.8
Navel radiation. Photo by Serge Cashman.

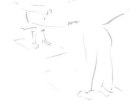

Chapter 6

The BMC theory is that the glands have a particular impact on the joints. DE integrates other systems discussing the crystalline aspects of the joints that are emergent through the fascia (Tensegrity) deriving from the work of Maurice Vogel (Burnham 2020) (see p. 88). Through lived experience the following relationships have been explored by thousands of somatic practitioners for over fifty years and found to be meaningful guides.

In this next boxed list the connection is made between each of the actions initiated from different body parts (diaphragmatic and cellular breathing, the navel, the head, the tail, the arms, the legs, or a single arm or leg) and specific glands.

Neurocellular Developmental Patterns with Glands and Joints

Respiration – thoracobody – sternum and diaphragm

Navel radiation – adrenal – sacro-iliac and knees

Spinal push from the head – pineal – occiput/back of skull/hearing

Spinal push from the tail – carotid – spinal vertebrae, hyoid, temporo-mandibular joint/jaw

Spinal reach from the head – mammillary – middle skull/smell/taste

Spinal reach from the tail – pituitary – anterior skull/eyes and orbit/intervertebral

Push of two arms – heart bodies – wrists/radius and ulna

Push of two legs – pancreas – head–tail, feet–toes, and hands–fingers

Reach of two arms – thymus – shoulder/acromioclavicular

Reach of two legs – thyroid – sterno-clavicular and sterno-costal/elbows/vocal diaphragm

Push of one arm (and then the other) – gonads – ankles and tibio-fibular/pelvic floor

Push of one leg (and then the other) – coccygeal – hip sockets/pubic symphysis

Reach of one arm (and then the other) – parathyroid – ribs, costo-vertebral

Reach of one leg (and then the other) – parathyroid – ribs, costo-vertebral

This section provides a prose description of the charts and lists above. In this scenario the lowest gland/chakra is first. This is important for grounding, particularly if embodying them while standing up. If one starts these various glandular stimulation exercises with the head glands without having the head on the floor, one might feel faint.

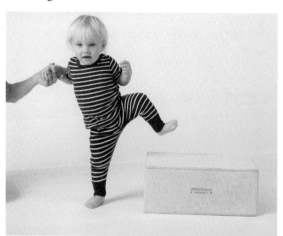

Figure 6.9
Body half, standing, pushing into root chakra, coccygeal body. Photo by Serge Cashman.

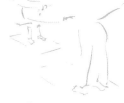

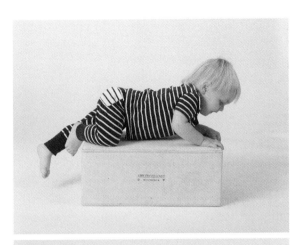

Figure 6.10
Body half, crawling. Photo by Serge Cashman.

The *coccygeal* body, together with the support of the perineal body in the center of the pelvic floor, "governs" the vitality of each hip joint and the pelvis. The gland can be stimulated by pushing from the foot through each of the joints of the leg into the hip joint – right into the acetabula (the hip socket) on that side.

The *gonads* "govern" the ankles and forelegs, and are stimulated by a movement on the belly where you push the arm on the same side to move the entire body backwards in space – known as the homolateral push of one arm (causing a lateral curve of spine).

The *adrenals* govern the navel region, as well as the femur, knees, and sacro-iliac joints, and are stimulated by activation of the entire body around the navel center – movement in and away from the core of the body.

The *pancreas* is at the center of a fully stretched out body. The pancreas governs the hands and feet, along with the extension of the spine between the head and the tail. The gland is stimulated by the push of two feet into the center of the body – as in a standing bounce or jump, and can be the center of an outstretched body like the shape called the Big X in Bartenieff Fundamentals.

The *thoracobody* governs the ribcage and diaphragm. It deepens breath when it moves away from the xiphoid process on the inhale.

The *heart bodies* govern the wrist and forearms, and are stimulated by pushing with two arms symmetrically toward the body center in order to move backwards in space. An example in the upright position would be symmetrically pushing off a hot surface, in order to quickly retreat.

The *thymus* governs the shoulders and is stimulated by the reach of two arms as in a child reaching out to a parent for a hug or to be lifted, or a frog reaching to hop forward to land on its front limbs. The limbs act symmetrically and the shoulders are kept open and wide by the width of the thymus.

The *thyroid* governs the vocal diaphragm, collar bones (clavicle) interacting with the breastbone and ribs, upper arm bones (humerus), and elbows. It is stimulated by the reach of two legs downward – as in footward, as in a child trying to wriggle down from the arms of a parent by reaching feet toward the earth.

The *parathyroid* glands govern the neck through to the lower back vertebrae and ribs including the vertebral–costal joints, and are stimulated by reaching for/toward something with one limb. This happens in walking, creeping, or crawling when one arm or one leg reaches for something, often crossing the body midline, and pulls the opposite limb with it.

The *carotid bodies* govern the hyoid, jaw, neck, and upper and lower back (cervical, thoracic, and lumbar vertebrae) and are

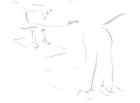
stimulated by the compressional forces from the tip of the spine up toward the head (the sequence of thrust from the tail through the spinal column comes up under the jaw, helpful in closing the mouth).

The *pituitary* governs the eyes and vision, and the spaces between the vertebrae. It is stimulated by elongation of the tail (downward or backwards). Actions include a 90 degree bow at the hip joint, crawling backward, or sitting down – with or without a turn.

The *mammillary bodies* govern the senses and smell. It is hypothesized that they are part of an anti-gravity response. They are stimulated by the reach and pull of the head – as in diving into water without the arms leading – or a flip.

The *pineal* governs the ears and hearing, and is stimulated by the yield and push of the head – an important action in childbirth and beyond. It is also impacted by the circadian rhythm.

Relating to Yoga

The above lists are powerful supports to practicing yoga. With embodied awareness of how to engage a developmental pattern one can often begin to see the patterns within all sorts of other aspects of everyday life, sports, and expressive and therapeutic movement. For instance, in order to jump forward from downward dog or plank into a folded shape one needs to put one's hands on the floor, push from the feet and pull the lower body into the new place. In other positions where the hands are not already planted on the ground, swing the arms and reach them out first, supported by the heart and thymus, then place the hands down. Jumping backwards from the feet is supported by having the upper body activated with thyroid support.

Yoga often teaches what chakras are stimulated by a movement. The DE approach recognizes that the activation of chakral energy by increased glandular awareness, and related neurodevelopmental movement, can improve your yoga ability.

The main point here is that there is access to the embodiment of the endocrine (hormone-secreting) glands through these developmental movements. Integrating these movements and their connections to the glands also links to efficient use of the joints. When they are performed with awareness, allowing for subtle sensations, the opposite is also true – the clear use of the joints can enhance the coordination of the movement, and support the radiant glandular energy inherent in engaging with asanas.

As described earlier, movement involves a wonderful interaction of compression and suspension of the body. When we move with a goal of maintaining equal joint space, the suspension and compression into the glands can become even clearer. One way to support the balanced use of each joint is to consider a crystalline structure around it, a sacred space all of its own. Laban/Bartenieff Movement Studies include the Bartenieff explorations of connectivity between bony landmarks. The bony landmarks are the places on the surface of the body that allow for contact with the bone and clearer activation of joints. As mentioned throughout this book, Bartenieff identified various key bony connections that, when felt or envisioned, encourage ease of muscular use. During the Sun Salutation it can be helpful to utilize the finger–scapula connection, heel–sit bone connection, scapula–sacrum connection (see Figs 5.4 and 5.5), and head–tail connection. The practice of breath support uses many joints in the ribcage such as the sternal–costal and costal–vertebral joints. Awareness of these connections can be applied to engaging with the Sun Salutation as a way to take care of your joints, by moving with awareness of the underlying developmental movement pattern to better manage joint challenges or pain, including activating your glands. The next chapter goes more deeply into joint health, maintenance, and healing.

Guided Sun Salutation with Developmental Movement and Glandular Cues

 Begin in standing.

Reach your arms up over your head: allow both arms to arc from hanging by your sides to forward using a homologous (symmetrical) reach of the upper with thymus (upper chest) activation as if seeking a hug, and then upward (as if a toddler wanting to be lifted). Feel free to continue upward and back "to see the sky" using the push of your feet from the pancreas into your diaphragm in the solar plexus region.

 Bending: keeping that reach of your arms going, bend forward from the hip joint. Hip flexion is ensured by allowing your tailbone to reach back (remembering the energy of your pituitary – third eye) as you fold at the hip joint. Bend your knees if you need to in order to make the hip flexion clear. Now curl downward from your tail, hollowing the navel and adrenal region, letting your head and your hands release toward your feet. Let all of yourself become small as in the condensing phase of navel radiation, feeling your adrenals and navel area relax over, resting on your thighs if your body allows for it and it feels good.

 Lunge back: reach your right leg back, feeling support from the throat (accessing the parathyroid). You can allow the right arm to reach forward in a counter-pull for stability or keep reaching it around into a twist to the opposite side to feel contralaterality.

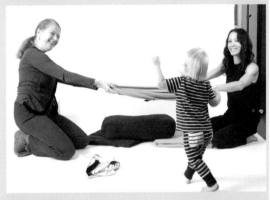

Figure 6.11
Contralateral, standing; notice twist in shirt. Photo by Serge Cashman.

 Downward dog: placing both hands down on the ground symmetrically (homologous) reach), stretch both legs back behind you. Feel the push of your two arms into the heart region and the push of two legs into your solar plexus pancreas region. Also feel the reach of your tail from your pituitary and the reach of your head from your mammillary bodies (from within the depth of the center of your head). If that is difficult to access, feel a push of your head from your pineal gland, the crown chakra, and use a push of your tail toward your head with an emphasis toward underneath your jaw – the carotid region.

 Plank: as you push with your arm symmetrically into your heart area, feel your feet reach

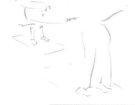

back from your heels, including the support of your thyroid in the mid-neck area.

 Fold knees–chest–chin: allow the adrenals and navel to soften as your knees, chest, and chin fold; again soften in the adrenals, while holding the breath.

 Upward dog/cobra: symmetrically, keep reaching both heels back from the thyroid as you let your head reach upright from the mammillary bodies.

 Downward dog: placing both hands down symmetrically (homologously), you may also press the hips down to feel the push of the tail towards the head and a reach of the head from there moving through all the glands of the spine. With both legs back behind you, feel the push of two arms into the heart region, continuing the push of two legs into your solar plexus pancreas region. Feel the reach of your tail from your pituitary and the reach of your head from your mammillary as you stay in this position.

 Forward lunge: reach your right leg forward, feeling the support of the parathyroid glands; this means that your neck is lifting up. You can activate more by reaching one leg back from the opposite upper parathyroid and reaching the same side arm forward and the opposite arm back, employing all the parathyroids with this reaching three of the four limbs (two arms and one leg) away from each other to expand in space.

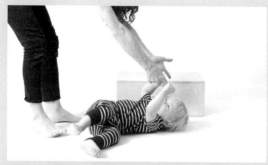

Figure 6.12
Contralateral, lying down. Photo by Serge Cashman.

Coming up: with both legs together fold the adrenal, softening over the thighs with navel condensation. Find the breath support by breathing in all body parts through all cells. Imagine oxygen moving to all parts of your being.

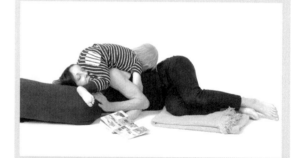

Figure 6.13
Giving in to gravity – time to yield. Photo by Serge Cashman.

 Then allow the tailbone and sit bones to point down as the head begins to reach up, while also radiating from the navel through the two feet. Feel the expansion from the head to the tail and out of both arms, as the legs straighten down into the earth. Allow the support of the pancreas to increase the expansion between all six limbs (head–tail–arms and legs).

 Arch: as you reach forward with your head and with your arms, travel as far up and high as you want, continuing to feel the thymus and mammillary bodies, as well as the pancreas, pushing into your solar plexus up under your diaphragm. Allow your arms to move with the support of your thymus as high and as far back as you are comfortable with reaching into the sky, while remembering your head and tail in a clear counter-pull lengthening the spine. This makes space between the vertebrae for the discs, including your neck, especially if you reach your heels into the ground from your thyroid.

 Ending: feeling your hand energy, bring the palms of your hands and fingertips to your heart and imagine your heart bodies while pushing your hands, pressing together.

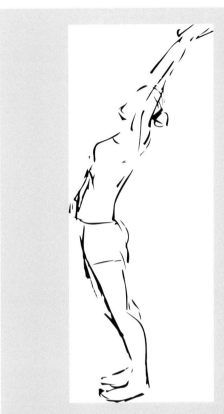

Figure 6.14
Reaching from the thymus, by Stewart Hoyt.

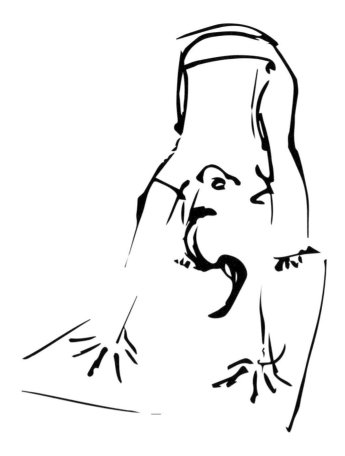

7 Considerations for Practicing the Sun Salutation – Preventing and Countering Pain

Introduction

To bring even more ease into movement, especially if experiencing weakness, imbalance, discomfort, or pain, learn some self-care tips to help out. A goal can be to understand how bodies work, what a positive use of alignment can be, and more about how the joints and glands interact to support movement ease. These "tips" focus on body areas and their related joints moving from the spine (inclusive of the head) and then outward from the chest through the arms to the wrists and fingers, and from the pelvis to the feet.

This process is psychophysical; therefore learning about your body structure (anatomy) and tuning in to your mental state can help you to reorganize the body. An example is learning about the primary and secondary curves of the spine. If you look at an anatomical chart of the

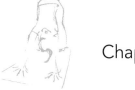

Chapter 7

spine you will see that the neck and lower back both have a natural arch; these need to stay in balance with each other. These sorts of relationships are important to know about and are part of a holistic perspective. Other important actions for joint health include decompressing joints by having good postural alignment and bodily use, balancing of muscle strength and flexibility, invigorating the organs, and engaging in diaphragmatic breathing.

Occasionally compression is also useful, particularly if ligaments are loose, as in a dislocation, and of course everyone needs hugs, which is also a type of gentle compression. Indeed, if in pain, a gentle, super-delicate and small squeeze of the tight muscle could bring relief after the squeeze is released. All of this takes self-awareness. One needs to be gentle and recognize the impact of gravity and how it can wear one down. The Sun Salutation is a great anti-gravity intervention. There are lots of benefits to actively flexing and extending the spine.

If new to movement, please move at a slower, smaller, and gentler pace and build up activity incrementally – maintaining self-awareness while moving and when at rest. If achy during or after, ask "does it last more than four days?" If so, it could help to "lay off" or "back off" – do less with more awareness. One of the best ways to avoid, reduce, prevent, or manage discomfort or pain is to learn about the body.

Use the activation of glands to help manage joint problems. Most people experience pain at some point in their lives. Pain is the body's natural signaling system that there is an imbalance. Often discomfort or pain results from the intensity of either physical drive (working too hard physically) or mental drive (pushing too hard). This pattern is exacerbated if compounded by self-criticism, which in turn can lead to exhaustion and even more pain. This is why Dynamic Embodiment[SM] (DE[SM]) guidance is often to

experiment with the Sun Salutation in a manner that is as gentle as possible and keeps you moving daily. In other words, rather than stopping one's practice or a certain movement, please consider the suggestions in this chapter for how to adapt the movement so that you can continue to move in a healthy and healing manner.

This chapter is full of adaptations for providing physical and emotional support for moving from asana to asana, and short examples of how to manage discomfort or pain. The more you explore these adaptations with full embodiment and self-compassion, the more likely you will be able to find your own variations and guide others in exploring. Focusing on the glands with some attention to muscles and bones is primary to this particular approach to the Sun Salutation. This guidance is chiefly about experiencing the Sun Salutation as it links to neuroendocrine awareness. It is unique to use embodied anatomy and developmental movement to experience each gland's relationship with specific joints. Many people find embodying the skeletal system with a focus on glands is a more concrete entry point to experiencing glandular consciousness.

The body is like a well-conducted orchestra with all parts simultaneously making a whole symphony. In this book, the glands are central, with the nervous system and bones being key inroads to sensing glandular energy. These are three of the seven major body systems as identified in Body-Mind Centering® (BMC®). To experience all cellular structures takes a full course of study or dedicated self-practice. There are other books that will help you investigate further (Bainbridge Cohen 1993, 2018, Hartley 1995).

The cause of pain may be located in any tissue. Indeed, DE asks you to get to know all seven different layers of tissue – from blood to organs to fascia to the awareness of them from the nervous system as well as the muscles, bones, and

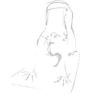

glands. Throughout this book there are passing references to the other four systems: the muscles, the organs, the fluids, and the soft tissues like skin, fat, and fascia. What is interesting to know is that how you move reveals a bit about which layers of tissue you more typically embody. Exploring the nature of each tissue provides an entry for varying the qualities of your movement and even your behavior. These are inroads to diverse expression and finding the style of behavior that accomplishes what you want, and that provide resources for shifting your physical habits to communicate better and to reduce emotional and bodily injury and discomfort.

Sharp Pain and Vulnerable Joints: Knees and Spine

If you experience sharp pain, that is when it is important for you to radically alter or desist that particular movement, especially in the knees and any part of the spine. Even a tolerable pain that is like a sharp needle can mean that a disc or cartilage is being damaged. The knee and spine are particularly sophisticated joints with many types of delicate tissues, such as complex ligaments, cartilage, and nerves, that can easily be compressed, torqued, or overly stretched.

From a BMC perspective, each knee joint is the site of interaction of four different convexities created by facets and discs (the meniscus), plus lateral and crossing ligaments. In yogic tradition the knee relates to the adrenal glands – our support for reserve energy. The spine is our core and is greatly impacted by posture, movement, our organ health, and our emotions. To reduce joint discomfort, work carefully with alignment, three-dimensional joint balancing, attention to the organs, decreasing overall inflammation, and getting enough rest.

This is true of the spine as well – a multiplicity of joints compounded by having articulating surfaces above and below each disc. The spine also allows for movement in all directions so it must be balanced with more care. If you have challenges in any of the spinal regions (neck, chest/thorax, lower back, or pelvis), you will learn about posture and of course the gland and chakra support for spinal flow. You will find it useful to integrate greater postural awareness, recuperative exercises, varied use of your body weight, and other resources besides the glands. Many will find relief from practicing the developmental approaches discussed in Chapter 6. If you experience pain in the knees or spine, please also read about glandular issues that may be related, in Chapter 8. In Chapter 10 there are additional resources about the use of light touch, visualization of realignment and space, support by breath, and the use of herbs such as arnica or other types of anti-inflammatories.

Acute Pain

If there is acute pain that needs a healing response, the DE approach combines light touch, visualization, and real or imagined realignment to bring space to a compressed joint, supported by breath into the area.

Of course, the common emergency first aid tradition is also useful. Its acronym is RICE:

- Rest

- Ice (or coolness)

- Compression

- Elevation.

In assessing when to get back to moving more rigorously or whether to begin with modification like staying in a chair, please talk with your physician. If needed, you can ask the presenting physician for permission to exercise.

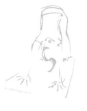

Chapter 7

Approaches to Joint Health

When there is pain or movement limitation, the somatic challenge is to find comfortable movement that brings blood to the area. This should often be as small as it needs to be for there to be no pain, referred to in DE as "moving under the pain." Next it can be useful to slowly and conscientiously experiment with movement that provides gentle traction for compressive pain (spinal discs, etc). On occasion, minimal compression may be needed (for example, to avoid joint dislocations). This is all a reiteration of the idea of experimenting with your movement options with gentleness, paying somatic attention to your sensations, and being willing to adjust your habits, rituals, and movement patterns. If even gentle movement hurts, it is advisable to find a skilled somatic or medical practitioner to guide you personally. If all else fails, active REST and breathing into the adrenals are useful. This is because becoming conscious of your body while engaging with slow and full inhales and exhales supports the magic that is described in the adage "time heals."

A colleague trained in both Laban work and BMC teaches senior citizens dance in upper Manhattan. She has been offering these classes for over 30 years. She says to them when they are feeling discouraged, "Show me what you can't do." And when they show her, that helps them notice that they are actually showing what they can do (Jones 1986).

Joint pain is often correlated with being overweight. Our experience is different. People of all sizes can find pleasure in yoga. This is embodied by the teaching of Michael Hayes, who, similar to our approach, says: "In Buddha Body Yoga, we take standard yoga poses and adjust, modify, and adapt them so that larger, overweight, or injured people are able to successfully practice" (Hayes 2021). DEPs also align with *Health At Every Size* (Linda Bacon), which offers important guidance as well.

Causes of and Help for Imbalances and Joint Challenges

What causes joint challenges? Of course, joint pain and imbalance can be caused by macro-trauma – an injury or assault from an external source. More often joint discomfort is caused by a series of micro-traumas such as repetitive use or ongoing stressors. Illness or infection that is acute or chronic can also be the cause of joint swelling, also known as inflammation, which causes immobility and discomfort. When the inflammation does not diminish, the joint dysfunction becomes chronic as well. This is typical with Lyme disease or lupus. Nerve damage is another cause of pain or numbness. This neuropathy can be a result of radiation, chemotherapy, or diabetes. If you have hot sensations or numbness in hands or feet, please have a neurological check. One can also explore what movements and sensations are felt. Lifestyle is a major influencer and that includes choices about how to best sit, stand, and move. Why? Because bodies are designed to move. One's mental state – feelings – impacts joints as well. Joints are where movement happens – articulations are for articulating! It is best to move joints in a "centered alignment" – with equal pressure in all parts of the joint instead of favoring one side or edge and causing imbalances. Emotions can cause shifts in posture, which in turn can cause off-center bodily positioning. Off-center postural positioning that becomes chronic can end up causing either intensified psychological expression and/or physical imbalances.

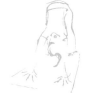

Joint Health Tips

It is useful to learn how to avoid or correct ongoing displacement or overly intensive static pressure in the joints. A goal is to reduce too much uneven movement and posture or to find the dynamic flow through varying postures. It is helpful to have choices and options. This shows up as being able to determine how to move with just the right amount of force for the task. It is easy to slip into doing too much – either by using too much muscular resistance (tightness) or by engaging in power moves without enough experience in modulating your own weight and maintaining a through-line in the center of the joints. This is the cause of many injuries from high-impact running or jumping, especially on hard surfaces like concrete, tile, linoleum or carpet over hard surfaces, and asphalt. It is important to know your pain threshold. If you don't feel pain, you may not know to avoid movements that are causing further wear and tear on the joints. You may need to regulate the external conditions that impact movement – how you dress, protect your feet, pay attention to your environment, or provide enough time for preparing, engaging in, and integrating your practice. You may even find that you can sustain many repetitions of the practice by taking the practice outdoors. Feeling good can come from what environment you are in.

Realignment

The best way to realign our joints and move them without pain is to learn anatomy (location and structure) and kinesiology (the study of movement). While three-dimensional breathing should be encouraged, it is important to also understand that every joint is three-dimensional. Focus on the concept of balancing the muscles around the joint. Most joints have muscles that are meant to act like perfectly coordinated reins on all sides of a joint.

Equal Joint Space through Somatic Awareness

Now that you have the concept of equal pulls on the joint, let's think about the space inside the joint as well. In order to avoid deleterious and/or painful joint use, (re-)establish "equal joint space" – a concept from BMC (Bainbridge Cohen 1993, Hartley 1995, Taylor 2018). Once you find the proper posture for a joint, you want to maintain it. It helps to actively use the muscles on all sides of joints in a balanced way but also to move with an attitude of lightness with groundedness. Some people find that the mindful state of being present or self-aware is reliable support for becoming grounded and more ready to be aware of joint pressures. Remember to enhance your kinesthetic sense, your somatic awareness. Your ability to become more self-aware of your body while moving will help you reduce or avoid joint problems.

Degree of Challenge

It is also important to choose wisely about how much you want to challenge yourself. It is important to act with practicality based on your level of fitness, your health conditions, and your motivation and energy levels. Without taking time to first know what is tight or weak in your typical alignment or posture, you might end up with muscle tension, spasms, strains, or pulls. If you are not used to practicing the Sun Salutation and also have not been doing any flexibility work with dynamic stretching, you might work too hard and end

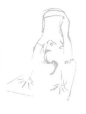

up with an overly stretched or twisted joint. A full twist of a joint with a movement done too quickly can end up causing ligamentous sprains and might even cause a bone fracture or a pinched nerve. Moving slowly as you learn a pattern or when you are ill or tired is a great preventative measure. Since pinched nerves are particularly common in the spine, it is important to know your spinal range. It helps to learn how to do a simple self-assessment or check-in of your alignment, especially for the spine.

Dynamic Alignment

Many people think of the spine when they think of alignment. Total body alignment does require the spine to find its natural curves and awareness of when there is a tendency to fall or pull backward or forward or sideways through the spinal joints. When attending to joints of the spine it becomes critical to focus on posture. It is helpful to learn more about what "good posture" is. For sure, this a changing construct and very much related to our own biological and cultural make-up. Keeping the idiosyncratic nature of all people's bodies it is still possible to just see what you learn by discovering your "plumbline." Plumbline alignment asks you to line up your ear over your shoulder, above your hip socket, through the center of the knee, and in front of your ankle, allowing your weight to then spread outward through your toes and heel. However, alignment is important in all joints.

Dynamic Alignment is a concept from BF that recognizes that alignment exists throughout the body and is a dynamic interaction of all body parts. It also includes the idea that the body is moving all the time and that alignment adjusts constantly according to what one is doing and what actions are being taken.

Learning about your plumbline alignment is a helpful assessment tool. Once you know your plumbline you can be aware of the subtle but healthy deviations that happen as you move about your day. If you have had a day at the computer, your head might slip forward. If you are tired, your stomach or shoulders might slouch. If your inner voice says pull your shoulders back all day long, your back muscles may be exhausted.

Alignment for Pain Management

So, how can you improve alignment and relieve pain? Movement habits (use of bodies, whether in static or active models), our emotions, and organ health can affect posture. Learning about your body structure (anatomy) and tuning in with your mental health can help you to reorganize your body! An example is learning about the primary and secondary curves of the spine. If you look at an anatomical chart of the spine you will see that the neck and lower back both have a natural arch. These are called convex curves as opposed to the head, chest, and pelvis, which are concave. These two convex curves are developed by most infants in the first six months of life, learning to lift the head when on the belly. This is one of the reasons that "tummy time" during the day is important. Once these curves are established, everyone needs to learn to at least be aware of them when dealing with the challenge of being upright. Crawling on hands and knees usually helps these curves. Striving for good spinal alignment can shift overall health and mental attitude. Once you have a sense of the curves it is a pleasure to "pretend you are a kid" and move on the belly and quadrupedally again. Notice if your mood gets playful, if you smile; if not that activity, what other experience is more supportive?

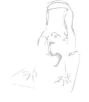

In exploring spinal alignment at rest on the ground, and then in coming up to sitting or standing, there is a good chance you have balanced your deeper abdominals. These practices can reduce joint pain.

When forgetting to pay attention to dynamic alignment (ever-changing posture), fixed curvatures can develop in the spine. The most common are called: kyphosis (dowager's hump), scoliosis (lateral curvature often beginning when we are teenagers), and lordosis (also known as a sway or arched back). These can be painful in and of themselves *or* be the cause of nerve pain. Some are genetic and others can be caused or exacerbated by diseases such as osteopenia and osteoporosis. Working with the somatic concepts of breath support, organ support, and movement awareness can help to slow down these postural deviations.

Good ways to prevent and reduce pain or to manage joint pain include the following principles:

1. *Know YOUR body*

2. Maintain equal joint space – bones aligned in the socket with no pressure in any direction

3. Recognize that the body *is three-dimensional* – move and systematically stretch and strengthen in all four directions while being aware of the compression that comes from gravity

4. *Be gentle and jiggle – move synovial fluid in the joints to keep it circulating!*

5. Pay attention to signals – *stay tuned in* by doing a body scan, listening to the joints whenever you can. As you are listening and noticing each part of the body from feet to head or head to feet, ask yourself:

Are you experiencing any discomfort? What are the sensations?

It is important to do this "check-in" before any workout including the Sun Salutation. It gives you baseline information to compare to each time you begin doing a similar movement. It is easiest to learn to pay attention to somatic cues when in stillness or moving slowly. Once you get familiar with perceiving your body signals in a still shape you can notice more while slowly moving, and then, with practice, you can perceive more even while moving quickly.

When in doubt, remember the "Core Concepts of Somatics" identified in Chapter 1: slower, and often smaller, movement can help you find a more relaxed way of moving. If this is still difficult, then lying down allows you to pay attention to your proprioceptive bodily cues and may also help reduce pain, depending on what the cause is. This proprioceptive information can help you make better alignment choices. Whenever possible, move at a range of motion and pace that is "under the pain." Once you find this pain-free zone, then explore new activity gently with equal proprioceptive awareness (this is moving somatically). This is not taking the "easy way out" – this internal focus actually challenges your mind and wakes up neural pathways. It also creates new signals and the body's responses stimulate new neural pathways – all of this adds up to giving your joints new options – finding new movement choices.

Interconnections – the Sun Salutation with Joint and Glandular Awareness

The Sun Salutation is a repetitive practice; hence you can cause injury from practicing it without awareness of your alignment.

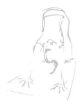

Chapter 7

As you deepen with somatic practice you will most likely want to get to know more resources. Iyengar yoga really focuses on alignment. The Alexander Technique helps move the weight of the head up and off the neck and torso in a healthy way. Embodied or Experiential Anatomy classes in Body-Mind Centering®-derived training teach these skills.

BF takes a unique streamlined approach to learning about the moving body. Recall that Irmgard Bartenieff was a movement specialist, trained in Laban concepts of movement analysis, and integrating them into her work as a physical therapist and as a dancer. She realized that people could pay attention to the body's organization, and that the best way to move more efficiently was to gain proprioception of our skeletal "body connections" and let the organization of our muscles flow from this level of motor planning. Irmgard was well aware of how humans learn to move as babies (see more about this in Chapter 6) so she would often begin with basics – breath coordination, then how our whole body centers around our core, and then back to posture – how does one organize the head in relationship to the tip of the spine, the coccyx or tail (head–tail connection). For grounding, she also identified other critical "connections," as previously discussed in Chapter 6 (see also Figs 1.4, 5.4 and 5.5). Recall that these include:

- Heel to sit bone

- Sacrum to scapula

- Scapula to fingertips.

And, in order to assist healthy joint functioning, you can also bring in the glandular energy of locate, vibrate, and energize, and of course you can move with these awarenesses. In order to bring vitality to a joint it is helpful to return to the concept of tensegrity and the fascia and muscular pulls that impact the joints. By invoking the images of space around a joint and finding the counter-pulls that make for a lovely crystalline form around the joint, one can feel interconnectivity through the entire body. When this whole-body awareness is present it helps the tensegrity, which in turn supports whole-body alignment.

You can also use props for support and clarity of alignment. Many in the somatic wellness industry began using balls (large physio and small super balls), mini-trampolines, rollers, and any of the other fun objects that help relieve tension and awaken sensation and awareness. The distribution of these products for health began heavily in the 1970s. Tuning forks, pillows, and balance boards are other tools that stimulate awakening through vibration, otherwise activating the body. Being on or off balance will contribute to dynamic alignment.

Ways of Working with the Psychophysical Self

There are many inroads to self care. The DE approach includes embracing the full psychophysical experience. For instance, there is a movement–meaning continuum: what does your movement style say about how you live your life? Understanding what space you move in can help you know when you need to do more exploring, intending or deciding about "what directions you will benefit from moving in now." Another example is that noticing how much effort you put into something may lead you to make better decisions about when to surrender, yielding into gravity, or whether to push up against it with strength, reach out to others, or pull yourself toward what you need or want. This also relates to whether you need to rest or activate your energy, and what will help you feel more balanced in a particular situation. This includes bringing the attention

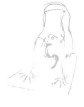

to exploring movement and consciousness with the joints and the glands.

One More Point of Awareness – Addressing Emotional Pain

Physical pain is best managed by providing many options for the body (many levels of support).

Social pain is seen as significant and influencing every person on the planet, historically and in the present. In speaking about social pain, pain that comes from either societal pressures or unjust norms, or from how individuals act due to those pressures, can be either constructive or destructive. If the pain causes chronic denial, or ignoring or hurting another person, this is destructive. If the pain is responded to with healthy action for interpersonal and personal growth in consciousness, that is constructive pain. Both hurt, but constructive (clean) pain moves through us and dissolves, and is ultimately more valuable, while destructive (dirty) pain hides out in our bodies until it rears its head again (Menakem 2017).

Spiritual pain can be eased by attending services or through meditation that accepts the body and perhaps the need to move to calm the mind and heart (versus sitting still in meditation).

This perspective sees that emotional pain can be addressed, for some people, by opening spiritually while staying physically grounded and doing the day-to-day work of clear, compassionate communication. It can be supportive to learn the DE approach to peaceable communication and embodied conflict resolution.

Learning "ways of sitting with discomfort," whether it be physical, emotional, social, or spiritual, has been critical during the Covid-19 pandemic and as all people focus on changes in behavior to prove allegiance to Black Lives Matter. By taking DE's neurodevelopmental plus glandular approach, people are empowered to ease stress, especially that which is event-derived or stems from psychosocial oppressions, especially acting in groups for social change.

Working with Pain and Depression

When handling ongoing chronic pain or the end of an acute macro-traumatic experience, it is suggested, in time, to bring in tiny movement that either brings blood to the area indirectly and/or provides some traction for compressive pain (spinal discs, etc.) or minimal compression for dislocations. One can use a towel, a ball, an apparatus for inversion, or other approaches to inversion.

For long-time intensive pain it is a common tool in somatic work to go into dialogue with the body – what is this body part's role, what is the pain protecting, what function has it been serving, how does the immobility or imbalance serve me now, what else could provide this role? There are many layers of tissue to consider – the cord, the nerves, the ligaments, the discs, the vertebrae, the muscles (small and deep/long and superficial), the digestive tract, and the glands. Any one layer or combination of layers may need this investigation.

This is all a reiteration of the idea of experimenting, paying somatic attention, and being willing to adjust one's body, mind, or emotions in order to find balance. The mental attitude of compassion and the practice of finding ease can be of service in many instances. Often rest and breathing into the adrenals are useful. The passage of time and deep oxygenation do heal.

Be alert to degrees of pain, if you or a student experiences:

1. intense emotional pain such as a trauma response. This is when someone "is triggered" or panicking; please have resources

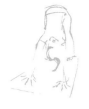

ready. (Signs: breathing heavily, sobbing, or not being aware of where they are/ being withdrawn). Potential resources include finding a trauma-informed yoga instructor or a trauma therapist, or having a private session with a somatic therapist skilled in trauma recovery.

2. sharp physical pain. That is the one time to **desist from movement** – change your posture, your alignment, your movement action, or its level or intensity until the pain is no longer happening.

Here is a general reminder for practice regarding embodiment to enhance doing the Sun Salutation with ease: movement stimulates sensation – expect to feel new sensations as you advance your practice. It is also important to begin to discern sensation as signals. Pain in particular is something all of us should listen to with our own bodies – using our proprioceptive, interoceptive, and kinesthetic senses.

Arnica or another type of natural anti-inflammatory allows you to still feel sensation while reducing the inflammation, instead of using steroids that mask the sensation. They can be useful to have on hand or in one's studio if you have chronic pain and or are experimenting with new levels of fitness, energy expression, or movement dynamics.

Adapting the Sun Salutation with Awareness of the Joints

Next is a section about each joint, providing information about ways to become more aware of each one and about its function. Learn specific ways to work with injuries and a variety of ways of caring for injured joints. Injury reduction concepts and some injury interventions

can be found here. Rather than working from top to bottom, or bottom to top, this chapter is organized developmentally, beginning with Navel Radiation – the second developmental pattern described in Chapter 6 – whereby the baby learns motor coordination from the navel region outward, first through the spine, then through the upper body, and finally through the lower. It can feel as if you are moving in a spiral, through the joints. After exploring and engaging in core support the limbs learn to coordinate. Moving upwards, the focus goes

Adapting the Sun Salutation with Awareness of the Joints

A. Joints of the core of the body

Lumbar spine (low back)

Pelvis: sacro-iliac joint (low back)

Spine

Neck

Head and jaw

B. Joints of the upper body

Chest

Shoulder girdle

Elbow

Wrist, hands, and fingers

C. Joints of the lower body

Ilio-femoral joint (hip sockets)

Knees

Ankles

Feet

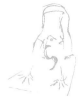

to the chest, shoulders, arms, wrists, and hands. Then, returning to the pelvis, the experiences move to the legs and feet. This is an invitation to how to do things differently, to find an organic embodied pathway that emanates from center versus the typical hierarchical model of moving from top to bottom, or linear model of bottom to top. This is also an embodied metaphor for how to be in interpersonal, social, and political aspects of life and society.

Here are ideas for how to continue with the Sun Salutation even if you have problems with that joint, providing activities for each and adaptations for most.

The Joints of the Core of the Body

Lower Back Pain/Lumbar Region

Garland pose: When you are experiencing low back pain, a good pose to drop down into is the squat (see Fig. 7.1 here). As you press your elbows into the inside of your knees, you can focus on reaching your crown away from your tail, and your tail away from your crown. This often does the trick in alleviating pain, as it releases the spinal vertebral joints, opening up the low back. You can try and see if this works for your body. Practicing it regularly is preventative. Feel your breath supporting you as you condense into this pose. Take it a step further and sense the earth below, allowing the energy of the root to bubble up through the 3rd and 4th chakras to help support an opening in the chest. There is more in the next chapter that works with restorative activity for the lower back as it relates to the adrenals and also to the rest patterns of the pineal.

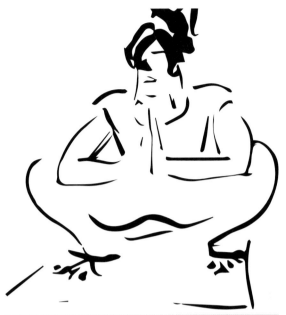

Figure 7.1
Rooting and grounding (garland pose), a drawing of Shakti by Stewart Hoyt.

Rest with legs up the wall, or Viparita Karani: use a pillow or folded blanket beneath your low back for 5–20 minutes. Let the weight of your legs pour into your sacrum, sacro-iliac joint, and the rest of your low back area, giving compression and massage. Allow the weight of your own body to open and soothe the area.

Martha's Personal Story: Easing Back Stiffness

After sleeping in a curled side-lying position for several hours I often wake up with my lower back overly flexed – no longer having its natural arch, or concavity. When my lower back feels particularly stiff or is in even a little pain, I baby it. My spine is important! How do I do this? I keep myself in that position

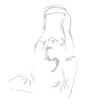

Chapter 7

and walk around, allowing my head to be low and my spine to be curved, noticing how it feels. Gradually my breath changes as I move through my morning rituals (toothbrushing, etc). I find little places to lengthen upward – pressing my hands into the sink as my head looks up. Then as the morning progresses I find my way into the Sun Salutation and play with the honest range of motion that I am capable of in that moment.

DE yoga remedy – Sun Salutation: One way to tune into the tone of the lower back is to allow it to yield its weight into support, and then to activate the deep muscles that support it, "it" being the many joints that articulate with the five lumbar vertebrae and the pelvic bones. Begin the Sun Salutation with a deep bow to the earth, hanging the full weight of the torso over the knees in order to breathe deeply into the adrenals. See how much you are able to surrender your weight. Depending

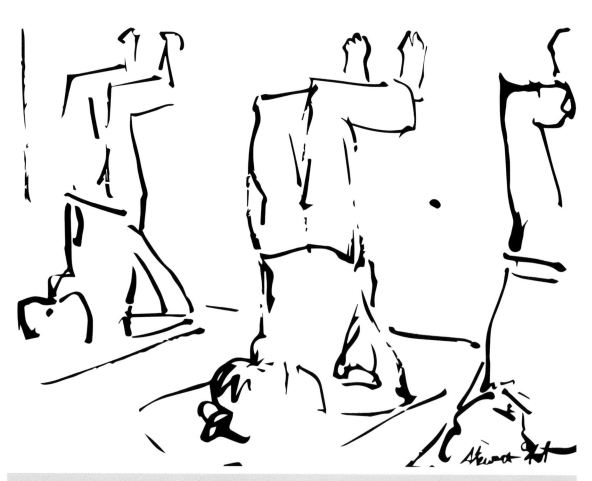

Figure 7.2
Heels over head, by Stewart Hoyt.

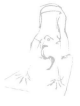

on your flexibility, body shape, and morphology, you may want to put a pillow between your thighs and your body to provide more support to relax into. Then, in order to check in with your deepest, largest muscle – your psoas – stretch one leg into a lunge. See how it feels and then further check to see what your range of motion is, gradually lengthening the lower end of the psoas by bending your knee to the ground or stretching the leg as fully as possible backward. You can further stretch the upper end of the psoas by bringing the spine in full extension upward (and even backward) toward the sky. You may place the knee on the ground/mat/cushion. Next explore the range of motion of your arms – either rising up vertically, straight up, out to the sides, or forward and up. See which feels best but most importantly do what you can to stretch the upper part of the psoas.

Yoga remedy: When moving into uttanasana in the Sun Salutation, try rotating your thighs inward. This usually opens up the low back, lengthening it and allowing you to deepen into your forward bend. Try this and see how this works with your body.

On all fours: An assessment of alignment – do the cat and cow, alternating between these to feel whether one direction is easier or harder than another. Moving the entire spine is important for the lumbar part: it interacts with the neck as the two parts of the spine that have become convex with the "secondary curves" that develop after birth while the infant elongates out of the fetal position. By flexing and extending the entire spine you loosen your lower back, and help to return to the root pattern of seesawing between the head and the pelvis, being curved and extended. Then recuperate in "neutral spine" – not overly flat but not curved or arched. Notice when you relax whether you are more in cat or cow. This

positioning can be used to determine if you are "holding in a gland," bracing it and not moving it or letting the energy move.

Pelvis Area

The pelvis is comprised of seven bones, three of which fuse during childhood – the ilium, ischium, and pubis – forming two pubic bones, on each side of the sacrum. The two pelvic bones and the sacrum can move where they come together at the sacro-iliac joints and pubic symphysis (the two pelvic halves are also known as the *os innominatum*). If any of these is out of balance it helps to go deeper into the pelvis and work with the DE principle called "Rearranging the Furniture," as if it is spring cleaning day, which we sometimes need to move the furniture to find the deeper dust. In the body we may need to move organs that get too stuck within their space. In this case it is important to pay attention to each of the pelvic organs, and glands. Specifically the ovaries/testes are the glands and the penis/vagina/uterus are the reproductive organs plus there is the bladder, rectum, and intestines. Give them a chance to move, jiggle, breathe, and reorganize. Integration can include initiating movement within the pelvis from the organs while using the cranio-sacral rhythm, which further helps to balance the autonomic nervous system. This exploration can be done seated or standing – beginning with the flexion and extension of the head, allow the rest of the spine to follow and feel how the pelvis responds. It works well to engage with this movement super-slowly with a sense of ongoing flow – eliminate any abruptness in your movement. This exercise can be experienced within a BodyMind Dancing^{SM} class when doing the cerebrospinal fluid spiral sequence within the fluid Phrase Dance^{SM}.

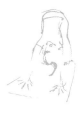

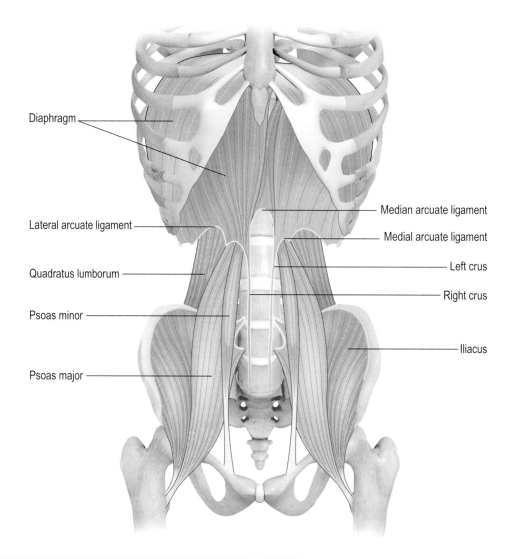

Diaphragm

Lateral arcuate ligament

Quadratus lumborum

Psoas minor

Psoas major

Median arcuate ligament

Medial arcuate ligament

Left crus

Right crus

Iliacus

Figure 7.3
The iliopsoas and diaphragm. The iliacus and psoas major connect to the lesser trochanter, while the psoas minor connects to the pubis. Also something to explore, some new science as taught by Bainbridge Cohen: the diaphragm's tendons, the crura, can connect as low as the pelvic floor, especially if you keep breathing into this area. Learn more about the "Unified Diaphragm" from BMC.

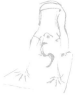

This work contributes to the larger DE principle of "being as big as you are."

Specifically for the sacro-iliac joint:

- Pigeon pose is important to release hip and sciatic tensions.

- Any other stretch for the piriformis will then reduce the pull on the sacro-iliac joint, such as rotating one of the legs inward or outward while stretching the front or the back of the muscle. One example involves stretches while you are lying on your back or seated in a chair – cross the leg with ankle over one knee and then pull the externally rotated leg closer to the chest or bring your chest to it. This stretches the area under the buttock, the piriformis, which is so important because the sciatic nerve runs through it.

- Derived from BF, DE's "Clearing the Back" works well for people who have fairly stretched hamstrings. It involves folding over at the hip joint, usually with straight legs, and hanging one's head and arms from the hip joints. Find bony leverage from one foot and, while keeping the knees straight (if you can), shift your weight predominantly from one leg to the other, meanwhile allowing the head and arms to swing to the opposite ankle. This often expands the lower back, releasing both gluteal and external rotator muscles. If your ligaments are too lax (often the case while pregnant or soon after giving birth), having another person palpate and support the sacro-iliac ligaments is important.

- Moving using the super-slow Cranio-Sacral evenly paced rhythm is a central modality of DE.

- Also important are breath work and working with the adrenals to rejuvenate. See Chapter 8 for more on this.

Spine

If you were on a desert island and could only do three yoga poses, the authors would strongly recommend a twist be one of the three: seated twists, supine twists, and forward-bending twists. They are a powerful and sure way to release the strong musculature of the back, to encourage it to breathe and have more space in it.

The spine is designed to flex and extend, laterally flex and extend, and rotate. Rotation is important to health and is an antidote to our "forward"-thinking society. It is great to learn about a variety of spinal twists. Twisting can be done "grossly" or in small areas. The spine is designed to twist in tiny segments at the deepest level, and in larger segments at a more superficial muscular level. Moving through the different layers of the muscles in turn supports "getting down to the bones." Bones can be closer to our core. When one leads from the bones precision and clarity of form help release muscular tension. More flexible muscles supported by balanced ligaments leave even joint space for the discs, allowing for more space in between the bones of the spine.

Rotation massages our organs, bringing fresh blood and lymphatic flow through different organs – like the stomach and liver, intestines, and lungs. Twists assist the fascia in being softer, less rigid. All this helps us in sitting and standing more comfortably. Twists move us into space and through different planes, breaking up the rigid forward–backward patterns that are so dominant in our culture. Twists demand our attention, bringing us into the present, especially when returning to

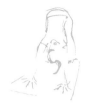

Chapter 7

the midline. This helps us settle into our centers and can support focus.

Spinal twists are also generally prescribed after backbends and shoulder stands, to aid the spine in breathing and finding resilience after the intensity of those poses. This is especially necessary for those who experience low back pain.

Rotation often most naturally comes from the head turning to observe what the eyes see, the nose smells, and the ears hear.

Neck

Extra care is needed for the delicate neck. It supports the weight of our brain and skull. When it is aligned well with the rest of the spine, this support is effortless. Often, the chin juts forward, or upwards, causing the neck to arch one way or the other. To remedy: bring your awareness into the back of your neck, slowly invite it to lengthen, reaching upwards into your skull like a flower reaching for the sun. This may immediately cause a drop in your shoulders, and a cascade of widening at the upper back, rounding of the chest forward and up, and fuller breath being taken into your lungs. Widening at the neck brings you into parasympathetic (see adrenal section for more information). The parasympathetic nerves emerge from the skull. Allowing the musculo-skeletal area around the brainstem to ease encourages increased blood flow to the brain, and importantly helps release the tension around the cranial nerves, which impact multiple regions of our body and attitudes. With these attitude shifts, classroom educators, researchers, and therapists report their patients/clients/elders settling into increased comfort. Comfort and agency are enhanced when those who have been silenced are invited to speak. An important nerve – the polyvagal nerve – also is activated when we align head,

heart, and the gut brain, the cortical with the parasympathetic – the thinking brain with the gut brain. Once settled, imagining the widening of the neck helps release neck tension through cross-fiber expansion and also activates the parasympathetic nerves, calming the nervous system and balancing engagement with both the intero- and extero-perceptions. Playing with the differentiation of "vertebral muscles" versus hyoidal muscles can really help neck alignment. Working with the glands sometimes just helps this happen automatically. Bonnie Bainbridge Cohen continues to work with the role of the surrounding space as support. When the neck hurts it is typical to freeze to protect. Another option is to slowly explore movement with a "sponging quality" – picturing the water inside and outside of cells and doing gentle tightening and releasing of the muscles around the area as if squeezing out a wet sponge and then allowing it to refill. If you are wondering how much to squeeze, explore within the range of motion that is comfortable to you, hugging into the areas with the joint limitation and then allowing for expansion. In the case of the neck, feel how this buoyancy can support the weight of your head (like an imaginary balloon or pillow) (Bainbridge Cohen 2018).

Add to this another nugget of a tip: bring your awareness into your pituitary gland. Imagine it growing a long tail that reaches downwards through your spine; sense and see it moving down through your sushumna and center line, all the way down to the tip of your tailbone. Stay with this for a minute. This will support your neck in being longer and wider.

Head and Jaw

Invite your head to bobble on the top of your neck. This can include softening through the

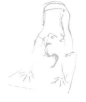

eyes and relaxing the tongue. Now feel the jaw, the temporomandibular joint, which is the first joint that gains control – newborns need to suckle and already know how – it is the relationship to gravity that is new.

DE remedy: Place your jaw/chin on your hands or table. Keep it stable as you raise your eyes up and allow the mouth to open – this will stretch the muscles of the jaw. As you bring your eyes down, your mouth will close.

Sun Salutation remedy: Open your mouth with initial arching into slight backbend from tadasana. Feel your rootedness into the rest of your body. This will connect you from your head through your spine into the pelvis and out of your chest through your arms.

Joints of the Upper Body

Chest

There is a general tendency in our culture to collapse the chest, as the shoulders bow forward and the head looks down at a computer or phone. The other extreme is to pull the shoulder blades together in an extremely upright but often rigid position, squeezing them together in the back. These involve overworking the muscle system, which can be another cause of fatigue.

Three tips:

1. Come to your center line, at the sternum. Breathe from here out to your side bodies, inviting the chest and upper chest to be wide, supported by the breath within.

2. Gently draw your two shoulder blades together in back: not too much, and see if it feels supported by the breathing you just instigated. There is a slight arch to the spine; try to be gentle and not overcorrect.

3. Next, do slow, luscious shoulder circles, by raising your shoulders up as you breathe in, and beginning to roll them back and down and around as you exhale. Repeat this several times. Revisit your breath and the scapulae moving towards one another.

Visit each one of these tips and weave in the others, for a holistic sense of a more supported open chest.

Mobilize the thoracic area – the rib joints – to change your entire posture: If someone has a locked set of ribs not only is breath impeded, but movement through the entire body is impacted. Kyphosis is when our thoracic spine takes on a chronic flexion – sometimes referred to as a "dowager's hump," which might relate to letting the heart retreat. One way to keep flexible is to remember to move all the vertebrae and explore the mobility of each rib. Then connect the ribs via the thoracic spine upward into the neck and downward into the pelvis. Here are some guidelines: the costovertebral joints are often neglected, as are the sternocostal joints – the joints that support flexibility in the ribs. By awakening movement in these joints, thoracic posture can be improved. Start with narrowing in the front of the body at the sternum/breastbone by moving the ribs forward, and then open and widen them with awareness that the costo-vertebral joints are closing in the back. Playing with the breath will bring in new movement through the area.

Shoulder Girdle

Finger pressing: Bring your hands to rest on a table in front of you. Press into the thumbs of both hands while sensing the connection in between your shoulder blades. Then press into your second fingers – you may be able to

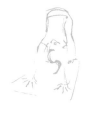

sense a connection ½ to 1 inch higher up in between the scapula's medial border and the spine. Now try the third finger, fourth finger, and pinky, sensing the connections a little higher up each time. Next bring your hands up to chest height, and press into each thumb and finger, again sensing this connection. See Figures 5.4 and 5.5 for the anatomy of these connections. Visualize your chest, torso, arm, and finger connection being a circle filled with light; see them as connected and talking to one another. Sense into the support that you feel in your torso, chest, and shoulder girdle now (Foster 2007).

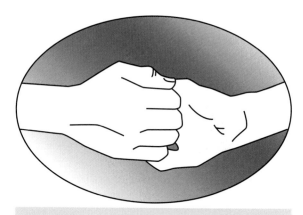

Figure 7.4
Ganesh Mudra.

> **Shakti's Personal Story: Finger to Scapula Connections**
>
> This is something I learned from Mandy Chan, DEP, when she and Dana Davidson, DEP, were teaching Developmental Movement for the Dynamic Embodiment℠ program in Brooklyn, NY, three or so years ago. Making these finger to scapula connections noticeably strengthened my spine's ability to sit upright in space, and countered the forward collapse that I sense happening from slouching/ computers/texting (see 'Finger pressing', p. 159). After class I remember unlocking my bike outside BAX (Brooklyn Arts Exchange) on Fifth Avenue. As I rode to my studio to work with clients, I pressed my fingers and thumbs into the handlebars, experiencing the conversation with my back. To this day, I practice this when I am riding; it effectively maintains a healthy and aligned posture during one of my everyday activities. This exercise is adapted from Bartenieff Fundamentals.

Integrating the Upper Body

Ganesh Mudra: This is a heart opener; it brings blood into the chest and activates the musculature of the ribs, sternum, shoulders, arms, and hands. Bring your hands and arms up to chest level, parallel to the ground. Bring one palm to face forward and one to face you; clasp your fingertips. When you breathe in, pull away, extending the elbows away from one another. When you exhale, relax. Repeat four times. Feel into the anatomical connections as you do this. Can you feel each fingertip to wing (medial to the shoulder blade) connection? Enjoy the fullness, life power, and strength that comes from doing this mudra.

Remedy = Dance: Begin slow movements into space from shoulder, chest, elbow, wrist, and fingers. Let them dance and integrate these newly activated connections.

Elbow

When in arm-reaching poses, like the first part of the Sun Salutation or warrior 2, activate your fingertips, wiggling them a bit. This activates movement in the muscles of your forearm and elbows, helping them to also be a part of the pose. This aids you in embodying the fullness of your arms by making clear skeletal contact between each part of your arm – fingertips to the forearm to the elbows connecting to the

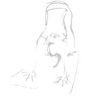

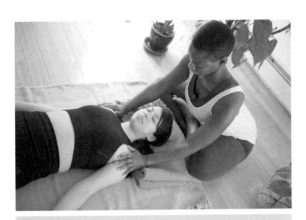

Figure 7.5
Widening the shoulders to stimulate the thymus.
Photo by Serge Cashman.

finger? There are three bones in each finger (the phalanges), and two in the thumb; try to press down through each of these sections.

Cupping: Bring a gentle cupping into your hand, by transitioning from pressing weight through every part, to pressing most of the weight just into the edges of the palm and fingers, an almost imperceptible rising up, or cupping, happening at the center of the palm.

You could use both of these – spreading your weight evenly and the cupping – at different times. Notice how they both help save your wrists.

Wrist injury adaptations: If your wrists are in acute or chronic pain, you may want to support your yoga asanas through a different base, like using your fists or forearms to support you

upper arm and armpits. Remember that your thymus sends energy out in this circle. Make the thymus/arm joint connection by reaching the arm out and feeling your upper chest and lower neck area for emotional and physical support.

Wrists

Our wrists are like our knees in a way, such a complex and strong yet delicate area that is often strained. First, here are some tips for how to care for the wrists over time, then how to do poses without them when acutely injured.

Cat/cow is a good pose to practice this.

Spreading your weight evenly: With your hands beneath your shoulders, notice how much weight is going into the palm of your hand. Notice which parts of your palm are taking the weight. Often it is the back of the palm, by the wrist, that is taking most of the weight. Consciously spread this out into the center of your palm, and the sides. Now how does this feel? Continue by pressing evenly into each finger. Pour weight down evenly to each finger. Notice if your fingers are arching up: are you pressing through each part of your

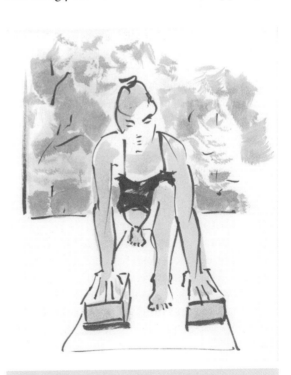

Figure 7.6
Use of blocks in lunge or anjaneyasana, by Stewart Hoyt.

in your Sun Salutation flow, instead of your hands.

Using blocks: Another tip for saving wrists is to use blocks in poses like forward lunge. If they are soft blocks this provides relief simply by presenting a softer surface. Pressing into more than one side of the block gives relief (pressing into the top and side of the block with your hand).

Incorporate some of these wrist relief suggestions into your practice at the first sign of wrist discomfort. Make this a habit that curbs the discomfort early on, and prevents it from becoming a chronic problem.

Joints of the Lower Body

Ilio-Femoral Joint (the Actual "Hip Joint")

This is the largest ball and socket joint in the body. It is designed for global movements – meaning circular. In order to maintain the health of this joint it is important to balance all sides of it. You can begin with the internal–external rotation in the legs of the movement, and then add in either a leg swing or a lunge as described above under lower back for the sacro-iliac joint and pelvis. Also test with some side-to-side movement, what Bartenieff called Lateral Weight Shift. Once standing or walking, it is educational to sense all the interconnected parts between the core of the body and how it expands out through the limbs. Then standing and lunging opens up the front and back aspect of the hip joint. Walking in big steps forwards starts to unlock the energy. Walking backwards also increases the range of motion with a focus on stretching the front of the thigh. Once walking or standing, reconsider the angle the foot position is in. You can stretch the small rotator muscles by leaning

forward as you sit with the ankle over the knee. Whether male or female or non-binary, it is good to practice the lunge to stretch the lower back, the yielding forward to stretch the lower back and muscles, or the leg rotation while walking as in Qigong. It is exciting to view the role of the hip in each of the standing poses. If you have tight muscles around the hips or too much flexion or slumping in the lumbar spine, you may want to sit on a block whenever on the floor for a prolonged amount of time – as in a seated meditation. Using the block when sitting opens up the hip joint by letting the knees drop open and down toward the floor.

Knees

A lot of what can be done in yoga to care for the knees relies on becoming aware of alignment. When you are in a forward lunge, or in warrior or triangle, be sure that your knee is tracking forward over your middle toe. This is the generally true alignment advice. It may be that for your body, your knee needs to track slightly to the left or right of center. That is something you can determine through your own self body knowledge in combination with a trusted bodyworker or yoga teacher.

Since the knees are truly complex in their design, representing four different concave and convex joint interactions in each leg with eight different places where compression is possible, one must learn to be discerning of one's alignment, discomfort, and pain.

The inability to bend the knee can be further exacerbated by conditions like a Baker's cyst, which is a protruding wad of fluid. These cysts happen when there has been an infection, inflammation, or an injury. It is often located in the back of the knee.

Tried and true knee care: Bend and unbend the knees 3–5 times when folding over into

Martha had undiagnosed Lyme disease for at least five years. While cleansing out the parasitic organisms called spirochetes that come with Lyme disease, it has been important to also stretch and condense, yield and push, push and reach, and locomote. She also rested a lot to heal the knee.

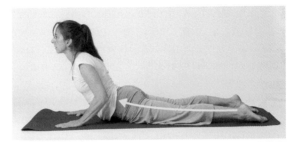

Figure 7.7

Map of the ankle to gonad connection. Photo by Serge Cashman.

forward bend or uttanasana for the first time as you start your practice. Do this consciously and slowly in rhythm with your breath. This rhythmic movement of large muscle groups gets the arterial blood flow going, which warms the tendons attaching the hamstring (and calf) muscles to the bones of the joint. This warming, increased blood flow allows the muscle to stretch with more ease. Repeat this when going into a downward dog or adho mukha svanasana.

Ankles

Activate the feet: Do this by pressing down into the balls of the toes, heel (calcaneus), and sides of the feet, which causes the feet to grip, like a bird holding onto a branch with its claw. This gripping causes a lift in the arch. This helps the muscles of the ankle to be rising upwards, rather than collapsing and then causing the ankle to tilt medially or laterally. After the exercise, remember to relax the toes and keep the arches lifted.

Cultivate your ankle to gonad connection: Do this over time to awaken the balance of muscles in the inner and outer leg, enlivening all parts of the legs. With a connection between each ankle to each related reflex point, you are helping the whole body to ground. The easiest way to do this is to shift your weight from leg to leg. Feel how the inner contents of your pelvis are transferring weight through your hip joints down toward your feet. Notice if your ankles feel flexible or stiff. Test how deeply you can bend them. Compare with a friend. See Figure 7.7 for map of ankle to gonad connection.

Remedy for ankle to gonad connection: The key here is movement of the pelvis. In particular, many people hold the pelvis in a locked position at the hip joint, which in turn affects the lower back. One can notice when on all fours or in kneeling whether the tops of the ankles are able to contact the floor – if not, explore moving your pelvis to release weight into the floor through your ankles. Often this requires letting yourself fully arch your back and let the sit bones reach back. Notice how both the pelvis and the ankles free up. Enjoy dancing with your pelvis to continue the feeling of freedom.

Remedy for tripping accidents: Do you have a tendency to twist your ankle, stub your toes, or fall off balance more than just occasionally? If so, you may want to spend time activating the push of one arm down into the pelvic bowl near the gonad reflex point (below the navel and slightly out to each side). Next, repeat that and allow yourself to move in space – downward or backward, feeling how your ankles respond. Are they stiff? Do

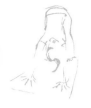

they adjust? Open up the connection of leverage through your arm into your body center down into your ankles. If you are on your belly you could feel like a fish (or mermaid) backing up.

Peripheral vision: Now use your arms to open up your peripheral vision – follow one finger of one hand with your eyes and let your body weight transfer, stepping as you look around. Keep feeling your feet and let your arms help with balance as you need.

Remedy for ankle impact: The ankle joint itself is mostly about forward and back movement of the foot or foreleg. However, together with the many bones of the feet the ankle area is able to make a circle. Slowly rotate the ankle as if painting a circle with the arch of your foot. Relax the toes as much as possible while you make the smoothest circles – even if they need to get smaller to be smooth. This exercise serves to learn how to reduce snap, crackle, and pop, eliciting more equal space in the joints.

Feet

Our feet hold us up all day; they support the weight of the whole body. It is especially important to take care of them. Throughout your Sun Salutation, practice pressing into what Daria Fain calls the *Nine Pillars of the Feet*. Activate each of these centers. This not only will be good for the health of your feet, but also it activates flow of energy throughout the body, instigates an upward cascade of alignment connections from ankle to knee to hip, and strengthens your feeling of grounding, your sense of connection to the earth. The latter lowers anxiety and calms the mind.

This a very simple but powerful practice. Press weight down through the nine pillars of your feet: the five toes, the base of the pinky and big toes, the center, lateral edge of the foot,

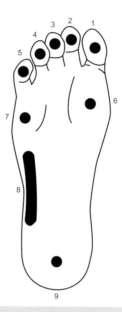

Figure 7.8
The Nine Pillars of the Feet.

and the heel/calcaneus. Feel the musculature active. Sense each pillar's connection down into the earth. Breathe into each of the pillars. This practice comes from Fain's teacher, Mantak Chia (see Figure 7.8).

Shakti's Personal Story: The Nine Pillars of the Feet

This is a Qigong image that I (Shakti) learned from SoHo Qigong teacher and dancer Daria Fain. I first learned this from her during the first months of the Covid-19 outbreak in New York City, while sheltering in place. She guided us into the nine pillars at the beginning of our two-hour online practice, and then we would visit it again and again, folding it into the other movements. I would often be surprised how quickly I had "left" my feet, due to the

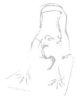

crisis and all the emotions raised. Coming back into the nine pillars would ground and calm me, all while practicing with 40 other dancers gathered online three mornings a week, from all over the world, from our living rooms, porches, and dance studios, united by our somatic practice while this virus changed our lives.

Integrating the Lower Body (Hip–Foot Connections)

To help integrate any work you have done in the lower body, from the joints of the hips to the feet, try this DE adaptation from Irmgard's Bartenieff Fundamentals, which has also been adapted to the pelvis–toe connection by BMC. While different people select different "connections," basics can be explored in this way.

As you stand and press into your big toe, see if you can get sensation in your pubic bone region. Pressure into the second toe often leads to sensation or connection to the hip socket while the third toe connects to the sit bone. The fourth toe can connect to the sacro-iliac joint and the fifth toe to the iliac crest (the large hip bone that people rest their hands on).

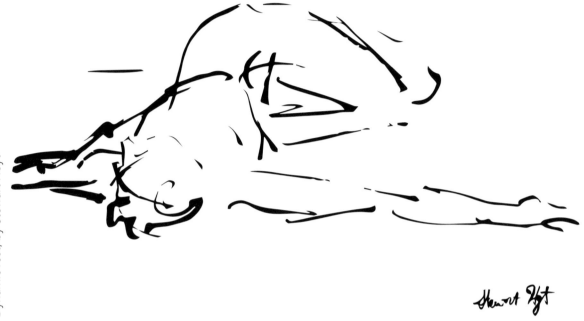

Dynamic rest, by Stewart Hoyt

Stewart Hoyt

8 Managing Glandular Challenges

There are many common health syndromes that relate to glandular imbalances. The four selected are adrenal exhaustion, sluggish thyroid, sleep irregularities, and immune weakness. These may be especially common in the Global North due to the lifestyle stresses that have been created by "westernization." They demonstrate a need for balance and we can learn from rich cultures where holism has managed to stay strong despite colonization by the North. The rituals of care from the Global South include lifestyle choices from different continents like being encouraged to take a siesta, squatting, balancing a basket of food on the head, sleeping on harder surfaces, or engaging in regular movement practices. These activities integrate various elements that are powerful for glandular balancing – keeping the spine strong, good rest, and movement. Dynamic Embodiment^SM (DE^SM) and

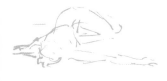

Chapter 8

Body-Mind Centering® (BMC®) work with the glands with these in mind, and so has yoga for thousands of years.

This chapter describes the glandular syndromes that many members of classes and private sessions in the United States are contending with, and ways to work with them using lifestyle practices. Here they are.

Common Issues

- Adrenals (core gland): exhaustion and chronic fatigue/Epstein–Barr. Focus on rest and recuperation, which also relates to the pineal gland and sleep patterns.

- Pineal (head gland): sleep patterns, difficulty sleeping or having to adjust to different time zones. Focus on circadian rhythm.

- Thyroid (throat gland): energy confusion, too much/too little work, and the need for expression and play. Focus on metabolism and energy protection.

- Thymus (chest gland): strengthening the immune system, dealing with immunity challenges. Focus on keeping healthy.

How does an imbalance present itself? Some personal stories help you notice that a particular gland is "out of whack." What can you do to balance? Experience ways of working that are typical of most forms of yoga and some that are specific to DE, as well as how they can be woven into your practice of the Sun Salutation. Humanity is also contending with climate crises, living on a planet that is out of balance. In Chapter 10 other types of supports are considered, beyond movement, such as the use of allopathic and integrative medicinal support, including herbs and entheogens.

A. Exhaustion and the Adrenals

Focus on rest and recuperation/becoming calmer and focused.

Common Issues

These include stress, sleep issues, weaker immunity, energy issues, city life, telephone addiction, irritability, and over-consumption of coffee and sugar.

Introduction

In this world where people even drive themselves intensely in a yoga class, it is important to learn new skills of recuperation and focus.

The adrenal glands are a storehouse for that extra spurt of energy needed in times of stress. As is common knowledge today, life and death stimuli are more rare (although cars, gun violence, and chronic abuse are indeed out there) than the *fears* of these and a multitude of other stressful concerns that can run rampant in the mind. When the mind is feeling under attack or when the body *is* under attack, the adrenals release up to three different hormones – epinephrine, norepinephrine, and cortisol. These are called the stress hormones. They direct our blood to reduce its flow to the organs of digestion (thus deactivating the parasympathetic nervous system) and outward to the muscles (activating the sympathetic nervous system beyond alertness into vigilance). The reason for this is that shunting of the blood is required to provide the oxygen needed to run away or self-defend – activities which require muscular action of the limbs and core. During this shunting process,

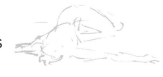

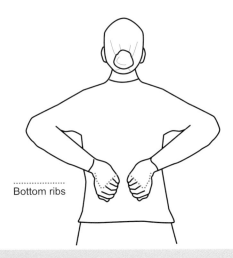

Figure 8.1
Locate the adrenals and kidneys.

the shift from a parasympathetic or balanced sympathetic–parasympathetic state to a sympathetic state known as the fight–flight–freeze condition, the ability to heal taxed cells and take in nutrition is greatly reduced.

Shakti on the Adrenal Glands: To Practice

This next section is written as if you were a student in class. Feel free to read through, then come back and do this part. Make yourself comfortable: sit on a meditation cushion, a yoga block, a folded towel, or a book.

This is how I teach about the adrenals.

In an anatomy book you'll see the adrenals sitting right on top of the kidneys, like two little caps or hats. Let's locate the kidneys in your body. Find the bottom rib of your ribcage, and trace it around to your back. Then make two fists with your hands, and place them with about half above the bottom rib and one half below (see Fig. 8.1). This is roughly where your kidneys are, on either side of your spine, next to (in line with) your spine.

One kidney is probably a little higher than the other. Some people have just one kidney. My mother was born with three. Now relax your fists and rest your arms/hands comfortably in your lap. Sense into this area, and picture/sense/feel the adrenal glands sitting on top of the kidneys. Again, there is one on each side, roughly in line with your spine.

Body Mind Centering/Dynamic Embodiment guides you to make a *ssssst* sound into or from the glands, almost like a bike tire being pumped up with air. You can imagine your adrenals being fortified, empowered, strengthened as you make this sound. This experience can help you to locate the glands kinesthetically within your body. Try it: on your next three out breaths, send this slow "*ssssttt*" sound into your glands. After your third exhalation, take a few normal, relaxed breaths and just notice and shifts/changes in your state of being.

Next I'd like you to try coming onto your back, with your legs curled into you, knees bent. Hug your knees into you, and sense your kidneys/adrenals being pressed into the ground. This is an "adrenal hug." This may be enough for you. Many experience this as calming, grounding, comforting. And you can also try rocking back and forth three or four or more times. Investigate; see how this feels.

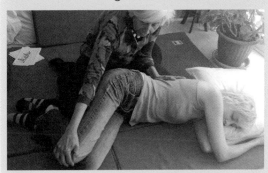

Figure 8.2
Linda Tumbarello side-lying adrenal hug with Dana Davison, photo by Shakti Smith.

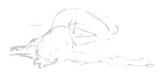

To try with a partner: locate their bottom rib in the back. Receiver, close your eyes and relax into the touch. Giver, bring your hands to the location of the kidneys, and intend warm, supportive energy for the adrenal glands. Rest here for 2–3 minutes.

Then switch roles, and take a few minutes to talk about it with each other afterwards. Also, notice how you and the room feel, before and after.

Last time I taught this in a group there was a palpable shift change in the room. The energy dropped in a feminine womb kind of way; at the same time it heightened and felt more connected. Everyone in the class could feel the shift.

Rule of Three

Now let's take a few moments to connect below and above, to practice our rule of three. Tune into your adrenals and trace a line or cord down to your ovaries. We're grounding the adrenals a bit, by connecting them to the glands below. You can place your fingers on your belly at the level of your navel; go down a few inches, and a few inches out to both sides. This is the rough location of your ovaries; let your fingers go intuitively to where they are. You may be one of many women who actually feel the ovaries each month, and know which is ovulating. If it is new to you, just trust your fingers to find the right location. Our body's wisdom, and your fingers' intuition, is so much stronger than some cultures lend us to believe.

If you have a male reproductive system, you can use the same energetic point. Bring your fingers to the navel; move 2 inches down and 2 inches out. Press gently here: this is the energetic point for your gonads. It is the top of the vas deferens, the duct that conveys sperm from the testicle to the ejaculatory ducts, and to the prostate gland and urethra.

In female bodies, the ovaries, like our kidneys, are likely placed one a little higher than the other. Sense in here for a minute. Often the ovary energy feels bright, a little zingy. You might feel it like this, or it could feel different for you. Just giving you something to "look" for. Good.

Now, let's trace the energy from the ovaries up to your adrenals, and then further up sense the energy internally, along your spine and sushumna, your energetic spine, up to the level of your heart. You can also place your fingers/hands on the outside of your body to trace these places physically. Put both hands on your heart for a minute. Sense into the reality that your heart has endocrine function. In DE the heart bodies are the emitter of endocrine function here, within the heart.

Take a few moments to rest here. See and sense the connection between these three places: your heart, adrenals, and ovaries. You can sense the connection between them, see/feel energy between them – visualize this as lines or perhaps a streaming of energy. The three being consciously connected by you will help them to be balanced, not over- or undercharged.

Some Yoga for Grounding

Press your sit bones into the earth, then reach up through your vertebrae, through your crown, to find a little height. Breathe in, bring your arms up, reaching gently towards the sky and, as you exhale, twist to the right, bringing your hands and arms down to the ground to support you. Sense into your kidneys and adrenals. How do they feel in this twisted position? Breathe in and out, for three more breaths. Inhale, and as you exhale come back to center, facing the front. As you inhale, bring your arms up again; sense into your kidneys/adrenals and notice

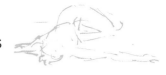

how they feel as you move into the twist to your left. Bring your arms down as you come into your position. Hold for three breaths. Then on an exhale come back to center. Take a moment to notice how you feel.

Kidney and Adrenal Wrapping

I (Shakti) understand that in Japan they sell a commercial item for warming the adrenals. As with India, I admire a culture that has endocrine health more intact in its mainstream culture. This item is placed on the back while you go about your day. Well, here's a version that you can make at home. Simply take a scarf, sarong, or pashmina and wrap it around your torso to cover the kidney and adrenals. Many visitors to my home or studio have arrived to find me dressed like this. Try it! Wrap like this for at least five minutes and notice how it makes you feel. This is a fine home remedy for supporting, calming, nourishing the adrenals. It counters fight or flight, and balances anxiety.

Dynamic Embodiment^SM Yoga Remedy for the Adrenals

Activity Descriptions

Body wrap: this is one of the many props that DEPs use as part of their practice. This particular one can be a warm woolen scarf or a flexible hot water bottle wrapped in cloth. This warms the kidneys and fosters relaxation for the adrenals.

Three-dimensional breathing and sounding (standing, seated, or lying down): with touch, breath, and/or sounding explore the three-dimensional capacity of the ribcage, and in particular this vast space of the upper body at the solar plexus.

Hands on kidneys, breathe into kidneys and adrenals: take time to locate the kidneys and bring this same three-dimensional breath into this area of the body.

Cat/cow: with hands and forelegs on the ground, explore extension and flexion using breath support. Specifically, breathe out fully while hollowing the front body and curving the back. Then breathe in before expanding and curving the back into convexity. (Notice your ankle–gonad connection too!)

Thread the needle: still in cat/cow lace one arm through the space between arm and knee to twist and stretch the rhomboid muscles and other areas of the back, volumizing the movement with lung support.

Triangle version of child's pose: start seated on your forelegs. Place your arms over your head, making a triangle with the index fingers and thumbs from each hand touching, keeping elbows apart. Bend over as if to bow and place your hands and forearm on the floor, keeping the triangles intact. Once in this position continue to practice three-dimensional breathing.

Adrenal breathing in "forward bend" of the Sun Salutation: whenever you fold over feel free to stay there and breathe. Feel your fetal energy. Expand into your kidney and adrenal region, enjoying expansion and release in your lower back.

Bartenieff Fundamentals open and closing, or Xs & Os (versions of this can be done seated or standing): lie down on the ground (it's OK to be on a mat or blanket if you like) and stretch out into an X shape, arms above your head and legs wide. With your exhale begin a curling-up action from your core – the area around your navel, front and

back – ending up condensed on your side (in a little O shape) with your head toward your knees. Stay there and complete your exhale fully. Then as you automatically inhale, coordinate your body to rotate, lengthen, and widen gradually, radiating out from your center by moving in all the above directions simultaneously.

Savasana (dead man's pose): lying down in the open X position – now the arms can move like a snow angel down to the sides of the body. Rest here and meditate. And, of course, practice yoga nidra.

B. Pineal (Head Gland): Sleep Issues and Pineal Imbalance (Melatonin)

Focus on circadian rhythm.

Common Issues

These include insomnia, macular degeneration, vision or hearing problems, sleep imbalances, and menstrual imbalances like dysmenorrhea and amenorrhea.

Introduction

The pineal gland is located in the upper back part of the ancient forebrain – in other words, it is nestled under the cerebral hemispheres (commonly referred to as the right and left halves of the brain). The pineal was considered a body – an entity that exists but which has no clear function or hormonal secretion – until 1959, when it was found in other animals. However, few in laypeople's circles knew of it or discussed it until the mid-1980s. I had been involved in sleep research as an undergraduate in the late 1970s and serotonin was being widely studied. Melatonin was not yet.

As is now well known, the pineal is indeed an active endocrine gland and releases the hormone called melatonin. Melatonin registers the circadian rhythm – letting the body know whether it is night or day.

BMC and DE picture a slightly upward inclined line from between the bridge of the nose to the soft spot on the back top of the head to visualize the connection between the pituitary and the pineal. We also feel that the mammillary bodies (one on each side of the midline of the upper brainstem close to the midbrain), which are along this axis, are glandular in nature. Their function(s) is linked to memory due to tracts to the hippocampus and the thalamus but the exact recollective memory functions continue to remain unknown.

> **Martha's Personal Story: Experiences with Light and Shifts in the Pineal–Ovarian Cycle**
>
> I grew up with a full moon every night. What? Well I lived on the third floor of a walk-up tenement in Manhattan where the street light was always on – beaming directly into my room.
>
> My period came within days of turning 12. That wasn't so strange. But, unlike my mother, I didn't have one each month. It was a really irregular, irregular "period" – in other words, no periodicity. It wasn't until about 25 years later that I met a man (now my husband) who liked room-darkening shades. After not many months my menses were coming every 28 days. Light makes a difference. A big difference. I have been asked whether or not it was simply having a regular partner that made a difference. That counts but I had lived with three other people during those 35 years

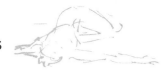

and this change didn't happen then. Others would say, "Well your sleep pattern got regularized." Nope – I was running a non-profit and doing payroll into the wee hours of the night, and then my doctoral homework and …. The light was what made the difference in me.

Now what does this have to do with the pineal? Remember that melatonin is released in response to the cycles of dark and light, as happens with the daily circadian rhythm. Research published in *Biological Research in Nursing* states "There is evidence of a relationship between light exposure and melatonin secretion and irregular menstrual cycles, menstrual cycle symptoms, and disordered ovarian function. In women with a psychopathology such as bipolar disorder or an endocrinopathy such as polycystic ovary syndrome, there seems to be greater vulnerability to the influence of light–dark exposure" (Barron 2007).

And it came back – fast-forward another 20 years, a time of perimenopause for me. I started to get headaches. Along with the headaches I started to have insomnia. Disturbances in sleep patterns, changes in menses, and issues with light returned. The impact of the moon on our cycles is worthy of learning more about. What is clear is the need to respect light and its impact on our physiology. *And* the benefit from celebrating darkness.

A nice side effect – the retina also benefits from darkness; the visual pigment in the back of the eye, rhodopsin, also requires an alternation of light and dark. Vision eases with a healthy retina. Consider issues like macular degeneration. There are stories about people who have greatly slowed down degeneration by "palming" – covering the eyes and relaxing or envisioning darkness or blackness as a way to meditate.

Shakti's Personal Story: Moon, Light, Sleep, and Menopause

How the Light of the Moon's Different Phases Affects Us

Another way to attune to monthly rhythms is to consciously watch the cycles of the moon change over the course of a month. In the city this is also a doorway into deepening your connection with nature. Some years ago I began calling the new phase of the moon "the dark moon." I picked this term up from shaman Lynn Roberts. To differentiate, the new moon is when you see that first crescent appear in the sky. The moon's light and gravitational pull affect not only the ocean and its waves but also our body's rhythms, and for women, our monthly cycles. During the dark moon I like to spend a little time outside, often on the roof of my apartment building in Brooklyn, appreciating the darkness. Then, when the crescent appears, I'm more apt to be touched by her beauty, and as she waxes over the next two weeks I can enjoy her growth.

This practice helps me know my own energy and mood rhythms. And I have recommended this to many clients. Seeing how the qualities of your mood intertwine with the phases of the moon can help you steer your own path to wellness. I notice an inwardness during the dark moon, and often a great amount of energy at the full moon. The police in NYC know that crime rates are always higher during the full moon – the statistics support this. My Iyengar yoga teacher, Eileen Muir, would speak of how she stayed up meditating during full moon nights because she couldn't sleep. I notice that I sleep less and wake up earlier during the full moon. And when I am in the country, I relish that light, that beautiful light of the

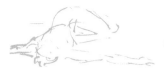

Chapter 8

moon, how it falls through a window and lights up a room. Or going for a walk out in it, being bathed in moonlight.

The Light and Sleep Connection

A decade ago I traveled to Jordan with some of my family. For two nights we stayed with Bedouin tribal members in the desert, near the edge of the Sahara. At night, during a new moon, the light of the stars was as powerful as the light of our full moon in the States. This showed me how distorted our sense of light is in the USA. I grew up in the woods, in the mountains of Vermont. But I had never experienced skies as dark and full of stars as I saw in Jordan, where there is less electric lighting due to the country being less developed. At 10pm I walked by starlight into the desert with my partner, Stewart, my Mom, and my older brother. And we all awoke with ease at 5am to watch the sunrise.

I'm sure that many of our culture's sleep issues would be solved if we lived more aligned with nature in this way. When I go camping I rise with the sun and go to sleep earlier in the night. We can recreate this in our homes with electric lighting, by turning out lights slowly as the evening progresses – even lighting candles instead in some parts of your home, and turning off electronic devices an hour before bed to allow your body to tune into the darkness, to allow melatonin to be released instead of suppressed.

Low lighting, or streetlights that have the light pointing downwards instead of up towards the sky, is growing in popularity, and is required in some cities, in some cases because of concern for bird populations and how city lights will disturb their ability to navigate their flight paths. A commercial building with uplighting filled my bedroom with light for a few months; when they switched to downlighting we could sleep in darkness again.

Reframing and Honoring Menopause

Perimenopause was brutal for me. In my mid-forties, I began waking up every 2–3 hours with heart palpitations and sweats, and all the quality of mood that comes with that (read irritability in here). My perimenopausal symptoms were exacerbated by the busy Brooklyn avenue I lived on, and also by the Kundalini rising that I had been experiencing already for decades. I found that when we moved to a different part of Brooklyn I began to sleep better as there was less light and less noise. What a difference. But even so, when menopause kicked in at age 50, I was not able to sleep for more than an hour for almost a year. I woke up every hour sweating. I was not able to read more than one page of a book during this time, as my mind was so agitated; I began to actually wonder if I would ever be able to read a book again. Luckily I shared with my older women friends, and they assured me that this would pass.

Valerian root tincture gave me a little help. But it wasn't until I began combining it with melatonin that I slept sometimes as much as 4 hours in a row. Chinese herbs, along with dark shades, and the weight of an eye pillow on my eyes, also helped to relax me into a deeper and longer sleep each night. Being aware of what I ate became even more important, avoiding spicy foods, especially before bed, and also sugars and chocolate. Tuning into our fine human systems, our bodies, really listening and paying attention to what they need, can genuinely help us find what we need for greater health.

One year into menopause I began to experience frozen shoulder in my left arm. This is quite challenging and can be difficult to treat. Even with my 25 plus years' experience treating clients and teaching the health practitioners at the Swedish Institute College of Health Sciences in New York

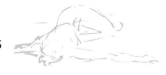

City, I didn't know about this symptom until it happened to me. Since then I have heard from other health practitioners, including many acupuncturists that they *think maybe* it's a symptom. I've heard enough corroboration to know now that it is one. Also see Martha's story above. I do wonder at the mysterious shroud that seems to veil helpful and useful knowledge around menopause. There still is shame for many women in speaking about this time in their lives publicly. If some of us feel comfortable doing so, well, it will only help others and our culture to evolve.

Menopause is a special time in a woman's life. Martha and I are both sharing our stories in part because we've noticed that women, still, do not share much about this time in their lives. The more we share our stories with each other, the more we can learn from each other, and find the answers each of us needs for comfort and health.

One of my colleagues at the Swedish Institute, Alix Keast, teaches a course on menopause for bodyworkers and acupuncturists. It's from Alix that I learned how to reframe this time – to truly begin to get that it is a time of turning inward, and wisdom naturally arising. It's a time to be honored. And interestingly, in cultures where this is the case, women experience fewer negative menopausal symptoms. Only 7 percent of Japanese women have hot flashes. Some studies say this is due to the amount of soy that they eat, but I resonate with there being a sociological aspect.

Menopause is a way for our bodies to help us live longer. Chinese medicine enlightens us to this process: now we are conserving blood rather than eliminating it. It stays inside more and transforms to the Shen, or spirit. Shen is the aspect of us that is spiritual. Menopause is that transition into the third aspect of a woman's life, the time of the crone (the Maiden, the Mother, and the Crone); or according to Alix Keast, it is "The second spring, the beginning of the second half of our life guided by spirit, the first half integrated as wisdom. It's the time to begin cultivating the inner self, a time of grace, connectedness, and understanding" (Weed 2002, Wolfe 1990).

Dynamic Embodiment^SM Yoga Remedy for Pineal

For activating the pineal: child's pose with rocking from head to feet.

The "on the floor" triangle pose "push from the head" from BMC: go into child's pose and place your arms over head with your thumbs and forefingers making one triangle and your hands and elbows another. Likewise in the lower body your big toes touch and your knees are apart. Feel these each as triangles. Once again, take care to shape your body in space while also adapting the position so that you are comfortable. Once you have done that, check in somatically. Is your weight distributed equally through each arm and each leg? What is your contact into the ground with your forearm and forelegs? As much as possible, seek symmetry – equal weight into each limb, being careful to avoid pain. This is a simulation of the starting position for the movement of a baby getting ready to be born and the practice (or re-practice) ground for the *"push of head and push of the tail."* In the BMC theory the push of the head stimulates the pineal gland. I have also found it is one of the best ways to relieve headaches. The rocking back and forth:

- massages the head/scalp

- loosens up the atlanto-occipital joint

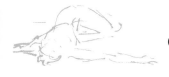

- provides stimulation through the bodies of the vertebrae of the spine.

Palming and/or blindfolded meditation: In order to sleep more deeply and with ease it is often recommended to meditate before falling asleep, especially if you have been having a hectic or challenging day emotionally. Covering the eyes or wearing a blindfold provides darkness, which is so important for the brain, the entire nervous system, and the retina of the eyes (sometimes helpful with macular degeneration). The use of an eye pillow brings in the weight that triggers a physiological relaxation response in the eyes. If one is traveling through diverse time zones it can be helpful to deeply rest, and especially rest one's eyes, while on the plane. Timing the rest may even reduce jet lag. Some people use essential oils (ylang ylang) and practice finger holds from Jin Shin Jyutsu to help reduce jet lag as well. Many people respond well to homeopathic jet lag remedies.

Use of pineal when pushing backwards into downward dog: there is so much physical benefit to the downward dog. Let's think about the additional benefits that result from engaging the pineal as well.

Even though the pineal responds to light, it is thought to govern hearing (both sound and vibration) and is powerful in settling the nervous system. The correlated developmental movement is pushing backwards from the head. Once you have learned this coordination (or relearned it since most of us used it while *in utero* or in our first movements as newborns) involving pushing off the floor, or wall (and originally our mother's womb), you can enlist it while standing without anything to push off but *space*. The sequencing of movement from head toward tail through the fullness of the spine and core is happening in subtle ways all day long.

In doing the Sun Salutation, this coordination can support actions that are or feel challenging or that are simple enough to keep practicing: for instance, whenever you want to move backwards (by stepping from the leg or the sit bones). You can start the movement from finding your crown chakra. Then sequence from that point down through the spine until you have shifted your weight to your feet. If sleep does not improve *or* if you are feeling happy but have an overwhelming experience of fatigue, please move on to exploring the peacefulness that can come from compression from the head to the tail.

C. Thyroid – Metabolism Issues

Focus on energy protection.

Common Issues

These include cold hands/cold feet, fast heartbeat, higher blood pressure, anxiety, sensitivity to heat, diarrhea, weight loss (often sudden), increased appetite, thinning hair, sweating, itchiness, trembling and shaking, irritability, and sleep problems.

Introduction

The thyroid gland sits nestled behind the Adam's apple in the center of the neck and performs the important function of determining our metabolic rate – just how fast the body operates.

The thyroid thereby sets our basal metabolic rate at which our more autonomic parts (heart, breath, organs, and other glands) function. According to BMC, embodied awareness of the thyroid opens up awareness

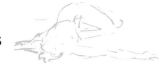

of the entire endocrine system, serving as its keystone.

When with children, teachers sometimes say "How hot is your engine?" The thyroid hormones help set into gear the activity of many other glands (together with direction from the pituitary gland). For instance, there is the pituitary–thyroid–gonad complex.

There are now a multitude of books on thyroid dysfunction and many inter-relate with Lyme disease, menopause, and immunology.

Martha's Personal Story: Thyroid Underfunctioning

Cold hands, cold feet. Do you like to put on socks to fall asleep at night? Yes, these can be familiar signs of thyroid imbalance. However, it took spending time with my elderly father and an excellent integrative physician to learn that there are other signs of thyroidal distress – fatigue, narcolepsy, itching skin, memory loss. What a variety of uncomfortable symptoms – hard to pinpoint but all about the overall rate of the body not working well. As you may recall, the thyroid sets the metabolic state of the body, helping determine whether one operates quickly or slowly – the life rhythm. And yet testing for the thyroid levels in the blood is often cursory – checking on Th1 and Th2 but not T3 and T4. It takes an investigative doctor to insist on digging deeper.

Sadly, my dad only learned of his thyroid imbalance a few weeks before his death. He began taking his medication just around the time he started experiencing mini-strokes, falls, and other more life-threatening consequences of being "out of whack." He suffered with what he called his "17 ailments" for years prior to that. Unfortunately, he could have lived more comfortably. He often was cold, especially at his extremities, he had terribly itchy skin, constipation was also an issue, and he would

fall asleep in the middle of the day – deep fatigue and memory issues.

Does this sound like getting old?

Or perhaps being dehydrated?

Or being perimenopausal?

Or related to Raynaud's disease?

Maybe, yes, since all of these are symptoms of an underactive thyroid: five of the 17 ailments (that he recognized as inconveniences not illnesses) that made an 85-year-old pretty uncomfortable and unwilling to travel any more. Hypothyroidism is more common than many might think (4.6 percent of Americans, predominantly women, have it) and yet still relatively unknown in the everyday world. There is also an autoimmune condition called Hashimoto's disease whereby one's body attacks its own thyroid, and this is becoming more and more widespread.

Overactive thyroid, also known as hyperthyroidism, can exhibit conditions such as thyroiditis, goiter, and Graves' disease. These all mean that the thyroid is working harder, producing more hormones, and the body's metabolism is speeded up because of it. Symptoms range from fast heartbeat, higher blood pressure, anxiety, sensitivity to heat, diarrhea, weight loss (often sudden), increased appetite, thinning hair, sweating, irritability, trembling and shaking, and sleep problems. An important word of caution: this condition asks that no more large stimulus be given to the gland. In particular, minimize vocal work and rather than engaging with the organ and gland hissing described earlier ("*sssst*"); instead, spend time in meditation, quiet singing (almost whispering), and/or restful movement.

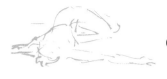

Chapter 8

Martha's Personal Story: Balancing the Endocrine System

As mentioned in the pineal section, when I (Martha) turned 50, I started to be perimenopausal and was feeling stiffening joints, tiredness, and occasional heart palpitations. As it turned out, not all of my symptoms were menopausal at all… It took me two years to figure out that the three times I had taken antibiotics for a tick bite hadn't held. I had Lyme disease – what some call chronic Lyme. But more to the point, my integrative MD discovered with his thorough blood tests that I also had chronic fatigue syndrome and Hashimoto's disease. The heart palpitations and anxious feelings were an anomaly – they more often show up with hyperthyroidal imbalances but it turns out they are symptoms of Lyme. I first learned I had Hashimoto's when I was tested for Lyme disease. I am thankful for the knowledge of yoga and the interaction with the glands in balancing my thyroid activation.

The heart palpitations became my most worrying feature since they didn't fit the low thyroid profile. To understand the science of this a bit more, here are more facts, as stated in MyThyroid.com: "The heart is very sensitive to even small changes in the levels of thyroid hormones.

The heart is a muscle and contains receptors for thyroid hormone, hence heart muscle growth and cardiac function may be influenced by too much or too little thyroid hormone. There is increasing evidence that even small changes in levels of thyroid hormone may be associated with measurable changes in how well the heart functions" (Biondi et al 2002, Schmidt & Ascheim 2006). As even small amounts of thyroid hormone can speed up the metabolic activity and oxygen consumption of your heart, treatment with even small doses of thyroid hormone may cause angina, shortness of breath, or palpitations and rapid heartbeats in some susceptible patients.

So now I live with "balancing my endocrine system" with more care than ever. I need to align with the circadian rhythm, exercise, and eat well (especially no gluten), and am forever thankful that I understand how the Sun Salutation – my daily ritual – and attention to the glandular activation within the Sun Salutation can help bring more balance to my body.

Dynamic Embodiment[SM] Yoga Pose Remedy for the Thyroid

- Throat chakra breath and awareness

- Standing or sitting: suspending from the thyroid by arching the neck back and up (see Chapter 1 on suspension and compression, p. 52)

- Fish pose (suspension)

- Savasana or Legs Up the Wall (compression)

- Shoulder stand (compression)

- Neck extension and shoulder circles (combines compression and suspension).

- Jumping back from being bent over – moving into plank (developmental).

Throat Chakra Breath and Awareness

Bring your awareness into your throat, allowing one hand to rest at your upper chest/throat area. Take three full complete in and out breaths. Find that yawning feeling in the back

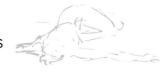

of your throat, to help this area be open physically and energetically. Sense this area's depth and width, its breadth. Begin to breathe light into this area, bringing in more fullness. See this light becoming blue, the first shade of blue that comes into your mind's eye.

Tuck your chin slightly, and lengthen the back of your neck. Invite your neck to gently reach up through the crown of your head towards the sky.

Come to lie down, near an empty wall or a tree. Consider bringing yourself into fish pose, which is beneficial for its thyroid stimulus. It opens up the whole upper throat and chest area (see Fig. 8.3).

Now lying on your back, shift into Legs Up the Wall (see p. 153 for instructions). Rest in this pose for 5–20 minutes. Allow it to do its natural magic. With this gravitational reversal your fluids and energy are all flowing downwards with a pooling at your throat and a reoxygenation of your brain. Enjoy this rejuvenative pose.

Standing or Sitting, Suspending from the Thyroid

Let's dig into what else is involved when simply being still, whether sitting or standing. When you are vertical, upright, it helps you extend your neck and with a little extra stretch it can position the thyroid (and parathyroids) within a tensegrity that helps activate these glands.

Align your spine and look up.

Attempt to find a "high point" from the Adam's apple and downward in the low region of your neck.

Hang from there. Hold the upward focus. You may even feel energy as vibrating or trembling. Include the focus of suspending from your thyroid in your practice wherever you can. Notice any pulls on your collar bone – either from along your breastbone or ribs and

out into your arm to or from your elbow – these connections with the joints are important and, together with thymus problems, may underlie issues like frozen shoulder (the nickname for menopause in Japan). What is important is to breathe into the sensations, allow for little changes of alignment and blood flow. If you have the experience of cranio-sacral work, allow for sensation of the cranio-sacral rhythm or the cerebro-spinal fluid to help balance each arm from throat through sternum to elbow – or if you have the resources schedule a cranio-sacral session. The goal is to feel energy circulating in your throat and vocal diaphragm. It may also feel like a pulse. Play with sound, if desired. Remember sound is vibration, and vibration heals and balances. Explore guttural and bird-like sounds; every possible use of the larynx helps awaken thyroidal activity.

Sounding with the Thyroid

Reminder: this is for low thyroid – hypothyroidism; see above for hyperthyroidism.

Protecting Energy

Is Hashimoto's a response to overactivity? It could be. Hence it is often a good choice to consider doing less, since resting more is a way to balance the thyroid active. Use the remedy from the pineal and adrenals. This can be integrated with spinal undulation initiating from the chin (from African dance and sometimes referred to or explored from a glandular perspective: for instance, during BodyMind Dancing, a loosely structured DE dance class that focuses on embodiment and self-healing more than learning steps). Now add in your choice of sounding from the throat and expanding energy through the arms – extending the elbows.

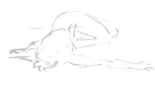

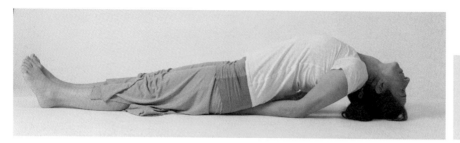

Figure 8.3
Fish pose/
matsyasana. Photo by
Serge Cashman.

Fish Asana: Also Suspending from the Thyroid

In the Fish, lift the chest from supine (lying on the back) and allow the head to extend backwards – with the crown of the head taking weight (on a book or block if needed) as well as the hips and legs and the elbows/forearms. The center of the neck is on stretch as in the standing or seated suspension described above. When the cervical spine is arching this becomes a "suspensional" stretch – meaning that an apex is created with a high point that lifts up against gravity. Tension is established at each end of the stabilizing sides and the high point of arch allows for musculo-fascial connectivity that in turn facilitates glandular energy flow along the whole line.

Integrated with the Sun Salutation

Do all of the above. Then, take time to move from mountain pose (asana #2 of the Sun Salutation) into the arching of your back. This round, make sure that you feel the throat as the apex of your "suspension bridge." Take time to pay attention to the subtlest sensations of your shoulders down to your elbows throughout the ritual.

Stimulating the Thyroid with Whole-Body Movement

Developmental movement: remember that the reach of two legs backwards or downwards is a thyroidal stimulant. Examples include jumping the legs out into plank position or reaching the heels down from being up on the toes. Other variations: reach the heels down and away from the head while in plank or upward dog, or reach the heels away from the sit bones in downward dog. For extra support, keep the energy active along your collar bone out through your elbows.

Allow what Bonnie Bainbridge Cohen calls the "nectar of well-being" to release through the skin, supported by pleasurable touch. Then breathe through your nose toward the roof of your mouth and feel how both skin and breath relate to oxytocin, while stimulating cranial nerve zero. You can feel this is nature – when the breeze touches your skin and the smell of plants, earth, and water stimulates the release of oxytocin, emerging from the anterior pituitary. Open your Third Eye to feel the pleasure of being alive.

Dynamic Embodiment^{SM} Yoga Remedy for the Sun Salutation

The primary focus is on reaching back with two legs for the thyroid and one leg for each (opposite) parathyroid. Feel the reach downward into the feet, from the neck region, when standing and when reaching away with the arms – especially during the backbend. In other words, take time to "suspend from the thyroid," lifting up from the apex of the neck to arch the back. As you continue, feel

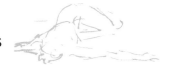

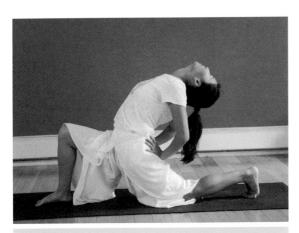

Figure 8.4
Suspensional support for thyroid and parathyroid lunge. Photo by Serge Cashman.

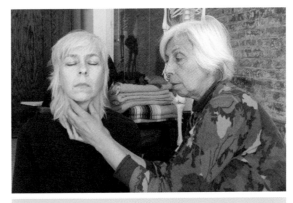

Figure 8.5
Accessing the thyroid – Linda Tumbarello with Dana Davison, photo by Shakti Smith.

the counter-pull of the "symmetrical reaching of two arms" with the downward "symmetrical reaching into the earth of two legs." This action is using both the thymus and thyroid in consort – balancing the metabolism while activating the immune system. The reach of two legs backwards can be a great tonifier for the thyroid. Knowing this, pay attention to the reaching of the two heels down toward the floor when in down dog – notice any sensations in the thyroid region. When reaching one leg back, feel the thyroid region and now pinpoint the opposite higher parathyroid and make a high pitched sound from there.

On days with more time one can engage with the fish (matsyasana, see Fig. 8.3) and also with other directly thyroid-activating asanas like camel (ustrasana pose).

Finally, attune to posture and "use" throughout the day, especially after hovering over a laptop for many hours. Here are some questions to ask:

- How can I feel my feet and lengthen and breathe, even through my neck?

- How do I sit at the computer, at the dinner table?

- How do I stand and walk? Do I enjoy my length? Am I comfortable with my height?

- Where can I move and sing? Sing!

These minute-by-minute uses of the body add up and impact our overall health. Little steps go a long way.

D. Thymus – Autoimmune Issues

Focus on keeping healthy.

Common Issues

These include strengthening the immune system, dealing with immunity challenges (e.g. AIDS/HIV, rheumatoid arthritis, chronic fatigue, candida, Lyme and other autoimmune illnesses), and lymphatic flow.

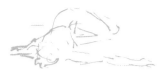

Chapter 8

Introduction

The thymus was thought to have no function beyond the release of growth hormones until the highpoint of the AIDS crisis when research began into this disease and discovered that the thymus also is a factory for T-cells – infection-fighting cells. Prior to this knowledge, recommendations were fairly common to remove the thymus after adolescence if there was a minor issue with it. What is really important is how it impacts the T-cells and amplifies the immune response – all important for fighting off invading substances. More research is needed on the links to melatonin and insulin. What is important is that this gland is *important*.

Martha's Personal Story: Understanding the Thymus

For a period of time in the late 1980s I lived with my female partner and a dear friend who was a gay male. We talked a lot about him donating sperm for us to build a family, providing semen for artificial insemination. Sadly he discovered he had HIV and we discontinued this dream, and even more sadly we lost our dear friend and potential father, from AIDS. It was a deeply tragic time, with so much loss. There was so little known about the disease and certainly about how to control it with drugs. Within the next few years people with AIDS taught us about an unknown function of the thymus gland: it *produces* killer cells – T-cells – not just adolescent growth hormone (AGH). If someone had a health problem in the manubrium area (top of the breastbone, where the thymus is located) it was not atypical for the thymus to be removed. The medical community did not know in the 1980s that the thymus was a primary body area for the production of cells that would fight off viral infections.

Shakti's Personal Story: Touch Aiding Heart and Thymus Awareness

I recently had the experience of helping someone who felt her heart was upset. I asked if I could put hands on her upper thoracic area (around the first rib circle and upper sternum = breastbone). She said absolutely. So I placed my left hand at the base of her neck on her spine and my right hand over her manubrium – the top bone of the breastbone. She instantly felt an easing up of her tension, fear, concerns.

I asked her – might you like more sense of safety and protection for your heart? She vehemently said YES, that is exactly what she needs. She reported that her heart actually feels okay but she does feel the need for protection.

I said – I want you to know that my hands are not on your heart – they would need to move down and to your left more (where one's left hand falls across the right chest during a "pledge of allegiance"). I asked if I could do that. She said sure.

As it turned out she quickly learned that her heart was quite open and receptive but that she needed more stimulus to her thymus – the gland behind the manubrium that is response for creating T-cells for fighting off bacteria and other foreign agents in the body.

She resonated deeply with the metaphor of the thymus's function – not just the production of growth hormone during adolescence – but also being the seat of our immune or self-defense system.

Needing protection is an age-old theme. It may stem from parenting that didn't include enough protection physically, emotionally, spiritually, or even cognitively. Or it can be born from disease and the need to produce but also balance the production of white

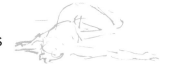

blood cells and other sorts of macrophages. One can have a weakened immune system for all sorts of reasons.

Dynamic Embodiment^{SM} Yoga Remedy for the Thymus

- Heart mudra and then work with heart, high heart chakra

- Immune system stimulation tapping

- DE thymus meditation/somatization

- Camel, upward dog, savasana

- Lymphatic warrior dance – hugging, squeezing, and elongating, stretching into *huge* kinesphere – includes claiming space – "My Space"

- Reach and hug – notice resistance to reaching out and especially reaching out for someone or something.

Reach and Hug

What is quite poetic is that the developmental movement that correlates with the thymus in Body-Mind Centering® (BMC®) refers to the arms reaching out symmetrically, like a young child reaching for a parent. This reaching out for what one wants or needs is a critical psychosocial milestone. As adults one can still practice reaching out for what is needed and wanted, including asking for a hug. In this way the natural desire for connection can be fulfilled by asking for what one needs; as long as one attunes with who to ask – ideally sensitive and caring people who respect your needs, avoiding anyone who is oppressive or abusive.

Interestingly, it is having the courage to reach out for our needs – whether facing adversity, or being shy, or needing support – that also strengthens our immune systems. Experiential: stand in front of a mirror – reach out to yourself. How does it feel to do this? Easy, silly, or hard? Or something else? Try it with a friend. Dance classes that include these reaches keep it more abstract – perhaps a nice way to begin activating your thymus more.

In BMC, and adapted for Moving For Life Cancer Recovery, the immune system is awakened by gently or vigorously tapping on one's upper central chest. The vibration, whether light or more firm, enlivens this energy center rather quickly.

Other activities and poses include starting child's pose and then shifting into "hang and hollow," an exercise of Peggy Hackney's (1998). "Hang and hollow" allows you to place your weight on your upper chest and into two outstretched arms until your hips come off your heels and your lower back is arched. In this scenario one can rest one's thymus on pillows and breathe, or breathe and sound until the vibration returns. It is a great time to notice

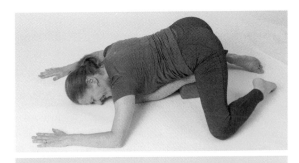

Figure 8.6
Frog pose with thymus support. Photo by Serge Cashman.

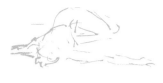

Chapter 8

how the collar bones (clavicles) feel and also to allow for width through the shoulder joint as well.

Martha's Personal Story: Confusing and Confluent

In doing anthropological research I have learned to wait for triadic confirmation – at least three points of agreement before postulating something new. For biologically based insights I am interested in the confluence of medical diagnoses, stories of lived experiences from others, and my own somatic experience. So when I turned 50 years old and was diagnosed with Lyme disease along with Hashimoto's disease and Epstein–Barr, I was fascinated by these interactions. At this time I experienced tennis elbow (epicondylitis). During the process of healing from these two diseases I felt strongly that they interact, sometimes overriding and sometimes working to help each other, and in that way getting confused. For a while the thymus and elbow became linked.

As I moved into menopause, I felt that the thyroid and shoulder are linked, perhaps because I experienced a frozen shoulder. During this time and after, I have heard dozens of women reporting the simultaneous medical diagnoses of frozen shoulders and thyroid problems. Some of the same as well as other women (and books) shared stories about their specific sensations and culture's responses to menopause or thyroid problems relating to corollaries with shoulder discomfort or immobility.

Hence, I have been dealing with both thymus and thyroid problems concurrently, along with the adrenals. Hashimoto's is an autoimmune problem of the thyroid. Epstein–Barr virus causes chronic fatigue, which also impacts the adrenals. I sometimes wonder how these two glandular health challenges integrate through me, especially through my joints.

Once my Lyme disease and Epstein–Barr were under control I experienced a frozen shoulder – I still had low thyroid levels. To this day I personally feel a strong pull between the lower neck and my coracoid process, along with a tiny bit of discomfort across the top front of my shoulder joint, specifically the bicipital groove of my humerus bone. I must breathe deeply into this area and make space there as I do all phases of the Sun Salutation. And I can also ask – has my thymus (in its attempt to fight viruses and parasite spirochetes) taken over some of the work of its neighbor, the thyroid? Or has my thyroid been attempting to shut down a bit and slow down productivity, do less, and let the thymus take precedence? Is this why my elbow hurt for a while and then uncomfortable sensations ended up lingering in my shoulder for a long time?

Once these conditions were managed I continued to add in my own memories of health challenges as well as medical data from diverse sources. Long before I was 50, I was teaching about the thyroid and how often it is linked to frozen shoulders amongst the women I work with who are dealing with cancer. In that class, a Japanese student reported that in Japan women informally refer to menopause as frozen shoulder since it is so commonly interconnected.

I imagine that if I'm experiencing huge exhaustion, both my adrenals and thyroid are impacted. The management of the Hashimoto's may well be supported by resting deeply. It could be that one affects the other or that there comes to be a confusion of their purpose (as happens with autoimmune diseases). Bodily functions become confused. It could be that related joints are confused as well. For instance,

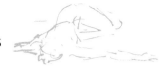

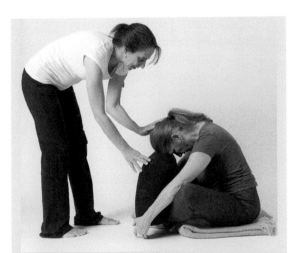

Figure 8.7
Support for the adrenals and pineal: deep rest of head glands, withdrawing the senses, extension of the arms with thymus and thyroid. Photo by Serge Cashman.

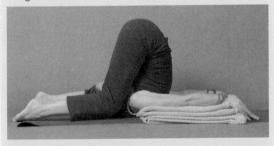

Figure 8.8
Adrenals and pineal. Photo by Serge Cashman.

I sometimes feel that my elbows are dependent on my thymus instead of my thyroid vitality, especially as I go to reach out with two arms. Similarly, sometimes I experience that the thyroid relates deeply to the shoulders (as in perimenopausal thyroidal shifts and frozen shoulders). Said another way, I sometimes need to engage the thymus as a great support through the elbows in order to fully extend the arms to do a complete reach. This extension is needed in protective extension and in

reaching for love – a hug or a lift, both courageous acts of self-care.

I find that both the thymus and the thyroid, as well as the shoulder joint and the elbow, support the early childhood movement of the reach of two legs to frog-jump backwards. Similarly, in order to reach down or back with two legs (often wriggling as a baby or jumping as a child), I feel not only the need for a strong connection between the throat and down the back through the legs but a need for grounding through the shoulder joint – to support the upper body weight. Our energy can rest, when there is less need for metabolic action when our self-defensive and growth-related hormones are not boldly triggered, when our cells are feeling safe.

What may be most important is the connectivity between the thymus and the thyroid. In Body-Mind Centering® a literal band of connectivity is perceived to exist there. For sure these two glands are in close proximity, and may work together either bio-chemically or as physical fulcrums of support. Once again, it's important to work with interactions with the glands and to remember that all cells have a neuroendocrine potential. Stay true to your own physical experiences and, if you enjoy being a detective, continue to investigate interactions between different lines of connectivity in the body – throat (thyroid) to elbow, upper chest (thymus) to shoulder for sure, and perhaps throat to shoulder and chest to elbow as well.

Conclusions about Managing Glandular Imbalances through Movement and Sound

There are many more challenges, syndromes, and illnesses that exist in the world – each can find support from the philosophy or practice

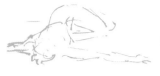
of yoga, especially when using the principles of DE:

- *Observe:* witness yourself, be present with the words and demonstration of the teacher, BUT always follow your own healthy and positive influences/thoughts first.

- *Support:* "feel into the experience," move small and slow to test the waters, constantly check in with your body's cues (proprioception) as you choose to "amp up," and take time for embodiment using sound, touch, and movement in order to stimulate your own awakeness – mindfulness comes from having feelings – of your breath, of your skin, of you – the you who lives in a body while alive on this planet. Celebrate it!

- *Options:* be as big as you are, knowing you can always retreat, condense, hide.

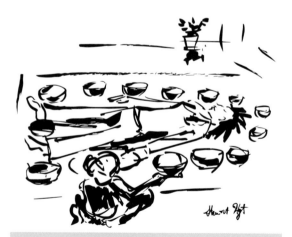

Figure 8.9
The sound is holding you, by Stewart Hoyt.

Vary dynamics until the experience is pleasurable (including your voice) and if you are truly comfortable in your body consider having some fun, getting playful, and even changing the dynamics to "stretch your comfort zone." In order to evolve as a species there is much unpacking of habits to do if we are to bring health to our society and planet. It is important to be able to sustain a certain amount of discomfort while look at the evil and imbalances in the world. Our own sustainability allows for observation versus engagement in the destruction and injustices in the world. This sustained focus can support us through lessons that hurt *and* changing our policies and the structures of our institutions.

Integration: Sliding Up the Wall

This action requires what DE calls the "symmetrical foot reach" or "foot reach and slide." The support involves compression in the head and throat, and can be described as *head gland compression.* Then, when initiating movement, all the head and throat glands from the pineal to the thyroid take weight as the lower glands activate to slide the heels upward. Along the way the coccygeal body, gonads (the ovarian pull is important for the menstrual cycle and testicular energy is grounded at the same reflex point), and adrenals come away from the floor and incline toward the wall, and the pancreas, thoracobodies, heart bodies, and thymus create a subtle slope, like a sling – another tensegrity. You can feel these connections of joints to glands energetically to make the movement easier: coccygeal–hip,

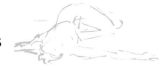

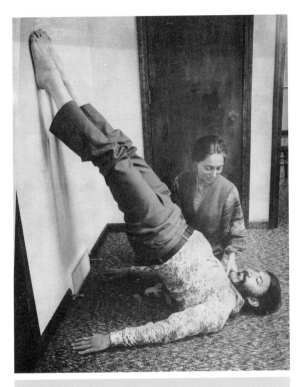

Figure 8.10
Sliding Up the Wall, as demonstrated by Leonard Cohen with Bonnie Bainbridge Cohen circa 1977, integrating all the glands, using compression and suspension. Springfield Union Staff Photo, by Vincent S. D'Addario. Shared by courtesy of Len and Bonnie Bainbridge Cohen.

gonad–ankle, adrenals – knees and thighs. The pancreas, thoraco, and heart bodies may want to slide up off the wall as well – that is fine – or they may remain part of the hammock with the neck being the lowest compressional point. This is all regulated by the mover and dependent on your:

1. coordination

2. flexibility

3. somatic awareness of spatial counter-tensions (more than strength).

Body-Mind Centering® – Sliding Legs Up the Wall

Beginning position: lie with sit bones close to the wall and legs approximating a 90-degree angle so your feet are up the wall (legs are usually predominantly straight – extended at the knee), with the back of torso and head relaxing on the floor (feel free to have a small pillow under your head if needed).

Task: glide the heels up the wall with a reach and pull from the feet. The reaching of the two feet simultaneously stimulates the thyroid gland with tensegrity (counter-tensional forces), and the positioning also compresses the thyroid due to weight pouring into the neck (like a mini shoulder stand, which has support from the wall). This exercise can be done with careful awareness brought to each gland as it moves off the floor – starting from the coccygeal body sequentially through to the thyroid.

9 Considerations in Teaching the Sun Salutation

Overview/Introduction

There is an interconnectivity in teaching about chakras, glands, yoga, self-healing, somatic education, therapy, and dance. Here you, as a teacher, can gain more resources for teaching classes. Methods are suggested for engaging the process of moving with glandular awareness and for guiding others through this practice. Some curricular structures are provided with sample themes and variations, and lessons built around emergent common needs/desires and motivations. Given the goal of making the Sun Salutation accessible to all who are interested, and the social somatic perspective that humans all have a multiplicity of needs and points of view, a shared goal is to strive to honor the wisdom of different people – culturally, racially, and in terms of all forms of identity. This is also true of personal bodily

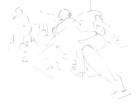

history. It is recommended that you, as an instructor, learn to accommodate lesson plans to meet your students. This includes social experiences as well as how personal life experience of illnesses and injuries shift perspective. It is ideal to be sensitive to students' abilities and also open to the wisdom that anyone with a disability brings to class. There are often needs for adaptation; it is a call for creative response. We build lessons around emergent common needs/desires and motivations. Enjoy the sample themes and variations.

Using Dynamic Embodiment[SM] (DE[SM])'s OSO model can support teaching. This means as a teacher you Observe keenly, Support

strengths and vulnerabilities, and optimize Options by being willing to provide new ideas and be playful. OSO involves engaging your creativity.

Observe: know who your group is, how to support them, and how to give them appropriate challenges, be present and mindful but also astutely observant of posture, facial expression, and their movement qualities, as well as your own gut feelings.

Support: learn more about your students' goals and motivations – spiritual, physical healing, and physical fitness, and if you are in your integrity in doing so, "meet them where you are." This is an invitation to be more focused on the ease of the class and to provide somatic cues that are culturally appropriate and meaningful. One way to begin this is to start to teach self-care strategies that can be used by anyone in the entire class. The life-threatening aspects of Covid-19 have made the practice of self-care really important. The silver lining is that there are now many free online resources available

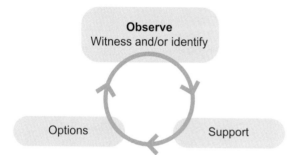

Observe
Witness and/or identify

Options

Support

For self-care ⟶ & others
Observe:
What do I/you do?
Tactile
Proprioception
Visual
Auditory
Gustatory

Support:
What works now?
What feels good?
What is supportive?

Options ⟶ Change
Options: Play, creativity & what choices?

Figure 9.1
Dynamic Embodiment[SM]'s OSO model.

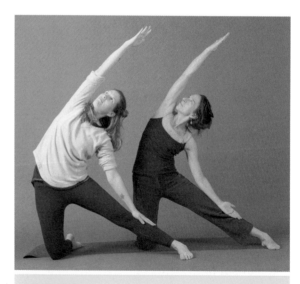

Figure 9.2
The art of creative yoga. Photo by Serge Cashman.

(DynamicEmbodiment.org; DrMarthaEddy .com).

Options: the most basic form of providing options is to invite students to participate with explorations and not force anything. Always remind them to follow their own body cues versus your signals. You are making suggestions for them to claim their own authority about what is best for them. If anyone is skeptical you can even encourage a few of those people to state where they are at. Whenever possible, provide each person within the group and the group as a whole with options, variations, choices. This allows for self-regulation and self-awareness. Learning to respect that in each other also helps with compassionate empathy.

Designing Classes: Chakra and Gland Focus

When teaching a somatic chakra yoga class in the DE style you are giving an opportunity to consciously experience the integration of the energetic and the physical. Guiding others to embody the chakras and glands is a way to guide empowerment, showing them how to ground themselves, how to come into their parasympathetic nervous systems when needed, and how to be more present in their human body. This chakral work settles expansion into the tissues. You can feel energy integrate into your body as you sense the neuroendocrine and chakral connections.

Let's start out with the simple structure of teaching one chakra per week for seven weeks. This provides a scaffolding that a teacher can augment with endless variations, and that the student can grasp with the enjoyment and pragmatism of integrating one holistic download of information per week, of letting that input settle in and digest over the course of seven days after each class.

Some Possible Class Structures

Below you will find two examples of class structures.

One Particular Chakra

a. Seven-week course, with one chakral area focused on per week

b. 1.5–3 hour workshop with focus on one chakra, one workshop per month for seven months

A Set of Chakras, and the Accompanying Glands

a. All seven can be addressed in one class

b. A set of three meeting the season or cultural moment with your teaching:

 i. Chakras 2–4 in spring detox with twists
 ii. During the first month of the BLM (Black Lives Matter) uprising in the USA after George Floyd's death, I taught heart and throat
 iii. During Covid-19: immune support with focus on lungs, thymus, throat (chakras 3–5)

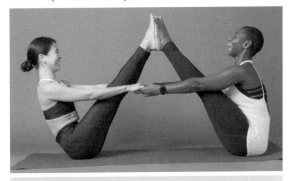

Figure 9.3
Rooted integration, two in boat pose. Photo by Serge Cashman.

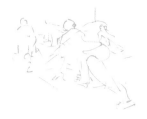

Chapter 9

Focus Points for Class Outlines Involving Any One of the Seven Chakras

 1 Root Chakra and Gland Focus

At this first class, introduce the neuroendocrine approach of working with the chakras, how glandular content provides a bridge between the physical and the energetic. Introduce benefits of working with glands and chakras over time (balance, overall health, alignment support, self-empowerment in healing). Introduce teaching suggestions of "suspending skepticism" and "embracing your superpowers of focusing awareness inside the body" to explore, activate, embody.

Suspending skepticism: does, the western scientific mind come into your head when you are exploring energetic work, causing you to doubt? For most of us it does to one degree or another. Now is a good time to invite it to sit on a nice pillow outside of your brain, while you focus the power of your brain at your third eye and enter into this exploration.

Embrace your superpowers: your ability to focus your brain (cultivated in practices like meditation) allows you to bring your thinking, your cognitive mind, to places inside your body. You can sense into them with your interoceptive awareness and see and discover what you yourself feel, sense, and know. When you visualize light in a particular part of your body, your mind thinks that is what is really there. Embrace it. Give yourself permission to explore. Later you can bring your scientific mind back in to evaluate. For now, be present with these experiences.

Choose anywhere from one to five class themes to weave in throughout your class. This is a great area to pour your creativity into.

Possible theme/s to weave throughout class: grounding, embodiment of feet and legs, awareness of sushumna, embodying bone, clear connection to nature, feeling/sense of roots connecting self to earth.

"Drop in" moment: meditation/centering/ checking on physical comfort and alignment, guided seated alignment.

Grounding: Chakra 1 – guided palpation and awareness of bony landmarks of pelvic floor attachment/kegels for pelvic floor awareness/ exploration/awareness of coccygeal body/mist red light into 1st chakra/see red lotus/yantra/ bija mantra/connect root to 2nd chakra with touch and awareness within/touch hand to earth to connect root to ground. Bring golden light up full sushumna to crown/anjali mudra here, fly arms out and down to sides while visualizing rainbow light egg forming around you to integrate all. Brush hands down face, tap thymus, pat down legs, slap/clap feet together a few times. To ground.

Asana: legs crossed, come into seated twist feeling root to crown connection/both sides/ janu sirsasana both sides/cat–cow to warm up/ movement at joints in cat–cow, dance/dog/ pigeon to open up pelvic muscles, both sides/ dog/stand – visit nine pillars. Begin Sun Salutation, both sides, adding in other poses should they support the themes you have chosen.

Upside down time/Rest: shoulder stand or legs up the wall/savasana/seated chant. End class together by chanting three ohms with hands in anjali mudra at the heart.

 2 Svadhisthana Chakra and Gland Focus: Gonads

Choose theme/s: water, creativity, flow, movement, pleasure, sensuality, low back health, 360 awareness at 2nd chakra, ovary/gonad connection to ankle/foreleg

"Drop in" moment.

Grounding: root chakra activation – brief or long, depending on your length of class.

Chakra 2: guided palpation and awareness of ovaries/gonad, gonad connection to ankle/bring in orange light/see orange lotus/yantra/bija mantra/30 seconds to breathe in and out and feel the effects of your practice so far on body, mind, emotions, and energy/connect 2nd chakra to 3rd with touch and inner awareness/touch hand to earth to connect root to ground. Bring golden light up full sushumna to crown/anjali mudra here, fly arms out and down to sides while visualizing rainbow light egg forming around you to integrate all. Brush hands down face, tap thymus, pat down legs, slap/clap feet together a few times. To ground.

Asana: legs crossed, come into seated twist feeling root to crown connection/both sides/janu sirsasana both sides/cat–cow to warm up/movement at joints in cat–cow, dance/dog/uttanasana for five breaths with thighs internally rotated to make room for low back/slowly unfurl spine to stand/nine pillars/drop into squat to open low back and strengthen spinal awareness/back to stand/standing twists with hands and arms moving freely and hands patting low back with each swing/standing do a power breathe into belly like kalabhati to increase fire in and awareness of belly/trace figure eights with sit bones or other belly movement/move into Sun Salutation with awareness of 2nd chakra power and flow, and your other themes woven into the practice.

Upside down time/Rest: shoulder stand or legs up the wall/savasana/seated chant. End class together by chanting three ohms with hands in anjali mudra at the heart.

3 Manipura Chakra and Gland Focus

Choose theme/s, some possibilities: three-dimensional breath at torso, at diaphragm, image of sun shining at 3rd chakra, detox for liver, twists for torso, personal power/confidence/esteem/fire.

"Drop in" moment.

Grounding: guided connection with root chakra.

Chakra 3: guided palpation and inner awareness of solar plexus, pancreas, diaphragm/kidney and adrenal *ssst* breath pump into adrenal/kidney/adrenal wrap/breathe into donut/toroidal shape of 3rd chakra area, yellow light/see a sun shining here, its rays spreading throughout student's body/yantra, guided visualization/bija mantra/30 seconds to breathe in and out and feel the effects of your practice so far on body, mind, emotions, and energy/connect 3rd chakra to 4th with touch and inner awareness/touch hand to earth to connect root to ground. Bring golden light up full sushumna to crown/anjali mudra here, fly arms out and down to sides while visualizing rainbow light egg forming around you to integrate all. Brush hands down face, tap thymus, pat down legs, slap/clap feet together a few times. To ground.

Asana: feet together, come into forward bend, dandasana, seated twist both sides, cat–cow, moving cat–cow/down dog/uttanasana/slowly stack vertebrae one at a time to come to stand/visit golden sushumna and rainbow egg/3rd breath of 3rd chakra/move into your Sun Salutation with fire and three-dimensional breath, balancing kidney/adrenal and visiting your other themes throughout.

Upside down time/Rest: shoulder stand or legs up the wall/savasana/seated chant. End class together by chanting three ohms with hands in anjali mudra at the heart.

Chapter 9

4 Anahata Chakra and Gland Focus

Choose theme/s, some possibilities: explore three-dimensional heart space with breath support, embodiment of legs/hips to support chest/neck/shoulders, giving and receiving pathways, Alexander technique golden threads lifting at front/back of heart, heart toroidal field, heart connections to lungs, diaphragm, pelvic floor via ligaments/crura, connect your heart to earth's heart.

"Drop in" moment: a little physical warm-up to begin: shoulder circles/clasp hands behind back, reach through fingers for stretch/lengthen neck, brush sternum to fingertips while sensing muscular and meridian connection/1 minute movement exploration of heart to wrist connection/Ganesh mudra.

Grounding: embodiment of root chakra.

Chakra 4: guided palpation and sensing into physical heart, heart beat, heart space, front and back of heart/sense into heart toroidal field, explore it with arms and hands/acknowledge heart bodies' presence/tap thymus/ mist green light into heart chakra/yantra/ bija mantra/30 seconds to breathe in and out and feel the effects of your practice so far on body, mind, emotions, and energy/connect 4th chakra to 3rd and 5th with touch and inner awareness/touch hand to earth to connect root to ground. Bring golden light up full sushumna to crown/anjali mudra here, fly arms out and down to sides while visualizing rainbow light egg forming around you to integrate all. Brush hands down face, tap thymus, pat down legs, slap/clap feet together a few times. To ground.

Asana: forward bend with soles of feet together/seated twist, both sides/cat–cow/ moving cat–cow/camel/move into your Sun Salutation with focus on heart in cobra,

integrate high cobra (arms straight) and visit your other themes throughout.

Upside down time/Rest: bridge/shoulder stand or legs up the wall/savasana/seated chant. End class together by chanting three ohms with hands in anjali mudra at the heart.

5 Visuddha Chakra and Gland Focus

Choose theme/s, some possibilities: communication, creativity, connection to 2nd chakra, thyroid, ether/space, breath support in lower chakra 4 supporting chakra 5.

"Drop in" moment.

A little physical warm-up to begin: lie down; guide torso breath cave; breathe into length, depth, and width of body/keeping shoulders on ground, bring head up to look at toes (Judith 1987). Seated: clasp elbows over head with hands, breathe into back of heart, heart mudra, shoulder circles, hold arms at "T" to body and do small arm circles to warm up area, breathe from heart up into throat, lengthen back of neck.

Grounding: connect with root chakra.

Chakra 5: guided palpation and sensing into throat, thyroid, and parathyroid. Move arms away from head and neck – side to side – to open up area, breathe into lower chakra 4 and explore how that supports chakra 5 to be full, explore throat space with hands inches in front of the body, move hands from throat to space into field to clear/mist blue light into throat chakra/yantra/bija mantra – spend some time with sound exploration at this chakra particularly/30 seconds to breathe in and out and feel the effects of your practice so far on body, mind, emotions, and energy/connect 5th chakra to 4th and 6th with touch and inner awareness/touch hand to earth to connect root to ground. Bring golden light up full sushumna to crown/anjali mudra here, slowly

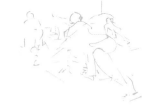

move arms out and down to sides while visualizing rainbow light egg forming around you to integrate all. Brush hands down face, tap thymus, pat down legs, slap/clap feet together a few times. To ground.

Asana: seated twist, cat–cow, cat–cow movement, fish pose, brief forward bend, downward dog. Move into your Sun Salutation with focus on the throat/neck/thyroid and visiting your other themes throughout.

Upside down time/Rest: bridge/shoulder stand (shoulder stand especially recommended for this chakra, followed by a supine twist) or legs up the wall/savasana/seated chant. End class together by chanting three ohms with hands in anjali mudra at the heart.

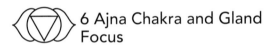

6 Ajna Chakra and Gland Focus

Choose theme/s, some possibilities: meditation, connection of inner wisdom to other chakras, spaciousness.

"Drop in" moment.

A little physical warm-up to begin: this bit of warm-up recommended to help ground and embody as coming into this high-vibration chakra can generate a lot of energy in the head: shoulder circles, head and neck circles.

Grounding: connect with root chakra.

Chakra 6: briefly move from root, through each of the chakras and glands thus far visited for alignment and support, even just saying the name of each with a brief pause in between, nadi shodhana for 3–5 minutes to draw senses inward, exploration of mouth cave (height, width, depth), press roof of mouth with tongue, move awareness up through bone to pituitary gland/third eye, anchor pituitary to coccygeal to assist in dropping of chin and lengthening of back of neck/touch ears to sense in between, then touch crown to sense this same place from

top of center line, touch forehead and occiput in back to sense depth with pituitary residing in the middle (see pituitary map, Fig. 3B.7), mist in purple light, yantra, bija mantra, 30 seconds to notice effects of practice so far/embody mammillary (this can be in lesson plan for 6th and/or 7th chakra) to support reach upwards through top of head and alignment supported via unified system of all glands and chakras/2 minute play with off-balance movements – moving head side to side/spirals/turns/2 minute meditation to sense into spaciousness opened up by mammillary exploration/a few seconds to breathe in and out, and feel the effects of your practice so far on body, mind, emotions, and energy/connect 6th chakra to 5th, 4th, and 7th with touch and inner awareness/touch hand to earth to connect root to ground. Bring golden light up full sushumna to crown/anjali mudra here, slowly move arms out and down to sides while visualizing rainbow light egg shape forming around you to integrate all. Brush hands down face, tap thymus, pat down legs, slap/clap feet together a few times. To ground. Grounding especially important with this chakra.

Asana: cat–cow, down dog, visiting any poses you have sensed/learned over the course of the five previous classes would be supportive for this group, move into your Sun Salutation with focus on the third eye and visit your other themes throughout.

Upside down time/rest: bridge/shoulder stand or legs up the wall/savasana/seated chant end class together by chanting three ohms with hands in anjali mudra at the heart.

7 Crown Chakra and Gland Focus

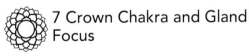

Possible theme/s to weave throughout class: crown and connection to oneness, awareness of sushumna, awareness of all seven chakras,

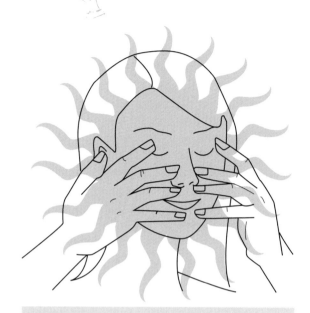

Figure 9.4
Bhramari breath/bee buzz breath – shanmukhi mudra.

connection to sky/cosmos, being a conduit connected to both earth and sky, pineal, nature connection.

"Drop in" moment.

Grounding: connection to root chakra, acknowledge that the 7th chakra brings us into connection, at the opposite pole of our bodies, to the sky. Here you, like a tree, are a channel between earth and sky.

Pre-asana breath and movement: 5 min of bhramari breath.

Bhramari breath is a good way to bring in some vibration and subtle movement to anchor the expansion that will come in the next section. Add in some movement like shoulder circles and a seated spinal twist.

Bhramari breath: find a comfortable and aligned seat. Bring your hands to rest on the top of your head, so that your thumbs can rest lightly on your ear flaps. An alternative position is to slide your fingers down from the top of your

head to rest lightly on your face, as in Figure 9.4. Close your eyes. Relax your jaw. Begin to hum. Relax your lips so that they are gently touching. This will allow for your hum to vibrate into your lips and your whole brain and skull. Do this for at least 5 minutes. Any tone is okay; it is recommended that you find one that feels good and that you can stay with. You are welcome to play and try different ones at first; notice how different pitches work or do not work to vibrate your head. This is also called bee buzzing breath. It is especially effective at focusing a scattered or spacey mind. It is grounding.

Chakra 7: brief visit with awareness and palpation to the chakras below, revisit/palpate map of pituitary (see Fig. 3B.7), move up to and embody the mammillary bodies, move into the pineal/engage in a developmental exploration of forward bends bringing top of head to touch the ground, push from top of head toward the hips/meditation to sense into past, present, and future all being in this moment, evoking the sense of timelessness that comes with pineal exploration (see Ch. 4). Now begin breathing into golden light of sushumna, from root to crown, up to rainbow lotus of crown yantra/bija mantra/a few seconds to breathe in and out and feel the effects of your practice so far on body, mind, emotions, and energy/connect 6th chakra to 5th, 4th, and 7th with touch and inner awareness/touch hand to earth to connect root to ground, briefly breathe from root to crown one more time, place your hands in anjali mudra at the top of your skull, slowly move arms up, out, and down to sides and to the earth while visualizing rainbow light egg forming around you to integrate all. Brush hands down face, tap thymus, pat down legs, slap/clap feet together a few times. To ground. Grounding is especially important with this chakra. Add in "windshield wipers" of legs and feet, shaking legs out.

Asana: seated forward bend, adding in some grounding poses here like janu sirsana or

pigeon, cat–cow, down dog, mountain pose with time to feel whole chakral system. Move into your Sun Salutation with focus on the crown, the unified chakra system, and visiting your other themes throughout.

Upside down time/rest: bridge/shoulder stand or legs up the wall/savasana/seated chant. End class together by chanting three ohms with hands in anjali mudra at the heart.

Tips for Teaching with the Chakras and Glands

These are some teaching tips from Shakti and Martha's personal experiences as educators.

Some Observations and Guidance for Teaching with the Chakras

- I (Shakti) have observed more than once a thickness in the room when guiding a group into the 2nd chakra. I try to leave more time for this chakra, as it seems we need it. The belly is where many of us hold our emotions. As a teacher or observer, you might notice the air, vibe, or energy of the room feeling chaotic, thick, cloudy, and/or confused. It can be helpful to first guide a group into some belly love by sending warmth and energy into the area through hands resting on one's own belly. Or some movement like belly dance, or hip movement while in table or cat/cow position.

- Take care when moving from chakra 3 to chakra 4. Many of us hold fear in the diaphragm; this causes it to be tight or blocked. Placing hands on the sides of the ribcage and inviting three-dimensional breathing here can enable a more fluid passage for awareness to move from the solar plexus up into the heart.

- I often spend more time with the throat chakra when teaching groups of women, as their voices have been constricted for hundreds of years. I will invite a longer or louder bija mantra time, followed by a longer, gentle integration time.

- As I write this, New York City is experiencing a heightened awareness of Black Lives Matter while sheltering in place during the Covid-19 pandemic. In my chakra yoga and healing movement Medicine Dance classes, participants have needed more time at the throat chakra, to help energy move, ideas integrate, expression be found – whether it's tears, sadness, anger, creative expression. Chakra yoga has been part of the healing for this time.

- When teaching the upper chakras and pituitary, mammillary, and pineal, it is useful to start with some asana, some physical practice, to get students in their bodies and grounded. Otherwise, depending on the energy of the day/in the room, folks might get real spacey, or be more challenged in paying attention. So weave in a little activity first, a few asana or other exercises like shoulder circles or movement, then bring in the upper chakra focus more deeply. And go from there into more asana and Sun Salutation. This leads to an experience that is expansive, centered, and grounded.

Some Guidance for Teaching with the Glands

This is a moment to consider what you might do to organize classes with the glands in mind.

Chapter 9

One organizational tool is to focus on one gland each class in a series of 12–16 classes.

Even with a single gland as your primary focus, please remember to refer to and activate at least three glands – one below and one above the focal gland as described in discussing "Teaching in Threes" (outlined in Chs 2 and 3). Consider beginning your series of classes with the glands located in the lowest part of the torso first and then review activation of the lower glands with touch, breath, sound, or vibration briefly during each subsequent class. This is one way to avoid any students fainting or becoming too chaotic from activating the glands.

Deepening Class Themes: Recuperation, Vibration, and Processing Emotions Including Grief

Another important way to focus a class is by themes. Three themes are selected below to provide examples of how classes that include glandular and/or chakral balancing can be used. They are quite different but equally important. Each is quite often used in a DE approach to yoga practice and can be integrated with your practice of the Sun Salutation. Theme 1 is Recuperative yoga; Theme 2, Vibrational focus practicing yoga integrating vibration; and Theme 3, Emotional focus – including awareness and balancing of emotions.

Theme 1: Recuperative Yoga

One of the huge themes of contemporary urban life (or at least in western cultures) is the over-exertion and push that come from a modern society. Millions of people do not have enough sleep, feel stressed all the time, and/or have little recuperation or recreation in

their lives due to the demands of the economic system on their lives (e.g. needing to work two jobs, or push to the limit in their job in order to keep it). Restorative yoga addresses the many physical and emotional discomforts that emerge as a result. However, you do not need to be teaching a Restorative yoga class in order to choose to focus on recuperation and nurturance in a class. Here are some focal points for classes based on different themes including that of recuperation. The following is a list of the three recuperative poses highly valued and often selected, followed by some enriching DE activities to use in recuperative classes:

- Child's Pose – complete inward phase of navel radiation, internal forward bend pose, and child's pose variations (arms forward/arms by side, over bolster).

- Savasana – supine tonic labyrinthine – stimulates active brain in rest.

- Legs Up the Wall (see description on p. 153).

- Constructive Rest position (with small book under head) – feet can be on the floor with knees bent or calves on a chair – with hips at 90 degrees. This is a classic exercise in Somatic Awareness whereby you lie on a hard surface with compensation for any jaw-jutting neck tension afforded by a small book under the head, and for the lower back by "standing on one's feet" while lying down. Take time to breathe deeply and to feel one's weight settle into the ground (see Fig. 9.5).

- The Four Dignities is a term used in the Tibetan Buddhist community for these different positions of meditation: lying,

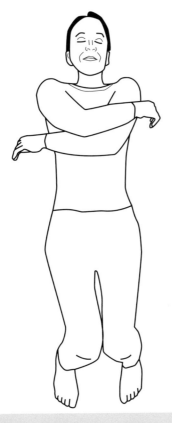

Figure 9.5
Constructive rest position.

- Lying down – for healing

- Sitting – for wisdom

- Standing – for power

- Walking – for envisioning.

If you need to rest more, feel free to meditate lying down.

- Apply gentle versions of DE's Hum Yoga^{SM} and Wiggle Yoga^{SM}; see next section for more information on these.

Theme 2: Varying Dynamics – Vibrational Focus

In DE, like most somatic practices, vibration and vocalization are key entry points to gaining greater awareness of sensation while still or in movement. DE brings together the sounding of vowels as taught by Irmgard Bartenieff (which she may have learned from yoga) and developed further by Bonnie Bainbridge Cohen during the time she was studying with Bartenieff. See Chapter 4, p. 107, for these vowel sounds.

DE's Hum and DE's Wiggle Yoga are two ways to apply these sounds and vibrations. DE's Hum Yoga is just that – humming while in different poses. It is typical to chant ohm at the beginning and/or end of numerous styles of yoga. In this style of yoga Martha uses humming both to warm up, as a deepening of breathing meditation, and to help loosen the muscles , organs, and glands while in an asana.

One can increase this further with wiggle – hence using both sound and vibratory action to stimulate organs and glands.

The use of the voice in humming provides a vibration that awakens the body from the inside out. Of course, the pitch can be played with. In Body-Mind Centering® (BMC®) pitches are

sitting, standing, and walking meditations. Cultural anthropologist Angeles Arrien (author of *The Four-Fold Way*, 1993), spent years visiting Indigenous peoples and studying their healing practices. She discovered that meditation happens in all levels and positions in space and that each has a different value. When working toward recuperation, lying down is perfect. However, stillness in each of these positions can be quite restorative and a wonderful way to end class – preparing the students for returning into activity (dealing with driving or public transportation, etc.).

selected that resonate the area that is the focus of the stimulation in much the same way as weighted pressure brings sensation. The pitch choice is easy – those glands that are lower in the body respond to lower pitches and the higher glands to higher pitches. To truly gain access to the full DE experience you would also be aware of the spatial pulls or tensions within the pose as you hum and continue to find the counter-pulls to sustain the pose. This comes from Bartenieff Fundamentals. The spaciousness is good for the joints *and* brings more sensation to the glands.

An Example : Spatial Pulls for Thyroidal Stimulus

When you are moving into a seated spinal twist: gently press down into the sit bones then stretch up through the crown on the "in breath." These are two opposite spatial tensions creating a counter-pull that helps you to sustain the pose with spaciousness. As you exhale and move into the twist, a new counter-tension comes from adding the horizontal (right–left) direction and plane (with front–back).

Let's look at the thyroid for another example: you can make space for it by raising the chin, allowing your thyroid (at the Adam's apple) to become a high point in the arch of the neck, and then also feel for the breastbone sinking down a bit, so once again you have both an upward and a downward pull – this seems to actually stimulate the gland. Maintain this counter-pull as you continue with any of your poses.

Applying Dynamic Embodiment^{SM} Humming to Sun Salutation

If you can hum in any one pose you can also hum throughout the entire Sun Salutation. It is fun to decide which glands you need/want to emphasize each day or week and use the pitch that supports that gland. Or you can refer to Chapter 4 to hum the yogic bija mantra for a chakral area of the body.

Applying Wiggling

The DE approach also includes "Wiggle Yoga." DE Wiggle Yoga is a two-phasic approach to one's practice that echoes dancing with DE concepts in BodyMind Dancing. It involves finding a shape and then letting go, being more inside the experience than focused on a shape. This involves establishing your asana and then gentle shaking, wiggling, or vibrating. The impact is often on the synovial fluid of the joints or in the organs. As learned in Chapter 3, this joint stimulation also brings in the glandular activity. By continually wiggling as you need to throughout the Sun Salutation you activate more small joints and awaken both fluids and glands throughout the entire body.

Wiggling activates what Movement Analysts call "being in shapeflow," a constantly changing versus held steady posture (and related state of mind). Finding your "shapeflow" or "shapeflow support" requires being less involved with relating to others and more intent on taking care of yourself. This mobile self-care time supports joint fluid circulation and can be helpful to break up fascial holding between the organs. Wiggling loosens up your body and in this way helps loosen up rigid mind states. Experiment with how it feels for your soul.

Theme 3: Working with the Emotions – Focusing on Grief and Loss

Humming and wiggling loosen up your movement potential and your organs. This loosening of the body can open the emotions that are

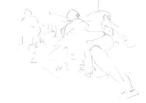

often sitting compactly in our torso. Shaking has been a long-known approach to letting go of trauma (Gordon 2019). While it would take another full book to talk about the DE approach to trauma recovery, this section focuses a bit on grief and loss. DE Yoga[SM] is linked to Moving For Life Gentle Yoga Moves – a system of yoga that was first developed for people who are scared by a cancer diagnosis, grieving about loss of a body part or movement capacity, or dealing with fear of severe illness, death, and dying. Everything shared above is useful in working with releasing the grief of loss or the fears of potential loss. Gentleness is critical. Key steps in this work include giving people time and support to: recognize grief in the body and heart; discover what the grief is about (for instance, any associations with the loss that intensify it); and accept all aspects of body sensation and feelings as important information (often about what one loves and thinks is most needed) and move the emotional energy. Other resources are shared, such as the Let's Reimagine End of Life Movement (LetsReimagine.org).

Working with Grief

As teachers in today's world, we need to be ready for a wide range of emotions being carried by students. The body holds feelings that even the person does not totally understand. As a teacher it helps to have comfort with being present for a wide range of emotions. In order to "be with emotions" one needs to be present oneself. Much of what has been shared above helps with presence. Grief is a particularly rampant emotion at present – since the time of Covid-19 and when attending to racial reckoning.

Breathing, vibration with sound or movement, and expression of emotion with words, movement, and relational exchange are all hugely important in "moving grief." There is also a mental clarity that can come from moving out of emotional intensity. And there are subtler ways to move grief that also are activating glandular balancing. Meditation is one of the most powerful resources in this realm. Meditation can cause healing imagery to arise, or use imagery to help shift a mind-state. Here is one example of these interactions and how it shifted stress, exhaustion, and loss. The DE approach to yoga and the Sun Salutation embraces this type of integration as well.

One colleague of Martha's, Jacqueline Wade, who was a loving and super-attentive caregiver to her husband when he developed Parkinson's disease, shared the following about how yoga and helped her with grief: "*I was dealing with a husband who was very ill from Parkinson's disease. I was also in a job that was very stressful at the time. Kundalini Yoga gave my life purpose and strength. My thoughts got clearer from the breathing and the chants. I loved the fact that I did not have to be physically fit to do it. Often Hatha Yoga hurts my body because I have four herniated discs. With Kundalini Yoga, it was about the breath, chants, meditation, and music which made me happy and at peace during the most turbulent time in my life. Kundalini Yoga is so positive. It is fuel to the soul. It also allowed me to reflect over my life. I could also feel my spine and inner strength growing, like a snake. The meditation made me more aware of my body and I was becoming more centered. I felt at peace and focused after I did it every day. It was a powerful life force. I felt connected to the universe. Since my husband recently passed away from Covid-19, I feel myself being drawn to Kundalini Yoga again. It makes me feel calm and sadness goes away. I feel inner peace when I do it and I feel my husband near me. I feel his love around me. I am thankful.*"

This can be inspiration for teaching classes that focus on adrenal calming, heartfelt emotional sharing, and/or thoracobody breathing. In particular the thoracobody sits near what one psychologist refers to as "the grief hole," the crevices in the solar plexus region. Moving the diaphragm, deepening the breath – whether sobbing, crying, or singing, are classic ways to move grief. Integrating release with regulated breathing that includes the moving of the xiphoid process away from the thorocobody on the inhale and toward it on the exhale is deeply healing.

There are two other branches of "somatic education" – somatic psychology and somatic bodywork. Any of these branches may take a social somatic approach – looking at social factors in body movement and awareness – and working for social equality and systemic change. Somatic psychologists are professionals who are especially skilled to help with deeper emotional and/or trauma experiences.

More Ideas for Class Design

You may also design a series of classes around one health or lifestyle issue or a few different ones. For example, you could develop a course containing 4–10 sessions focusing on:

1. adrenal burnout (see Ch. 8 for ideas for getting started)

2. thyroid imbalance (see Ch. 8 for ideas for getting started)

3. sleep issues (see Ch. 8 on the pineal gland for ideas for getting started; also, this could include some yoga nidra immune strengthening, with some focus on the thymus and all the glands above which work together holistically to support our immune system function)

4. heart opening (see class design above for heart chakra and glands)

5. sexual energy (see class design above for root and 2nd chakras and glands)

6. caregiver burnout or grief – focus on heart and throat chakras and/or all seven for balance and rejuvenation, and add in many recuperative poses/exercises (see Recuperative section above)

7. working with emotions – anger, impatience – partner work to help with feeling of connection, and feel compression into the thoraco-lumbar region to activate sympathetic nervous system (frame for expression of anger/impatience), focus on the breath, woodchopper exercise from Polarity yoga is excellent for release and easily folded into a yoga class

8. getting stronger – muscles and bones – alignment and power (refer to Ch. 7 for ideas to get your class scaffolding going)

9. inflammation – wiggling and giggling are the best therapeutic modality for any person with inflammation (see Ch. 7 for more ideas and information on this)

10. stiffness – towards the beginning of class incorporate ample time for movement exploration of each of the joints; this will activate synovial fluid and bring in circular and multidirectional movement that can continue to be applied throughout class. This can be done at first in in cat/cow, DE Wiggle Yoga, or Hum Yoga.

And of course you may find that you want or need to combine two or more of the above into one class.

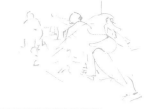

The Arc and Feel of a Class

As you develop the arc of your class, please get in the habit of observing yourself kinesthetically and your group visually and with attunement. Here are some tips:

- Attune to the energy of the room when you arrive/begin. This includes noticing what season it is – fall, winter, spring, or summer, the current weather and/or astrology, current events or climate change issues for your town or city, the world (i.e. on a hot summer day you could add Sitali Moon cooling breath; during Covid-19 era classes or climate emergencies add in parasympathetic calming asana and other activities – see adrenals in Ch. 8). Has recent rain caused a barometric pressure drop that you want to feed with a restorative pose or counter with some stimulating activity?

- Follow the mood and energy level of the group (help them take care of their needs). Tune in to what people are bringing into the room, i.e. are folks mostly coming from work and depleted, or is this a bright and perky Saturday morning crowd? Sometimes there are patterns like aching joints or a similar injury in a group. Look, listen, tune into your intuition, and feel free to ask questions or even do a "check-in" with the whole group at the start of class.

Starting Class Seated in a Circle

One yoga colleague, Heather Sanderson, makes time at the start every class with a circle – whether teaching Yoga Nidra, Restorative, or a Dynamic Flow yoga class. She invites the whole class to sit upon a circle of bolsters to check in, and those who wish to speak are welcome to say a sentence about how they are, report anything to Heather that they'd like for her to know; it is understood that anyone can "pass." Then she guides the whole group gracefully back to their mats for the rest of this class. This format has created a deeper sense of community (and safety and comfort) in her classes, and helped her get to know her students' needs.

- Be yourself – people choose classes because of the teacher. Feel free to go with your style or follow your own mood to a moderate extent – mostly to transmit your enthusiasm about yoga but also your pleasure; even if your mood is a bit melancholy you can show how yoga helps!

- You can choose to keep it lively! It is exciting to vary rhythms and dynamics. You can start with a class that is mostly about softening and being slow, and then move into amping up, perhaps when practicing the Sun Salutation ritual or before or after. This wakes folks up – brings in mental alertness.

- When you start with "amping up" to a higher level of intensity, remember that this could be great if the goal of the class is muscular strengthening. These connections can support "power yoga." It works well to find a time in the arc of your class for a deep dive into a cool-down and meditation; or a yoga slow-down and internal focus of shoulder stand/bridge/supine twist/savasana. A gentler variation to shoulder stand is

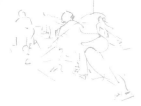

legs up the wall on a block followed by a bridge.

- When starting with a gentler class and staying with that general tone, still be careful to vary the dynamics within the gentleness in order to keep your students engaged. Your choice may be to bring them into deeper layers of relaxation and trance throughout a restorative and Yoga Nidra-type class, then arc them out of it with a gradual wake-up progression beginning near the end of the class (gentle movement out of yoga nidra, shifting positions towards sitting, engaging in humming or ohm, verbal interaction to transition to going back out onto the street).

Online Teaching Tips

With online teaching there are many considerations. Three tips:

1. positioning of teachers to see different views of the body – it can be useful to use two yoga mats for these classes, laid out in a cross design to allow for easy shifting from frontal to profile view for the student

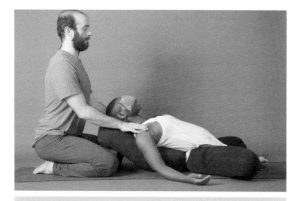

Figure 9.6
Hands-on support for deepening yoga. Photo by Serge Cashman.

2. adapting home space for safety and comfort

3. creating a sacred container: use of meditation, feeling the group support/community building, and building the "group energy" – find out how you can connect with each other's heart or other energies, even online.

Adapting Class for Different Age Groups

When designing lesson plans inclusive of the Sun Salutation in teaching, it is important to know your student group and to be ready to *adapt poses for different populations*. Of course, taking workshops on these topics is most likely the most effective as you get observation and interpersonal practice.

Central to DE: remember to use the OSO model. This means take time to observe the people in the room who you will be working with (even if on Zoom). If you are planning a new class, in a new location, ask in advance to visit the space and meet whomever you can. If you are meeting people for the first time then observe quickly – scanning the people who are present, engaging with everyone, even if they are hovering at the door.

Also be careful not to make assumptions. Get into dialogue about what you observe and find out the facts (Eddy 2004). This is especially important for cultural sensitivity. For instance, if everyone has white hair or is hooked up to an IV, don't assume they all want to move slowly – everyone comes to class with different histories, different energy levels, and different goals. To quote Martha's mother, "we are all aging" and one of the best ways to keep the body young is by being playful. This also fits with enhancing vitality and continuing to

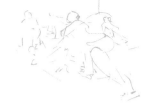

move in every possible way. Hence, observe carefully and you will find older people with joint diseases – Lyme, lupus, and fibromyalgia – mixed up with extremely spry older adults. Whether dealing with early onset of aging (due to illness) or simply aging because of the passage of time, whether working with older adults or cancer patients, it is important to know about osteoporosis, arthritis of the joint capsule, and osteopenia, as well as potential disc injuries. For spinal recuperation from flexion and extension integrate asanas beyond the Sun Salutation, like spinal twists (unless you have disc problems). Rotations, even within sagittal (forward and back, up and down) movement, whether big or small, can awaken different tissues of the body.

If someone in your class has osteoporosis, it is important to talk with them before class begins, to understand what their limitations are and what their doctor has prescribed. Some people with osteoporosis are exercising a large range of motion within their joints, others may not be ready to bring any but the most subtle movements into their spine due to their susceptibility to bone fractures. Respect their limits/boundaries and help guide them into exploring within their comfort zone.

Some of the material in this book can be adapted for working with children, particularly Hum and Wiggle Yoga. Children wiggle out of things, squirm around, want to jiggle. Go for shorter-length classes for kids.

In this chapter we have given you some outlines, lesson plans, and tips for applying the chakras, glands, and developmental movement to your teaching of yoga and the Sun Salutation. All the best to you with your teaching.

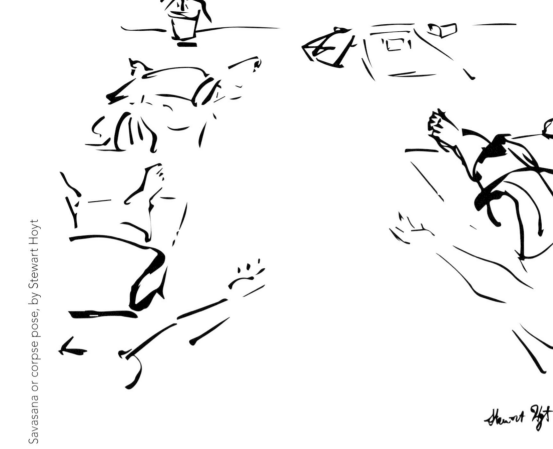

Savasana or corpse pose, by Stewart Hoyt

10 Get Moving with Glandular and Cultural Awareness, Supported by Nature

Introduction

Living with complexities and controversy is a pulse within our world dialogue at present. The body is complex; much is mysterious. By learning to listen to the body and not getting caught up in fear or confusion, it may be possible to get through challenges that are exacerbated by the worrisome machinations of the human mind.

Each individual is unique. Genetic and biochemical factors influence our physical bodies. In his book, *Radical Healing* (1996), Dr Rudolf Ballentine, one of the first doctors to integrate yoga into his practice, shares how healing happens on different levels – from the physical to the etheric body with subtle shifts in consciousness at each level. It depicts the molecular to the physical with biochemical and energetic circuits as elements in between.

Living with complexity and mystery is also part of the Dynamic Embodiment ^{SM} (DE^{SM}) model of engaging with yoga – part of the observe and support phase of the work is to embrace controversies – or conflict – within the body (joint pain or other discomfort), within oneself, or from the broader forces that impact the body – with family, with medical personnel about health, and in society in general. The calm that comes from yoga can help for seeing the interconnectedness between conflict and growth. The philosophy underlying this book has included two DE principles: (1) maintaining an improvisational mind and (2) being keenly aware of injustices in the world. For instance, the discussion of the process of moving with glandular awareness and living with the complexity of controversy is a natural outgrowth of Martha's doctoral research (Eddy 1998) on best practices in teaching embodied conflict resolution. As humans, in life, there can be situations of misunderstanding often based in concerns about scarcity of getting our basic physical or emotional needs met. Ideally every yoga class can be a brave, courageous space where people can drop down into their inner beings and feel the resources of the transcendent while also finding motivation for social good. Examples can be finding pathways for obtaining food (whether that means having a job, being able to chew, finding the time to shop or prepare food, or dealing with anorexia, to name a few) or being in the community (being kind to one another, getting to know neighbors who are outside of your current circles, etc.). Both the mundane and the transcendent are part of being human. It is our choice to claim each.

As part of this it is also vital to understand the importance of sleep, naps, and rests (and the dream life they afford) that exist within the cycle of an action – check out napministry.com. Along with rest, find other forms of sustenance:

food for the body, for the mind, for shifts of mood. In this chapter, love of the healing power of foods and herbs is included to whet the appetite.

And there is another type of food: brain candy. With feelings of being sad, hurt, or angry, once identified and acknowledged, tension is often relieved; this sometimes resolves trauma and most often shifts emotions. With this shift one is freer to explore ways to act that seek to rectify the challenges at hand – whether they be the systemic oppression of people of "other" genders, sexual orientation, economic status, ethnicity, race, or an intersection of any of these. Finding the support needed to acknowledge, be able to sit with, and, when appropriate, move through these feelings is the goal. The support can be the magic of the universal forces or the caring that comes from social engagement with someone you trust, or spending time in a personal individual practice. Engaging with nature integrates many of these potentialities.

Martha's Personal Story: My Experience of Lyme Disease

As an example of how many of these levels of healing come together, let's address the epidemic of Lyme disease. While coronavirus has been recognized as an epidemic, Lyme disease has remained mysteriously underplayed. And yet there have been people who have been mentally or physically inhibited for life by Lyme; while people rarely die from Lyme *per se*, they do die from related neurological and cardiac problems.

As mentioned in earlier chapters, Martha has been diagnosed with Lyme since 2013. She had experienced symptoms since 2008. They were easily confounded with what seemed like perimenopausal mood shifts, headaches and jaw tension, joint pain, organ

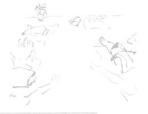

anomalies – from stress incontinence to heart irregularities and eye pain, memory issues, and concentration challenges, as well as overall fatigue. Working with Lyme demands a multilayered approach.

Antibiotics are one solution, but the need for constant antibiotics and their impact on the gut require that a larger-scale approach be taken. Herbal antibiotics are strong, though not as intense. They can give just the right amount of support to help control the disease if other supports – allopathic and lifestyle – are included.

1. Keep moving

2. Come to terms with a parasite living within you (and propagating prolifically)

3. Address the physical symptoms

4. Figure out how to go about your day as a creative human being who is managing challenging physical symptoms

5. Consider whether herbs will assist, expedite, or complete the healing and find advice for which ones will get to the core of the problem (there are as many different protocols as there are people with Lyme since symptoms can vary so much)

6. Get tested for allergies including food allergies

7. Eat well (for instance, even with a healthy diet, this might become a time to stop eating gluten completely)

8. Include heat therapies such as in infra-red saunas or cold treatment for joint pain

9. Include bio-electrical devices/treatments that do battle directly with the creatures living within

10. Help others struggling with similar symptoms but who do not have access to these options

11. Find experts to support the healing – integrative MDs or others trained in functional medicine, naturopathy, acupuncture, osteopathy, and chiropractic.

Most important was a movement practice and a spiritual practice. For Martha, engaging with the Sun Salutation from a DE perspective got her through the three-month period of having her dominant hand and arm immobilized with a frozen shoulder. Soon thereafter she also experienced the humility of potentially never being able to bend her knee again. It turned out that she had a most unusual experience of a Baker's cyst. When the cyst was identified and about to be drained she was rushed to the emergency ward to be tested with a Doppler for a blood clot. It turned out she was not at risk for an embolism but that the cyst was blood-filled – the cyst was ejecting a cystic form of a spirochete. During the periods when she couldn't easily open her jaw, turn her head, move her arm behind her back or walk equally with both legs, the same healing protocols helped and they were a combined approach:

- Slow the movement down and feel what is still possible to do

- Don't let go of rituals that are healing – return to meditation and meditative movement (including playful joyous movement) as soon as possible and figure out how to adapt the movement (this book is all about that)

- Move in the rhythm of the slowest part

- Keep checking for other complicating syndromes – glandular imbalances are common.

On days when it was hard to move, the process of finding out what still could be done and feeling thankful for that were critical. The practice of somatic dance and the practice of the Sun Salutation were touchstones throughout this process, and continue to be.

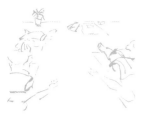

Chapter 10

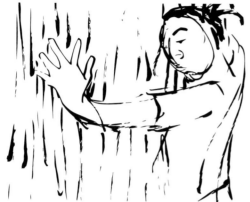

Figure 10.1
One with tree, by Stewart Hoyt.

The inclusion of stories is to honor how often information sticks best when the informational model includes activities, personal sharing, and the forging and preserving of healthy relationships. Support can come from nature. Humanity is of nature; any moments that open us up to feeling connected within ourselves and the outdoors reinforce relationship, creativity, and revitalization. These support healing. Healing resources from nature range from everyday foods to fancy foods, the use of herbs, and purging using synthetic or natural drugs.

Of the Earth: From Food and Herbs to Nature as Healing Forces

The sheltering in place that Covid-19 necessitated created unexpected inward time for most of the world. The stopping of modern life and its pollution gave us the stark contrast of cleaner and quieter skies throughout the world. Indigenous peoples across the planet are trumpeting the cry for all of us to tune in to change

our habits to care more for the earth, and all peoples everywhere (Kimmerer 2013). This is a feminine energy rising, from the earth itself and in all of our bodies, that says that all people, animals, and plants matter. All beings are connected. It feels right to us, in writing this book, to emphasize the importance of treating both your body and the earth well by healing yourself with the right diet and practices for you that also impact the earth in positive ways, and by honoring, thanking, and treating the earth well for the bounty that she gives us. We recognize that, like the breath, the earth is one of the constants in our lives. The quality of our connection with the earth affects the state of our wellness. Shamanism teaches us many ways to strengthen and deepen this relationship – us and nature. Ultimately you have hit the jackpot when you realize that you ARE nature – as in fact we are. We are part of nature too. Some of the earliest yogic practices came from animist traditions – ones that are and were deeply connected to nature. Yoga grew in cultures in the Global South that began as people from different sectors celebrated the beauty of their part of the earth. A Sri Lankan colleague shares how, in her country, the first spirituality arose from the closeness each community felt as they lived in and amongst the forest, the sea, the grasses, the mountains. Part of what has occurred with the development of yoga in India has been a reinforcement of the caste system. This is something to be challenged. Most important is to reconnect to the appreciation of "being nature" as well as depending on nature – at all levels of existence, recognizing our equality and interdependence. When you understand this depth of interconnectedness on a deeper level, you know that how you treat your body is connected to how you treat the earth. Wake up to loving yourself more, treating yourself better, eating well, and you will find that you can't help but care more

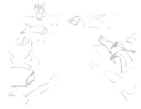

deeply for the planet. Connecting with nature, feeling her life force, can help you honor and treasure your life force and your body. We have cut ourselves off from our bodies and from the planet for far too long. New and rising multicultural, feminist, decolonial, and narrative psychology perspectives echo this cry. Indigenous people from all over the earth are saying that Covid-19 is in fact part of this wake-up call, that the earth created it, and that this is an opportunity for us to heal – ourselves, our societies, and the earth itself. Arkan Lushwala, Andean ceremonial leader, offered this wisdom in April of 2020 during the pandemic, about the pandemic: "In a deep primordial part of ourselves, many of us have been waiting for something like this to happen, something powerful and sacred had to intervene in order to stop the destruction of the sources of life. The earth herself has now done so. Viruses, like everything, are made by the earth ... Our earth, Pachamama, would not be doing what she's doing unless there was time to change. The capacity that nature has to regenerate is extraordinary. Extremely powerful, and sometimes surprisingly fast. But we have to listen. The earth is telling us that the moment for change is now" (Lushwala 2020).

The content and practices in this book are all avenues that lead us into deeper awareness and embodiment of ourselves. Listening is intrinsic. Enhancing the ability to listen within, and engage in self-care, can allow for listening to each other, to animals, to trees, and to the earth – waking up on a deeper level, to caring for the earth. And by listening to the earth while moving in interaction with her elements, and by feeling that interaction, healing happens. And on some level, at the same time, these collective efforts heal the earth. As you have found in this book self-care includes proprioceptive and kinesthetic attunement to your body in stillness and movement, sound healing, alignment with caring relationships,

healing from childhood mishaps or wounds, and also the foods we eat. Hence, here you can learn about herbs and entheogens, other resources for moving energy profoundly. Finally, the boxed text at the end of this chapter on integrating the practices of this book with nature guides you through four days of practice to nourish your body, have fun doing it outside, and grow your relationship with the earth.

Nature Connection

Both Martha and I (Shakti writing) have found herbs to be constant companions over the past decades. Learning about herbalism, using plants for teas and cooking and medicinally, is a practice that helps one attune to the earth. Upon moving to Brooklyn from a small cabin in the woods at Earthdance Movement Retreat Center, Shakti found the practice of herbalism one of the major avenues that has improved her health and helped her grow her sense of nature, and her ability to feel it while living in the urban environment. This connection is priceless. I (Shakti) am able to feel the life force of trees and other plants in the city in such a way now that I feel nourished by them. I don't need to leave the city as often as I used to. And I now teach Nature Connection practices to others, as a major component of my somatic bodywork and movement practice, to help them also be healthy and thrive in the city.

Tea/Infusion to Support the Nervous System

Infusion of 2 parts oatstraw, 2 parts linden, 1 part tulsi

Put a handful of this mix of dried loose herbs in a mason jar

Chapter 10

Fill it with boiling water

Let it brew for 8 hours

I (Shakti) like to bring this tea in a thermos or water bottle to work, to sip throughout the day. This nourishing infusion calms and soothes, and supports the nervous system. Oatstraw is an herb for any time of uncertainty, anxiety, depression, or grief. It improves libido, evens moods, and builds energy, supporting the pancreas and liver. Linden and tulsi partner nicely with oatstraw to ease anxiety and calm the nervous system; linden brings in a little sweetness, tulsi uplifts (Weed 2019).

Different Forms of Herbs

Herbs can be taken in many forms – in tea (as above), in food (as one finds turmeric in food from South Asia and common herbs like parsley, rosemary, sage, and thyme, too), in tinctures and elixirs (droplets), and in titrated forms like homeopathy. Plant life provides multisensory experiences – adding smell, taste, and touch (in preparing to use them) to our predominantly visual–auditory lives. Our purpose here is mostly to emphasize that engaging with Sun Salutation goes hand in hand with herbology. Personal experience of conscious use of herbs and food can powerfully enhance and assist embodiment practices.

Herbs can include flowers – like yarrow for liver cleansing and rose for the heart. Flowers can be used in a more subtle way, in the form of a flower essence – a distilled tincture made from flowers. This is another form of herbal and energetic support for the body. Essences work with emotional states, soul development, and mind-body health. All people can benefit from the support of the vibrational nature of plants. Rescue Remedy, one of the Bach flower remedies, is probably the most well-known blend. Take a few drops under the tongue at times of trauma, or when simply needing a little (or a lot of) emotional and/or nervous system support. The use of flower essences can help you grow awareness of your subtle body, and thus support awareness of your chakras and glands.

Herbs and other plants can be a powerful yet more gentle alternative to modern medicine. An approach to health that also attunes you to the earth, through learning about them, and incorporating them into your everyday life.

Psychedelics

There is a renewed rise in the 21st century of psychedelics to help in healing trauma. Hence, it would be remiss not to mention this. These biochemical resources are moving towards approval by the US Food and Drug Administration (FDA) to aid our armed forces in recovering from post-traumatic stress disorder (PTSD). The Multidisciplinary Association for Psychedelic Studies (MAPS) is heading phase 3 of these clinical trials using MDMA and psilocybin. It is only a matter of time before psilocybin, ayahuasca and other psychoactive plants become available to all to benefit from, should they be needed (FDA 2018). Note that even chemical compounds like LSD and MDMA were originally derived from plants or also found in nature. At the time of writing this book psilocybin and some other plant medicines (ayahuasca, iboga, cactus) have become decriminalized in Denver, Colorado; Ann Arbor, Michigan; Somerville, Massachusetts; Washington DC; and Santa Cruz and Oakland in California. This is the first step towards legalization. Decriminalization means that penalties for possession (that in the USA lean unjustly on BIPOC populations) and

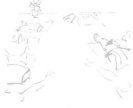

use are deprioritized and the city can no longer spend funding towards that end. Use is legal in the Netherlands in Europe. Both authors recognize psychedelics as an invaluable resource for continued healing of trauma to the human body and psyche, not only for severe cases, but also for everyday use, for healing for people that are well.

Psychedelics are in some ways an extension of herbal medicine. They have been found to be useful for health for millennia, by Indigenous cultures around the world. Why talk about them here? US illegalization in the early 1970s halted the great strides made by government-sanctioned research regarding help with mental disorders including addiction, largely for alcoholism. Researchers were having a great deal of success. These entheogens were found to hasten psychological processes, accelerating therapy (Grof 2019). The 50-year ban is beginning to lift. New research helping with PTSD, depression, addiction, and cancer is helping to deepen the connections. Studies are privately funded in the US so far; it is only a matter of time before big pharma joins in. Europe is ahead of the curve, with government-funded studies in Germany and Basel, Switzerland.

Psychedelics or entheogens open people to experience their embodiment and have been found to be tools for healing trauma. With the experience of a variety of different psychedelics, and in particular ayahuasca, psilocybin, and MDMA, people report the following four experiences (Hernandez 2020):

1. Allowing the body to move spontaneously releasing held tension and trauma (personal, social and historical)

2. Feeling the body in a new way – an experience of being inside the entire body and not just in the head; this new corporeal perspective can provide support for being, imagining, and acting in ways less conditioned by social and personal habits

3. Communicating with ancestors or spiritual forces

4. And with these sometimes comes gratitude.

This means that for people for whom being in the "head" is the only way to be, the impact of the entheogens/plant medicine shifts a person to feeling sensations guiding experience instead of remaining caught only in the intellect. And why is this hard for so many? It is easy to be caught in a paradigm that dictates this. "Newtonian Cartesian science has created a very negative image of human beings, depicting them as biological machines driven by instinctual impulses of a bestial nature. It did nothing to foster genuine recognition of higher values, such as spiritual awareness, feelings of love, aesthetic needs, or a sense of justice" (Grof 1985, p. 26). Psychedelics, herbs, and somatics are all key pieces in shaking off this image/mindset and potentially shifting us into a new paradigm.

Entheogens bring in the "oneness" factor. They lessen polarity on all levels. As feminism is rising in western culture, many are waking up to the idea of "the white man's perspective" not being the only way of being. These medicines awaken interconnectedness with all people and all species, and the idea of the earth and sky and water as being sentient. This can help cross racial and other divides. "With psilocybin, most people have claimed to have a long-term feelings change in their connectedness to nature, that the feeling of connection doesn't go away after the trip is over, it lasts for weeks, months, even the rest of their life" (Buller with Gandy 2019).

Many people who are "kinesthetically inclined" or relaxed in their bodies, at ease about movement, or who have gained skills like Authentic Movement where one can listen to the body versus direct it, may not need this experience for this end. However, for those who don't have these skills, psychedelics may be of benefit.

It is beyond the scope of this book to go into depth about entheogens/psychedelics but as it is a cutting-edge arena of healing that is gradually becoming more and more available worldwide, it feels important to include this reference to it and to relate it to movement and chakra balancing. Over the next five to ten years, we will be witnessing how these natural substances can be used for healing across the world in different ways.

Issues of Racial Equity

It is also important to note that these benefits have an important place in health equity. There is growing exposure to the fact that psychedelics can be used for overcoming years of systematic oppression by improving health and well-being and by helping people recover from racialized trauma. In a period when the BLM movement is burgeoning, more information is needed about how Black people are impacted by research, knowledge, access, and lack of access to psychedelics.

At the first showing of Horizon Media's new film *Death, Dying, and Psychedelics* in January of 2021 in NYC, the creators spoke about the need for access for BIPOC, acknowledging that there are many factors skewing psychedelic access including:

- who has the money and the time to pursue a PhD

- who has the freedom to experiment with psychedelics as a young person without fear of arrest and possible incarceration

- the likelihood of white clinicians being partial to working with white clients in studies (Stovall 2019)

- judgement about being involved with psychedelics (especially given the fear stirred up by the "war on drugs" in the USA) within the BIPOC community.

Stephanie Hope, DNP, RN notes (personal communication, January 29, 2021) how most studies happen in clinical settings, and that this factor is a deterrent to participation. She suggests that research expand into experiencing entheogens in a community context. This is in alignment with hundreds of years of history of Indigenous communities and current values with feminism and the BLM movement. Perhaps with this simple but profound adjustment, cultural and racial diversity will happen at a faster rate (FDA 2018).

"Drug policy reform is a central tenet of the fight for black lives. In order to understand this, we need to recognise the varying ways that drug policy is used to criminalise, incarcerate and kill Black people in the UK criminal justice system … Our ideas and misconceptions about drugs, addiction and criminality mean that, as a nation, we condone drug policy that is punitive rather than health-centred and fact-based" (Barton & Robinson 2017).

Initiatives within organizations such as MAPS are designed to bring attention to the huge number of intersectional issues, most notably between drug use and racial oppression, considering factors such as the racial injustice that arose from the "war on drugs,"

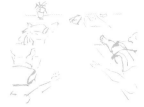

and the impact of poverty, mass incarceration, and issues of easing off harmful drugs. A critical fact in the USA is that Black people are incarcerated eight times more often than white people. Another theme is the positive use of, yet lack of access to, helpful psychedelics for BIPOC because of these racially oppressive forces. There is a dire need for research on the use of psychedelic drugs in overcoming trauma that is sensitive to racialized trauma.

Camille Barton, somatic educator, diversity consultant, and activist, states: "I was honored to do this, as I believe that psychedelic research has the potential to heal trauma and create positive social change in the world. More work has to be done to ensure that systemic patterns of oppression, including racism, stop being reproduced in the psychedelic research community… I found it peculiar that so few studies discussed included people of color (POC) or those from the LGBTQ community. People from these demographics have disproportionately higher rates of trauma than white people in the USA." Barton also discusses the Grady Trauma Project, describing how it "conducts research in Atlanta, [where] African American populations have higher rates of PTSD than veterans returning from Iraq, Afghanistan, or Vietnam. Therefore it was disappointing that only a single community forum on intersectionality and trauma in POC communities was programmed." (Barton 2017, p. 1).

Change is happening, with movement toward a healthier, more inclusive system, albeit slowly. In 2018 Dr Monnica Williams at UCONN, the University of Connecticut in the USA, ran an MDMA-assisted psychotherapy trial for People of Color diagnosed with PTSD. In August of 2019 MAPS held a conference to train 50–100 therapists to be clinicians in future MDMA trials for PTSD; all participants were People of Color (Joiner 2020). Up to the date of the conference 285 clinicians had been trained by MAPS, with just 10 percent of those being People of Color. The stage is being set for more equity and access for all in the dynamically growing and changing world and community of psychedelic use (Michaels et al 2018). Pharmaceutical medicines have stabilized over the past 50 years; however, we have not seen great change in the drugs themselves or in the benefit to individuals' lives. Entheogens may be the breakthrough needed for mental and physical health. Our hope is that knowledge of entheogens, together with the power of movement, and especially the asanas of

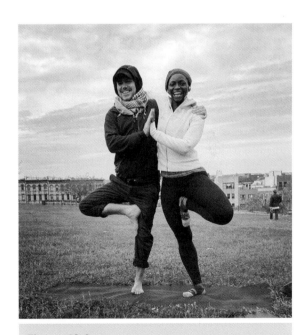

Figure 10.2
Tree pose together and outside. On the left is Serge Cashman, our photographer. Photo by Serge Cashman.

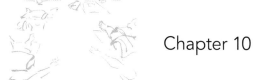

the Sun Salutation done with awareness of the neuro-endocrine system, will contribute to this potential for both healing and dismantling oppressive forces.

How to Integrate the Information from This Book

Slow down to feel yourself (Eddy 2016, Kourlas 2021) – Embody! Embody! Embody! Our experience is that by paying attention to your body you get to spread your thinking, and feel how your intelligence – "your brain" – occupies all parts of your body. Gia Kourlas (2021) expounds on this in the *New York Times* during the Covid pandemic.

Take care of yourself throughout the year with attention to seasonal alerts. Explore your movement process with a priority on focusing on the weather, your moods, and what demands you are experiencing. It is important to achieve calm while being active as a mover. It helps to remember meditation – your mediation practice can be an embodied movement practice if you find that movement meets your goals for calmness, centering, spiritual alignment, or focusing. There is no need to leave the body to meditate: aligning with the body in a true somatic experience and with physical focus can deepen the meditation.

Embodiment through yoga as ritualized in the Sun Salutation can be done with reverence, exploring the body as a temple or giving thanks. This approach reconnects us to the original purposes of yogic practice.

It is great to remember that movement and meditation are sources of healing and recuperation.

Engage with your practice of Sun Salutation with ease and flow.

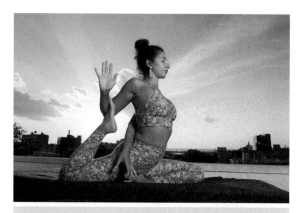

Figure 10.3
Yoga in the urban outdoors. Photo by Serge Cashman.

Conclusion: What To Remember, What to Forget

It can be overwhelming to digest lots of information. If nothing else, this book aims to lead you to a desire to explore your own needs, desires, movement, lifestyle choices, and your body's responses to each of these.

Being free to forget – to enter into the beginner's mind – actually makes room for integration, especially in practical and real ways. With this perspective of always approaching an experience newly you can practice the art of trusting – trusting that what you need is available to you, that what life dishes out can be dealt with, that resources may be difficult to obtain but there is always something that can support us in any given moment. Books can be handy as reminders of keys to unlock our own wisdom but ultimately choose to perceive, act, and reflect. Sharing with others can be helpful. If any information is overwhelming to you, let it all go. Give yourself permission to let go of your bias towards rational, methodical thinking and find ways to let your body sense/intuition be a leader.

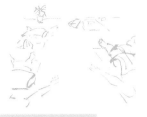

We Offer, as a Closing Practice, Doing Yoga Outside

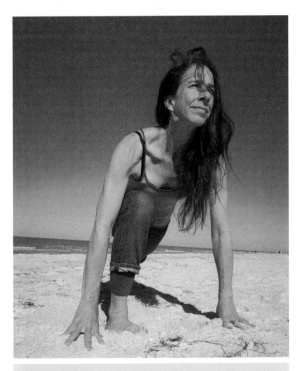

Figure 10.4
Yoga outside, photo by Stewart Hoyt.

Four Days of Sun Salutations Outside: Integrating Nature into Your Practice

Ah, so you know you have four days ahead of you where you have time to be outside each day, doing your Sun Salutation practice. Make this into a mini-retreat.

Each day practice the Sun Salutations upon rising. Below is some guidance on how to connect with nature in your practice – nourishing your body, strengthening your bond with nature, and being a conduit of nature's energies for the benefit of all around.

Nature Connection

Find your spot, barefoot if possible, and take at least a minute to close your eyes, with your hands in anjali mudra. Exhale your breath down your spine and through your feet, into the earth. Inhale the earth's energy up into your body with each breath in. After three or four breaths, shift your exhale to moving from your spine, up through the top of your head to the sky and stars above. With each inhalation, bring the star's healing life force back to you, breathing it deeply into your body and whole being. Do this for three or four breaths, longer if you like. You might notice the mingling of earth and sky energies in your torso.

When you are ready, open your eyes. Ground by feeling your feet touching the earth, even pressing your toes into the soil/sand/grass.

Begin your Sun Salutation Practice, expanding your awareness to encompass your inner body and the elements of nature around you. Enjoy the light, wind, smells, and visual beauty while being aware of your physical sensations, thoughts, and emotions.

Tips for Each Day

The following are some tips to help you focus on a different system or concept each day. This focus will help you deepen your experiential knowledge. Chances are your practice will reverberate into your day. Enhance that if you like by keeping the gems or harvest (see box) of your practice with you throughout the day, even consciously continuing to investigate the practice's focus.

217

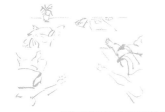

Chapter 10

Nancy Stark Smith and 'Harvest'

Nancy Stark Smith, "first woman" of Contact Improvisation, regularly used this word at the end of her classes. She liked to gather all the participants together in a circle after moving, investigating, dancing, to discuss what was learned, stumbled upon, discovered – what questions arose. Martha and I both studied with her. Nancy passed during the writing of this book, and we honor her memory. See https://libguides.smith.edu/c.php?g=1125759&p=8212030.

Day 1: Awareness of Glands

After Nature Connection

Do a 3–5 minute run-through of the glands, from coccygeal to mammillary, noting and feeling the physical location of each as you move up the spine. Tune briefly into the energy of each one. As you go, you might notice this affecting your physicality/energy/mental state/emotional state. Pause when you are finished, to scan for what effect this has had on you.

Shakti Noticings

(To help you be aware of the changes in you) Strength, connections inside enhanced (ankle to ovary, sense of whole spine, heart to wrists, collar bones feeling wider, sternum and scalp to fingertips), more aligned, skeletally, posturally, as well as energetically in a grounded body way vs. expansive chakra way. Spinal bones shift. What are you noticing about your body?

The Practice

Do your Sun Salutation practice today with the glands in your awareness. Explore some of the connections that have felt significant to you as you read this book – perhaps choosing just two or three to focus on, like anchoring your pituitary gland by reaching downward using the tail and feeling your eyes relax in the back of your head, relaxing any excess tension in your eyes or vision. You may also choose to sense your coccygeal body as you push from one foot into the pelvic floor. This will bring some buoyancy to your stance. Finally reach as far back with your leg as you can while keeping your balance and feel the sensation in your throat around the parathyroid gland of the opposite side. This awareness can help your head relax back more (resulting in the head jutting forward less).

Integration

Take a few notes, list the gems you found, and/or make a drawing at the end of your practice, to integrate what you have discovered, and help you continue evolving your awareness over the course of your day.

Day 2: Awareness of Chakras

After Nature Connection

Do a 3–5 minute run-through of the chakras, from root Muladhara to crown Sahasrara, noting and feeling the physical location of each as you move up the spine. Tune briefly into the energy of each one. As you go, you might notice this affecting your physicality/energy/mental state/emotional state. Pause when you are finished, to scan for what effect this has had on you. How is this the same as or different from your gland focus yesterday? Perhaps take a moment to write and include something about what is different or new in your experience

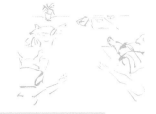

Shakti Noticings

(To help you be aware of the changes in you) Physical "pops" in the spine as the chakra awareness affected my skeleton. Energetically aware in a more expansive, finer-energy and soul-connected way vs. the physicality that the glands ground one in. What are you noticing?

The Practice

Do your Sun Salutation practice today with the chakras in your awareness; explore some of the concepts that have struck you in this book (seeing the color of each one, chanting the bija mantras… perhaps choosing just two or three to focus on).

Integration

Take a few notes or make a drawing at the end of your practice, to integrate what you have discovered, and help you continue evolving your awareness over the course of your day.

Day 3: Awareness of Back Body

After Nature Connection

Come into a seated position, for a 3–5 minute exploration of the back body. First tune into your alignment by bringing your awareness into your spine, the bones of your spine – the vertebrae, and the spinal cord and sushumna within. Try shifting, from your spine, forward and backwards, and side to side, finding the position that feels the most centered. Generally, most people tend to lean forward some. Our thoughts, goals, future thinking, and backpack wearing all support this habit. So let's take a few minutes to embody the

back body. If there is a rock or a tree nearby to lean against, use that to help you feel your back. Its touch will awaken your proprioception. Then bring your awareness into your sacrum, sensing into that bone. Move up into your low back; take a few breaths into your belly, noticing how the low back billows into your back space, then scan up into your kidneys/adrenals, then ribcage and back of heart. Pause at the heart to imagine you could breathe directly in here. Become aware of the nature around you, and breathe that in between your shoulder blades. Allow nature to help you feel your back space and plump up your heart. Then bring your awareness up the vertebrae to your neck, the base of your skull, the back of your skull.

Now telescope out into the big picture, feeling your back body from head to heart to tail. Begin to breathe into the width of it, from center to edges, from spine to shoulders, spine to lateral sides of ribcage, spine to outer hip bones. Include the backs of your legs and buttocks in this exploration.

Shakti Noticings

(To help you be aware of the changes in you) Embodying my back body usually flattens the back of my neck, in a good way: I grow taller. Feeling into the width of my back brings my awareness deeper inside: I grow calmer, more peaceful, and quieter. You may notice the sensing into the width of your back body also brings you into peripheral vision with your eyes. What do you notice?

The Practice

Do your Sun Salutation practice today with your back body in your awareness. Can you keep this awareness in you during the whole of your Sun Salutation practice? Like a meditation, anytime your awareness

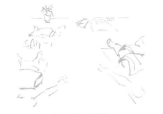

wanders, bring it back to feeling your back body. Intermittently breathe in nature through the back of your heart, as you move through your poses. Invite her to help clear and revitalize your chakras; invite her to help you stand and move through your poses more effortlessly. Invite yourself to cultivate this relationship with nature.

Integration

Take a few notes, list the gems you found, and/or make a drawing at the end of your practice, to integrate what you have discovered, and help you continue evolving your awareness over the course of your day. Let this practice settle through your body. Notice your resonance with nature.

Day 4: Bring it All Together

Try not to use this book today. Plant your feet into the earth, connect with the sky, acknowledge your own heart and spirit with a bow of your head. Begin to flow into your practice, doing what you remember, and what you loved most, what felt good. Allow your body and mind to come into a state of flow. Perhaps you will make something new up today. Creativity arises, and self-healing, when we stop taking notes/following the program. Let the soundscape of nature be your music as you fall into your practice today.

For a basic structure, take a few minutes now, and choose the aspects of the nature connection practice that resonate the most, to begin with. And choose three aspects of the Sun Salutation practice from the last three days that stood out for you, that you loved, were intrigued by, sparked you. These aspects can be your scaffolding – dive in and see what else arises.

Shakti Noticings

(To help you be aware of the changes in you) I like the extra push to dive in on my own and see what is true for me, to be the baby bird spreading its wings after learning from its parents. You might notice to what degree you resist or like this "mission." I noticed that my 3rd and 4th chakras wanted attention, so I scaffolded my Sun Salutation practice around those two, while feeling into the back body, and embodying heart bodies, thymus, and adrenals, and bringing in a little pancreas to help me feel the depth of my torso, from front to back, and back to front. What else did you notice about your practice today? How do you feel in your mind, your heart, your body?

Integration

Take a few notes, list the gems you found, and/or make a drawing at the end of your practice, to integrate what you have discovered, and help you continue evolving your awareness over the course of your day.

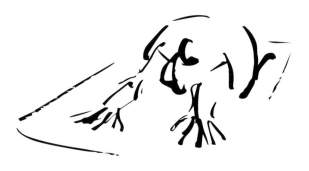

Figure 10.5
Gratitude to the earth, by Stewart Hoyt.

Remember to absorb and integrate; remember what feels good and have fun.

References

Alzaga, A., Salazar, G., & Varon, J. (2006). Breaking the thermal barrier: Dr Temple Fay. *Resuscitation, 69*(3), 359–364.

American Thyroid Association. (nd). Thyroid History Timeline – American Thyroid Association. <http://www.thyroid.org> Accessed October 4, 2020.

Anand, M. (2013). Conversations with Mona Anand, May 2013.

Aposhyan, S. (2007) *Natural intelligence: body-mind integration and human development.* Boulder, CO: Now Press.

Arrien, Angeles (1993), *The four-fold way: walking the paths of the warrior, teacher, healer and visionary.* San Francisco, CA: HarperCollins.

Avalon, A. (1974). *The serpent power.* Mineola, NY: Dover Publications, Inc (originally published in 1919, Luzac and Co., London).

Azikiwe, N. (2017). Melanin myth #7: melanin and the pineal gland. <https://keyamsha.com/2017/05/08/melanin-and-the-pineal-gland/> Accessed June 2, 2020.

Bach, J.F. (1979). Thymic hormones. *J Psychoimmunol, 1*(3), 277–310.

Bacon, L. (2010). *Health At Every Size: The Surprising Truth About Your Weight).* Dallas, TX: BellaBooks.

Bailey, A. (1934). *A treatise on white magic: the way of the discipline.* New York/London: Lucis Publishing.

Bailey, A. (1947, updated 1972) *Esoteric healing.* New York: Lucis Publishing.

Bainbridge Cohen, B. (1993). *Sensing, feeling and action: the experiential anatomy of Body-Mind Centering.* Northampton, MA: Contact Editions.

Bainbridge Cohen, B. (1992, updated 2003). *The basic neurological patterns and their governing endocrine glands.* Curricular materials. El Sobrante, CA: School for Body-Mind Centering.

Bainbridge Cohen, B. (2011). *Embryology.* Course materials. El Sobrante, CA: School for Body-Mind Centering.

Bainbridge Cohen, B. (2013). *The endocrine system* (DVD and online). <https://bonnie-bainbridgecohen.com/collections/embodied-anatomy-videos/products/endocrine-system?> Accessed June 10, 2021.

Bainbridge Cohen, B. (2018). *Basic neurocellular patterns exploring development movement.* El Sobrante, CA: Burchfield Rose Publishers.

Bainbridge Cohen, B. (2020). Phone interview with Martha Eddy. Aug 20, 2020.

Bainbridge Cohen, B. (2021). Phone interview with Martha Eddy. Jan 8, 2021.

Bainbridge Cohen, B. & Mills, M. (1980). *Developmental movement therapy.* Sebastopol, CA: Mills–Thysen.

Ballentine, Rudolf (1996), *Radical healing: integrating the world's great therapeutic traditions to create a new transformative medicine.* New York, NY: Three Rivers Press.

Barron, M.L. (2007). Light exposure, melatonin excretion, and menstrual cycle parameters: an integrative review. *Biol Res Nurs, 9*(1), 49–69.

References

Bartenieff, I. (1980). *Body movement: coping with the environment.* Philadelphia: Gordon and Breach.

Barton, C. (2017). The elephant in the room: the need to address race in psychedelic research. *MAPS Bulletin (San Jose, CA), 27*(3), 1.

Barton, C. & Robinson, I. (2017). Drug policy and the fight for black lives. *Vice* (online), Nov 2, 2017. Accessed May 22, 2020.

Batson, G. & Wilson, M. (2014). *Body and mind in motion: dance and neuroscience in conversation.* Bristol: Intellect.

Bendix, E. (n.d.) *Endocrine glands.* Available at: <https://bodymindcentering.movingmoment.com/endocrine-glands/> Accessed April 28, 2021.

Beaulieu, J. (2016). *Polarity therapy workbook* (2nd ed). Bookbaby Publishers.

Biondi, B., Palmieri, E., Lombardi, G., & Fazio, S. (2002). Effects of subclinical thyroid dysfunction on the heart. *Ann Intern Med, 137*(11), 904–914.

Blair, L. (1976). *Rhythms of vision: the changing patterns of belief.* New York: Grand Central Publishing.

Bradley, K. (2008). *Rudolf Laban.* New York: Taylor and Francis.

Bradley, K. & Parker F. (2020). E-Correspondence on Bartenieff and vowels. CMA List Serve, Feb 17, 2020, 3:20pm.

Brown, W. (2018). *Scientists show that water had memory.* Orange County, CA: Resonance Science Foundation (resonancescience.org).

Buhner, S. (2005). *Healing Lyme: natural healing and the prevention of Lyme borreliosis and its coinfections.* Silver City, NM: Raven Press.

Buller, K. (2021). Co-founder of Psychedelics Today, Interview on psychedelics. By phone, January, 2021.

Buller, K. with Gandy, S. (2019). Breaking Convention series: Psychedelics and our connection with nature. *Psychedelics Today,* July 9. <https://psychedelicstoday.com/2019/07/09/breaking-convention-series-sam-gandy-psychedelics-and-our-connection-with-nature/> Accessed June 14, 2021.

Burnham, L. (2020). Interview on glandular–skeletal interactions (by phone). June 25, 2020.

Cavassa, D. (2020). *Irmgard Bartenieff and sounding with vowels.* LIMS/Denison University: CMA List Serve. Feb 17, 2020, 6:15PM ET.

Chalam, M. (2000). *Spiritual art and mythology of India: anecdotes and symbolisms.* San Diego, CA: Unique Arts International.

Chronobiology.com (nd). *Melatonin history.* <www.chronobiology.com/melatonin-chronobiology/melatonin-history/> Accessed June 12, 2020.

Conti, A., Maestroni, G.J., Cosentino, M., Frigo, G.M., Lecchini, S., Marino, F., Bombelli, R., Ferrari, M., Brivio, F., Roselli, M.G., Lissoni, P. (2000). Evidence for a neuro immunomodulatory and a hematopoietic role of the Luschka's coccygeal body. *Neuro Endocrinol Lett, 21*(5), 391–403.

Dale, C. (2013). *The subtle body practice manual.* Boulder, CO: Sounds True Inc.

Davison, D. & Michalak, L. (2017). Breath is metamorphic: somatic anatomy of the breathing gland bodies. *Currents: Journal of the Body-Mind Centering® Association, 19*(1), 47–53.

Deak, T. (2008). Immune cells and cytokine circuits: toward a working model for understanding direct immune-to-adrenal communication pathways. *Endocrinology, 149*(4), 1433–1435. <https://doi.org/10.1210/en.2008-0170>. Accessed June 14, 2021.

Dell, C. & Crow, A. (1977). *Space harmony: basic terms.* New York: Dance Notation Bureau Press.

Diamond, D. (ed.) (2013). *Yoga, the art of transformation.* Washington: Smithsonian Institution.

Diehl, M. (2019). *Beyond biomechanics - biotensegrity: the new paradigm of kinematics and body awareness.* Hamburg, Germany: Tredition GmbH Self-Publishing.

Doidge, N. (2007). *The brain that changes itself: stories of personal triumph from the frontiers of brain science.* New York: Viking Press.

Ducharme, J. (2019). Spending just 20 minutes in a park makes you happier. Here's what else being outside can do for your health. *Time Magazine,* Feb 28, 2019.

Dynamic Embodiment Curricular Materials Sessions and classes with Somatic Movement Therapist Linda Tumbarello, Martha Eddy, Dana Davison, Lissa M, Many Chan, et al.

Eddy, M. (1993). The use of Kestenberg movement profile in gender analysis. *Movement Studies: Cultural Diversity,* 1, 5.

Eddy, M. (1998). *The role of physical activity in educational violence prevention programs for youth.* Teachers College, Columbia University. Ann Arbor, MI: UMI Research Press.

Eddy, M. (2002). Somatic practices and dance: global influences. *Dance Res J,* 34(2), 46–62.

Eddy, M. (2004). Body cues and conflict: LMA-derived approaches to educational violence prevention. *Movement News,* 29(1), 12–16. New York: Laban Institute.

Eddy, M. (2009). A brief history of somatic practices and dance: historical development of the field of somatic education and its relationship to dance. *J Dance Somat Pract,* 1(1), 5–27.

Eddy, M. (2010). The role of the arts in community building. *Currents.* Northampton, MA: Body-Mind Centering Association.

Eddy, M. (2015). The ongoing development of "Past Beginnings": neuro-motor development somatic links with Bartenieff Fundamentals, Body-Mind Centering® and Dynamic Embodiment[SM]. Updated from 2012. *Somatics Journal.*

Eddy, M. (2016, 2017). *Mindful movement: the evolution of the somatic arts and conscious action.* Bristol: Intellect Press.

Eddy, M. (2020). *Dynamic Embodiment as applied biotensegrity.* BioTensegriTea Party #21, Aug 14, 2020. <https://www.youtube.com/watch?v=Dbpy3U2SHik> Accessed June 10, 2021.

Farhi, D. (2000). *Yoga, mind, body, and spirit.* New York: Henry Holt, and Company.

Fay, T. (1947). The importance of pattern movements in the rehabilitation of cerebral palsy patients. *Temple Fay: progenitor of the Doman–Delacato treatment procedures,* edited by James Wolf. Philadelphia: Temple Books, pp. 98–108.

FDA (US Food and Drug Administration). (2018). Breakthrough therapy. <https://www.fda.gov/patients/fast-track-breakthrough-therapy-accelerated-approval-priority-review/breakthrough-therapy> Accessed June 14, 2021.

Feldenkrais, M. (1989). *The elusive obvious.* Capitola, CA: Meta Publications.

Fernandes, C. (2015). *Moving researcher: Laban/Bartenieff movement analysis in performing arts education and creative arts therapies.* London: Jessica Kingsley Press.

Feuerstein, G. (2003). What you may not realize about yoga. *Yoga International,* August/September.

Finger, A. (2005). *Chakra yoga: balancing energy for physical, spiritual and mental well-being.* Boulder CO: Shambala Press.

Foster, M. (2007). *Somatic patterning: how to improve posture and pain through movement.* Longmont, CO: Educational Movement Systems Press.

Geissenger, A., Webb, J., Sage, P. (2002). *A moving journal: Sound,* 9(3), p. 19.

Goetze, J., Bruneau, B., Ramos, H., Ogawa, T., Kuroski de Bold, M., de Bold, A. (2020).

References

Cardiac natriuretic peptides. *Nat Rev Cardiol*, 17(11), 698–717.

Goldman, E. (1994). *As others see us.* Lausanne, Switzerland: Gordon and Breach Science Publishers.

Goleman, D. (1995). *Emotional intelligence: why it can matter more than IQ.* New York: Bantam.

Gordon, J.S. (2019). *The transformation: discovering wholeness and healing after trauma.* New York: HarperOne.

Gore, A.C. (2013). In: L. Squire et al (eds), *Fundamental neuroscience* (4th ed). Cambridge, MA: Elsevier/Academic Press.

Grof, S. (1985). *Beyond the brain: birth, death, and transcendence in psychotherapy.* Albany, NY: State University of New York Press.

Grof, S. (2019). *The way of the psychonaut. Volume one: Encyclopedia for inner journeys.* San Jose, CA: Multidisciplinary Association for Psychedelic Studies.

Gutkowska, J., Jankowski, M., Mukaddam-Daher, S., McCann, SM. (2000). Oxytocin is a cardiovascular hormone. *Braz J Med Biol Res*, 33(6), 625–633.

Hackney, P. (1998). *Making connections: total body integration through Bartenieff Fundamentals.* London: Gordon & Breach.

Haines, S. (2019). *Politics of trauma: somatics, healing and social justice.* Berkeley, CA: North Atlantic Books.

Hartley, L. (1995). *The wisdom of the body moving: an introduction to Body-Mind Centering.* Berkeley, CA: North Atlantic Books.

Hayes, M. (2021). <https://www.buddhabodyyoganyc.com/> Accessed June 6, 2021.

Helms, J. (1990). *Black and white racial identity: theory, research & practice.* Westport, CT: Praeger Publishers.

Hernandez, A. (2020). Interview – YouTube publication forthcoming.

Hinson, J., Raven, P, Chew, S. (2010). *The endocrine system* (2nd ed). Edinburgh: Churchill Livingstone/Elsevier.

Iyengar, B.K.S. (1979). *Light on yoga.* New York, NY: Schocken.

Joiner, W. (2020) Who will benefit from psychedelic medicine? *The Washington Post Magazine*, September 21, 2020. <https://www.washingtonpost.com/magazine/2020/09/21/psychedelic-medicine-will-it-be-accessible-to-all/> Accessed June 10, 2021.

Jones, Eileen (1986), personal communication.

Judith, A. (1987). *Wheels of life.* Woodbury, MN: Llewellyn Publications.

Kanakis, M., Rapti, N., Chorti, M., Lioulias, A. (2015). Asymptomatic glomus tumor of the mediastinum. *Case Rep Surg*, 2015, 631625.

Kelemen, G. (2015). *The universality of the vortex-sphere archetype.* Timisoara, Romania: Transilvania University Press of Brasov.

Kestenberg Amighi, J., Loman, S., Lewis, P., Sossin, M. (1999). *The meaning in movement: developmental and clinical perspectives of the Kestenberg Movement Profile.* London: Taylor and Francis.

Kimmerer, R.W. (2013). *Braiding sweetgrass.* Minneapolis, MN: Milkweed Editions.

Kourlas, G. (2021). 'Slowing down to feel': moving our minds around our bodies. *The New York Times*, Jan 22, 2021. <https://www.nytimes.com/2021/01/22/arts/dance/somatic-practices-during-the-pandemic.html> Accessed June 14, 2021.

Laban, R. (1948). *Modern educational dance.* London: MacDonald and Evans (2nd ed 1963, revised by Lisa Ullmann).

Laban, R. (1984). *A vision of dynamic space* (compiled by Lisa Ullmann). Laban Archives.

Lauterwasser, A. (2011). *Water sound images: the creative music of the universe.* Eliot, ME: Macromedia Publishing.

Lewy, A.J. (2003). Clinical applications of melatonin in circadian disorders. *Dialogues Clin Neurosci*, 5(4), 399–413.

Lidell, L. (1983). *The Sivananda companion to yoga*. New York: Penguin.

Lieberman, J. (2018). *Luminous life: how the science of light unlocks the art of living*. Novato, CA: New World Library.

Little, T. (2016). *Yoga of the subtle body*. Boulder, CO: Shambhala Publications, Inc.

Lushwala, A. (2020). *Resilience and possibility in these times*. Webinar with Pachamama Alliance, April 13, 2020.

Maman, F. (2008). The tao of sound: acoustic sound healing for the 21st century. Czech Republic: Tama-Do.

Martin, J.V. (2001). Neuroendocrinology. In: N.J. Smelser, P.B. Baltes (eds), *International Encyclopedia of the Social & Behavioral Sciences* (pp. 10584–10588). Oxford: Elsevier/Pergamon.

McCracken, M. (2020). Dancing is good for your brain: hitting the dance floor isn't just fun — you might whirl your way to better balance and a better mind. *AARP*. July 2020 <https://stayingsharp.aarp.org/articles/dancing-good-brain/> Accessed June 14, 2021.

Menakem, R. (2017). *My grandmother's hands*. Las Vegas, NV: CRP Press.

Michaels, T.I., Purdon, J., Collins, A., Williams, M., et al (2018). Inclusion of people of color in psychedelic-assisted psychotherapy: a review of the literature. *BMC Psychiatry*, 18, 245.

Monroe, M. (2011). *Yoga and scoliosis: a journey to health and healing*. New York, NY: Springer Publishing Company.

Netter, F.H. (2018) *Atlas of human anatomy* (7th ed). Philadelphia, PA: Elsevier.

Northrup, C. (2012). *The wisdom of menopause: creating physical and emotional health during the change*. New York, NY: Random House (revised ed).

Olsen, A. (2002). *Body and earth: an experiential guide*. Lebanon, NH: UPNE.

Oxford Dictionary. (2020). Definition of neuroendocrine [online]. Oxford University Press. <https://www.lexico.com/definition/neuroendocrine> Accessed March 9, 2020.

Pert, C.B. (1997). *Molecules of emotion: why you feel the way you feel*. New York, NY: Scribner.

Pert, C.B. (2007). *The physics of emotion*. <https://www.6seconds.org/2007/01/26/the-physics-of-emotion-candace-pert-on-feeling-good/> Accessed June 10, 2021.

Pert, C.B., Ruff, M.R., Weber, R.J., Herkenham, M. (1985). Neuropeptides and their receptors: a psychosomatic network. *Journal of Immunology*, 135, 820s–826s.

Porges, S. (2011). *The polyvagal theory: neurophysiological foundations of emotions, attachment, communication, and self-regulation*. New York: Norton.

Saraswati, S. (2006). *Kundalini tantra*. Bihar, India: Bihar School of Yoga.

Scarr, G. (2014). *Biotensegrity: the structural basis of life*. Pencaitland, UK: Handspring Publishing Ltd.

Schmidt, U. & Ascheim, E. (2006). Thyroid hormone and heart failure. *Curr Heart Fail Rep*, 3(3), 114–119.

Schmidt, N., Richey, A., Zvolensky, M., Maner, J.K. (2008). Exploring human freeze responses to a threat stressor. *J Behav Ther Exp Psychiatry*, 39(3), 292–304.

Shrestha, S. (2013). *How to heal with singing bowls: traditional Tibetan healing methods*. Boulder, CO: Sentient Publications.

Singleton, M. (2017). *The roots of yoga*. London: Penguin Classics.

Society for Endocrinology. (nd). Melatonin. *You and Your Hormones*. <https://www.yourhormones.info/hormones/melatonin/> Accessed June 10, 2021.

References

Stovall, N. (2019). Whiteness on the couch. *Longreads*. <https://longreads.com/2019/08/12/whiteness-on-the-couch/> Accessed Jan 2, 2021.

Studd, K. & Cox, L. (2019). *Everybody is a body*. Parker, CO: Outskirts Press.

Swann, C. (2016). In: M. Eddy (ed.), *Mindful Movement*. Bristol: Intellect Press.

Taylor, M. (2018). *Embody the skeleton: a guide for conscious movement*. Pencaitland, UK: Handspring Publishing Ltd.

Transcriptions of Yoga Classes with Dr Martha Eddy.

Vann, S.D. (2010). Re-evaluating the role of the mammillary bodies in memory. *Neuropsychologia*, 48(8), 2316–2327.

Vann, S. & Nelson, A.J. (2015). The mammillary bodies and memory: more than a hippocampal relay. *Prog Brain Res*, 219, 163–185.

Weed, S. (2002). *The new menopausal years*. Woodstock, NY: Ash Tree Publishing.

Weed, S. (2019). *Abundantly well: the complementary integrated medical revolution*. Woodstock, NY: Ash Tree Publishing.

Wolfe, H. (1990). *Second spring: a guide to healthy menopause through traditional Chinese medicine*. Boulder, CO: Blue Poppy Press.

Wurtman, R. (1985). Melatonin as a hormone in humans: a history. *Yale J Biol Med*, 58(6), 547–552.

Permissions

Back cover
Photo of Shakti by Tara Eden.

Title page
Drawing by Stewart Hoyt.

About the Authors
Shakti and Martha. Photo by Serge Cashman.

About the Artist
Shakti and Teresa at Popham Beach, by Stewart Hoyt.

Introduction Opening figure
Rooting and grounding, a drawing of Shakti by Stewart Hoyt.

Chapter 1 Opening figure
Rooted strong with open heart and focus, by Stewart Hoyt.

Figure 1.1
The ten senses as taught at the Center for Kinesthetic Education, NYC. @Martha Eddy www.wellnessCKT.net

Figure 1.4
Bartenieff body connections, by Stewart Hoyt.

Chapter 2 Opening figure
Warming up in cat/cow, by Stewart Hoyt.

Figure 2.2
Brow chakras, Rajasthan, 18th century (author unknown).

Figure 2.5
Chakra positions in supposed relation to nervous plexuses, from Charles W. Leadbeater's 1927 book *The Chakras*.

Figure 2.6
Shakti, by Hrana Janto. Permission generously given to us by the artist. Shared by courtesy of Dave Sheppard and Hrana Janto, *www.hranajanto.com*

Figure 2.7
Caduceus, by Rama, 2004.

Chapter 3A Opening figure
Thyroid compression in shoulder stand, by Stewart Hoyt.

Figure 3A.1/3B.1
The endocrine system as taught in Body-Mind Centering® and Dynamic Embodiment℠. Based on original drawing by Amanda Latchmore.

Figure 3A.2
Compressional support underlying suspensional support. Photo by Serge Cashman.

Figure 3A.3
"Thymus reaching" of the arms with whole-body glandular support. You can see this from the aliveness throughout the body. Photo by Serge Cashman.

Permissions

Figure 3A.4
Open hands and heart help us connect, by Stewart Hoyt.

Figure 3A.5
Activating interoception through grounding and centering, by Stewart Hoyt.

Chapter 3B Opening figure
Space supports our presence, by Stewart Hoyt.

Figure 3B.2
Coccygeal thrust from tail to head. Photo by Serge Cashman.

Figure 3B.3
Radiating out from the pancreas/solar plexus, by Stewart Hoyt.

Figure 3B.4
Suspensional support of thymus and thyroid in camel. Photo by Serge Cashman.

Figure 3B.5
Find the carotid bodies in the "neighborhood" of the carotid arteries, drawing from the book *Gray's Anatomy*, first published in 1858.

Figure 3B.8
Reach of the head from the mammillary. Photo by Serge Cashman.

Figure 3B.9
Contralateral twist for parathyroidal activation. Photo by Serge Cashman.

Figure 3B.10
Opening up to claim space – a tensile and glandular experience, drawing by Stewart Hoyt.

Chapter 4 Opening figure
Breathing, by Stewart Hoyt.

Figure 4.2
Third eye/pituitary. Photo by Serge Cashman.

Figure 4.3
Turtle: an example of harmonic patterns in nature, this photo from book *Water Sound Images: The Creative Music of the Universe* by Alexander Lauterwasser, permission given by Jeff Volk for Alexander Lauterwasser.

Figure 4.4
1088 Hertz: Chladni sound figure at specific frequency; there are hundreds of such figures exhibiting the patterns of animals, this photo from book *Water Sound Images: The Creative Music of the Universe* by Alexander Lauterwasser, permission given by Jeff Volk for Alexander Lauterwasser.

Figure 4.5
Seven-element structure: "standing wave", as found in seven-petaled flowers, seashells, this photo from book *Water Sound Images: The Creative Music of the Universe* by Alexander Lauterwasser, permission given by Jeff Volk for Alexander Lauterwasser.

Figure 4.6
Water–Sound–Image with 14 spiral arms formed in a water bowl of 20 cm diameter. Frequency/102.528 Hertz: we can see this pattern in shells, cactus and other forms in nature, this photo from book *Water Sound Images: The Creative Music of the Universe* by Alexander Lauterwasser, permission given by Jeff Volk for Alexander Lauterwasser.

Figure 4.7
Multi-element/ "standing wave" 91.8 Hertz, by Alexander Lauterwasser, this photo from book *Water Sound Images: The Creative Music of the Universe* by Alexander Lauterwasser, permission given by Jeff Volk for Alexander Lauterwasser.

Figure 4.8
The dimensional spectrum relationship, by Gabriel Kelemen, The Universality of the vortex-sphere archetype, 2015. Permission given by Iulia and Gabriel Kelemen.

Chapter 5 Opening figure
Ritual, by Stewart Hoyt.

Figure 5.2
Knees – chest – chin, Ashtanga Namaskara, salute with the eight limbs. Photo by Serge Cashman.

Figure 5.3
Reach through top of the head, mammillary; reach through the arms, thymus. Photo by Serge Cashman.

Figure 5.4
Fingers to scapula connections – front view. An interactive influence between Bartenieff's general idea that relating the fingers to the scapula would support movement efficiency was refined by Bainbridge Cohen to include specific correlations between each finger and each part of the scapula. These are taught in both the Laban/Bartenieff and the Body-Mind Centering® systems now. Drawing by Marghe Mills-Thysen, Certified Teacher of BMC, depicting these relationships.

Figure 5.5
Fingers to back of scapula – back view (depicts index to acromion process, middle to socket, ring to blades of scapula and pinky to wing). Drawing by Marghe Mills-Thysen.

Figure 5.6
Lunge with parathyroid support for reach. Photo by Serge Cashman.

Figure 5.7
Playful spirit in integrative plank. Photo by Serge Cashman.

Chapter 6 Opening figure
Thymus/heart bodies soaring, by Stewart Hoyt.

Figure 6.1
Spinal reach from the head. Photo by Serge Cashman.

Figure 6.2
Spinal reach from the tail. Photo by Serge Cashman.

Figure 6.3
Push of two arms. Photo by Serge Cashman.

Figure 6.4
Reach of one leg. Photo by Serge Cashman.

Figure 6.5
Hunter changing levels. Photo by Serge Cashman.

Figure 6.6
Crawling on all fours. Photo by Serge Cashman.

Permissions

Figure 6.7
Symmetrical reach for mother's hands. Photo by Serge Cashman.

Figure 6.8
Navel radiation. Photo by Serge Cashman.

Figure 6.9
Body half, standing. Photo by Serge Cashman.

Figure 6.10
Body half, crawling. Photo by Serge Cashman.

Figure 6.11
Contralateral, standing; notice twist in shirt. Photo by Serge Cashman.

Figure 6.12
Contralateral, lying down. Photo by Serge Cashman.

Figure 6.13
Giving in to gravity – time to yield. Photo by Serge Cashman.

Figure 6.14
Reaching from the thymus, by Stewart Hoyt.

Chapter 7 Opening figure
Downward dog with spread fingers, by Stewart Hoyt.

Figure 7.1
Rooting and grounding, a drawing of Shakti by Stewart Hoyt.

Figure 7.2
Heels over head, by Stewart Hoyt.

Figure 7.5
Widening the shoulders to stimulate the thymus. Photo by Serge Cashman.

Figure 7.6
Use of blocks in lunge or anjaneyasana, by Stewart Hoyt.

Figure 7.7
Map of the ankle to gonad connection. Photo by Serge Cashman.

Chapter 8 Opening figure
Dynamic rest, by Stewart Hoyt.

Figure 8.2
Linda Tumbarello connection adrenal hug with Dana Davison, photo by Shakti Smith.

Figure 8.3
Fish pose/ matsyasana. Photo by Serge Cashman.

Figure 8.4
Suspensional support for thyroid and parathyroid lunge. Photo by Serge Cashman.

Figure 8.5
Accessing the thyroid – Linda Tumbarello with Dana Davison, photo by Shakti Smith.

Figure 8.6
Frog pose with thymus support. Photo by Serge Cashman.

Figure 8.7
Support for the adrenals and pineal: deep rest of head glands, withdrawing the senses, extension of the arms with thymus and thyroid. Photo by Serge Cashman.

Figure 8.8
Adrenals and pineal. Photo by Serge Cashman.

Figure 8.9
The sound is holding you, by Stewart Hoyt.

Figure 8.10
Sliding Up the Wall, as demonstrated by Leonard Cohen with Bonnie Bainbridge Cohen circa 1977, integrating all the glands, using compression and suspension. Springfield Union Staff Photo, by Vincent S. D'Addario. Shared by courtesy of Len and Bonnie Bainbridge Cohen.

Chapter 9 Opening figure
Group in lunge, by Stewart Hoyt.

Figure 9.2
The art of creative yoga. Photo by Serge Cashman.

Figure 9.3
Rooted integration, two in boat pose. Photo by Serge Cashman.

Figure 9.6
Hands-on support for deepening yoga. Photo by Serge Cashman.

Chapter 10 Opening figure
Savasana or corpse pose, by Stewart Hoyt.

Figure 10.1
One with tree, by Stewart Hoyt.

Figure 10.2
Tree pose together and outside. On the left is Serge Cashman, our photographer. Photo by Serge Cashman.

Figure 10.3
Yoga in the urban outdoors. Photo by Serge Cashman.

Figure 10.4
Yoga outside, photo by Stewart Hoyt.

Figure 10.5
Gratitude to the earth, by Stewart Hoyt.

Index

Index

Finger, Alan, 40, 99
Follicle-stimulating hormone (FSH), 62, 82
Food and Drug Administration (FDA), 212

G

Garbhasana, 37
Garland Pose, 153
Gender, 22, 71, 72, 107, 208
Gland–chakral–joint relationships, 133c
Gland–joint connection, 135–136
Glands, 132
   and bodies, 58–59
   location of, 59
Glandular
   complexes, 62
   energy, calming, 63
   secretion, 54
   system, 49
Global North, 23, 26, 167
Global South, 23, 26, 167, 210
Glomus caroticum, 80
Gonads, 90
Grief, 198, 200, 201, 202, 212
Grof, Stansilav, 213
Growth hormone (GH), 82

H

Hartley, Linda, 3, 5, 70, 97–100, 144, 147
Head gland compression, 186
Health syndromes, 167
Heart glands, 76–77
   BBC/DE history of, 77
   BMC/DE quality, 76–77
   function of, 76
   history of, 77
   hormones of, 76
   locations of, 76
Herbalism, 106, 211
Hinduism, yoga in, 37
Hip–foot connections, 165
Hormonal surge, 60
Hormonal system, 49
Hyperthyroidism, 177
Hypophysis, 50
Hypothyroidism, 177, 179

I

Ida, 42
Ilio-femoral joint, 162
Iliopsoas and diaphragm, 156
Imaginary crystalline space, 109
Insulin, 74

Interoception, 10, 56, 57, 63f
Ishta yoga, 40
Isvara pranidhana, 36
Iyengar, B.K.S., 1, 36, 37, 150, 173
Iyengar Yoga, 150, 173

J

Jainism, yoga in, 37
Joints, 132
   chest, 159
   health, 146
   pain, 146
   space, 147
Judith, Anodea, 106, 194

K

Keast, Alix, 175
Khumbhaka, 37
Kidneys and adrenal glands, 41
Knees, 162
Kundalini energy, 42–45

L

Laban/Bartenieff system, 53
Laban Movement Analyst, 130
Lateral Weight Shift, 162
Lauterwasser, Alexander, 101
Luschka's body, 69
Lushwala, Arkan, 211
Luteinizing hormone (LH), 62, 82
Lyme disease, 178

M

Maman, Fabien, 103, 104, 106
Mammillary bodies, 83–84, 92, 138
   anatomical history of, 83–84
   BBC history, 84
   BMC/DE quality, 83
   function of, 83
   hormones of, 83
   locations of, 83
Mandelbaum, Richard, 106
Manipura Chakra, 42c, 96c, 98, 193
Master gland, 50, 62
Melatonin, 84, 172
Messages From Water, 102, 104
Moods, impact on, 61
Moon Salutation, 36
Muir, Eileen, 173

Muladhara Chakra, 42c, 96c, 218
Multidisciplinary Association for
   Psychedelic Studies (MAPS), 212, 215
The Mysterious Kundalini, 39

N

Nauli kriya, 37
Neck, 158
Nerve damage, 146
Nervous system
   chakras and glands, 37–40
   and glands, physiology of, 49–50
     neuroendocrine hub, 50
Neuroendocrine awareness, 48–49
   integrating somatic influences, 49
Neuroendocrine cells, 49
Neuroendocrine hub, 50
Neuroendocrine system, 47–48
   activating glands, 52–53
   body connectivity, 57–58
   emotional and behavioral connections, 56
   foster greater interoception, 56–57
   locate and move, 55–56
   neuroendocrine awareness, 54–55
   suspend to stimulate, 53–54
Neuroendocrine tumors, 48
Neuroendocrinology, 48
Neuromotor Developmental Coordination
   (NDC), 134
New York Times, 216
Nine Pillars of the Feet, 164
Niyamas, 36
Non-binary, 162

O

Online teaching, 204
OSO model, 23, 24, 25, 190, 204
Overactive thyroid, 178

P

Pain and depression, 151
Pain and vulnerable joints, 145
Pancreas, 73–74, 90–91
   BMC/DE quality, 74
   function of, 74
   history of, 74
   hormones of, 74
   locations of, 73–74
Parathyroid glands (PTH), 79–80, 92, 137
   anatomical history of, 79
   BBC history of, 80
   BMC/DE quality, 80